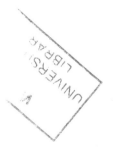

Protecting Childhood in the AIDS Pandemic

Protecting Childhood in the AIDS Pandemic

Finding Solutions that Work

EDITED BY ■

JODY HEYMANN

LORRAINE SHERR

RACHEL KIDMAN

Oxford University Press, Inc., publishes works that further Oxford University's
objective of excellence in research, scholarship, and education.

Oxford   New York
Auckland   Cape Town   Dar es Salaam   Hong Kong   Karachi
Kuala Lumpur   Madrid   Melbourne   Mexico City   Nairobi
New Delhi   Shanghai   Taipei   Toronto

With offices in
Argentina   Austria   Brazil   Chile   Czech Republic   France   Greece
Guatemala   Hungary   Italy   Japan   Poland   Portugal   Singapore
South Korea   Switzerland   Thailand   Turkey   Ukraine   Vietnam

Published by Oxford University Press, Inc.
198 Madison Avenue, New York, New York 10016
www.oup.com

Oxford is a registered trademark of Oxford University Press, Inc.

Library of Congress Cataloging-in-Publication Data

Protecting childhood in the AIDS pandemic : finding solutions that work /
edited by Jody Heymann, Lorraine Sherr, Rachel Kidman.
    p. ; cm.
Includes bibliographical references and index.
ISBN 978-0-19-976512-6 (hardcover)
I. Heymann, Jody, 1959- II. Sherr, Lorraine. III. Kidman, Rachel.
[DNLM: 1. Acquired Immunodeficiency Syndrome—psychology.
2. HIV Infections—psychology. 3. Child Health Services—organization & administration.
4. Child Welfare. 5. Child. 6. Health Policy. WC 503.7]
LC classification not assigned
618.92'9792—dc23   2011032185

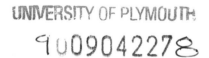

9 8 7 6 5 4 3 2 1

Typeset in Minion Pro
Printed in the United States of America on acid-free paper

To Margarita and all children living lives affected by AIDS.
To Jonathan and all those with a vision for and a drive to make the world do more
for children affected by AIDS than we have done in the past.
To Ari, Ilan, Jasmin, Yoni, Liora, Avrill, and Cheryl.
To Rachel's parents, who encouraged her, and to Sean, who believes in her.

CONTENTS

PART FOUR Getting Delivery Done Well

ACKNOWLEDGMENTS

No books are the product only of the authors and editors listed in their table of contents. This is particularly true of any academic work that brings together research and program leaders on a complex topic. Policy-makers and program leaders who write about their successes and challenges draw on the great expertise and experiences of field staff running programs and implementing policies. The research itself only occurs through the commitment and contributions of research teams making every step of the studies described possible. In the case of an edited volume, the number of contributors who make all of the work possible expands geometrically. We are deeply grateful to all the researchers in the field and at campuses, and to the program staff in community-based, national, and global organizations who contributed behind the scenes to the chapters.

The editorial team worked from three different countries. With the geographic distance and schedules of all involved, this book never would have come into existence without the indispensable, expert management of the entire process by Gonzalo Moreno. Gonzalo managed all the contributions, followed up with all authors on everything from chapter edits to references to logistics, coordinated the efforts of our editorial team in three countries, and gave critical insights into how accessible chapters would be to engage readers from a variety of fields. The quality of the process and resulting book were improved in countless ways by his immense contribution.

Many edited volumes arise when there are funds to support authors to come together on a topic. This book arose out of the deep commitment of everyone involved. Chapter contributors took time out of immensely busy schedules running large research endeavors and service programs on the ground in countries around the world. There were no special funds, only a profound commitment to changing how successfully we address the needs of children affected by AIDS. We are deeply indebted to all of the authors who found time—that often simply did not exist in their schedules—not only to contribute, but to revise chapters in response to feedback and to collectively pull together the most comprehensive volume we could achieve on moving from evidence to action on children affected by AIDS.

As editors, we each had many people in our hearts and minds during the editing of this book. Jody went to medical school in the 1980s, at the time when the world was just beginning to learn the biology of AIDS. But she spent time with two extraordinary teachers in 1990. Early in the year, she cared for Margarita, a 7-year-old dying of HIV before there was any effective treatment, who taught her about living with the disease with immense grace and courage. Toward the end of the year, she worked on an initiative Jonathan Mann conceived to develop plans for how global organizations could speed the availability and affordability of HIV treatment and vaccines in low-income countries—years before there was widespread global action on meeting this critical need. She would like to dedicate the book to Margarita and to all children living lives affected by AIDS, and to Jonathan and all those with a vision for and a drive to make the world do more for children affected by AIDS than we have done in past. No work is ever carried out without support. Lorraine would like to support Jody's dedication by adding her own children and sisters to the list of inspirational people who give her the courage to go on during decades of work on HIV treatment, care, and coping: Ari, Ilan, Jasmine, Yonatan, Liora, Avrill, and Cheryl. Rachel would like to dedicate this book to her parents, who encouraged her, and to her husband Sean, who believes in her.

ABOUT THE EDITORS

Jody Heymann is Founding Director of the Institute for Health and Social Policy, and a Canada Research Chair in Global Health and Social Policy at McGill University. Heymann established and leads the first global initiative to examine social policy in all 193 UN nations. This initiative provides an in-depth look at how social policies affect the ability of individuals, families and communities to meet their health needs across the political, economic and social spectrum worldwide. An internationally renowned researcher on health and social policy, she has authored and edited over 190 publications and has led the development of a unique graduate and undergraduate multidisciplinary training program that bridges research and policy development with students gaining experience in 24 countries.

Heymann developed some of the earliest models that examine the critical health consequences of whether HIV-infected mothers in countries in sub-Saharan Africa and elsewhere in the world breastfeed. This work was used by the World Health Organization and others to help lay the ground work for intervention programs in the field that seek to minimize infant mortality from both HIV infection and the diarrheal disease and respiratory infections that can accompany bottle feeding. Heymann also developed one of the first studies to underscore the importance of chemoprophylaxis for tuberculosis among HIV-infected patients in Africa. Her HIV-related work over the past decade has focused on what can be done to decrease the health, economic, and social consequences of the AIDS pandemic, and she has led a series of seminal studies around meeting the urgent needs of children affected by AIDS.

Deeply committed to translating research into policies and programs that will improve individual and population health, Heymann developed and chairs a five-year initiative, *Population Health: Moving from Evidence to Action*. She has worked with leaders in North American, European, African, and Latin American governments as well as a wide range of intergovernmental organizations including the World Health Organization, the International Labor Organization, UNICEF, and UNESCO.

Lorraine Sherr is a clinical psychologist and Professor in Clinical Health Psychology at the Royal Free and University College Medical School, where she is head of the Health Psychology Unit. She has been involved in studying HIV infection and the psychological aspects of the disease since the beginning of the epidemic in the mid 1980's. She is currently executive editor of the international journals *AIDS Care* and *Psychology, Health and Medicine* and co-editor of *Vulnerable Children and Youth Studies*. Sherr has published over 170 articles in peer-reviewed journals, written, edited or contributed chapters to over 40 books, and held numerous research grants looking into aspects of health psychology and HIV/AIDS in the United Kingdom, Europe and Africa.

Sherr was completing her clinical psychology training when the AIDS epidemic emerged in the 1980s. From the early days she became a tireless advocate for the importance of integrated approaches highlighting the crucial role psychology played in prevention of HIV, treatment, care and coping. The child in the family was a living example of this philosophy and she has tried to contribute to the understanding of children within their family context. She has also been an advocate of evidence-based policy and a supporter of evaluation. There has been a dramatic move in this direction, and the current focus and attention of children as well as good mental and emotional health are evidence of the efficacy of this approach. Indeed this text is seen as one such contribution to the enhanced quality of provision and understanding for children.

Sherr has acted as co-chair of Learning Group 1 on Families for the Joint Learning Initiative on Children and AIDS and sits on the steering committee of the International Coalition on Children affected by AIDS. She has sat on the Strategic and Technical Advisory group for the World Health Organization HIV section, and has provided psychosocial evaluations for international organizations such as the World Health Organization, UNICEF, Save the Children, the Norwegian Agency for Development Cooperation, and UNAIDS. She was appointed a Churchill Fellow for life for her work on HIV and AIDS in obstetrics and pediatrics.

Rachel Kidman recently joined the faculty at the Tulane University School of Public Health and Tropical Medicine, after completing her graduate work in social epidemiology at the Harvard School of Public Health and at McGill University. At Tulane, her research focuses on the development of appropriate social interventions to help protect the welfare of children affected by AIDS. She is currently conducting longitudinal studies designed to identify children's priority needs and to evaluate the impact of community-based programs for this vulnerable population in KwaZulu-Natal, South Africa. Prior to this appointment, she investigated health and educational disparities among children affected by AIDS in Malawi, and documented the extent of private and public support available to these children. Under UNICEF Malawi, she conducted research on programs serving vulnerable children and their families in order to recommend practices that could be replicated or scaled-up as part of a national initiative. In Botswana, she similarly conducted case studies of community programming for orphans in order to highlight best-practices.

Michelle Adato is Director of Social and Gender Assessment at the Millennium Challenge Corporation. Prior to joining MCC in late 2010, she was a Senior Research Fellow in the Poverty, Health, and Nutrition Division of the International Food Policy Research Institute (IFPRI). For 7 years, she was the co-leader of IFPRI's global research program on Large-Scale Human Capital Interventions, evaluating the impacts of health, nutrition, education, and social protection programs, and for 3 years, she was the theme leader on AIDS, Community Resilience, and Social Protection of IFPRI's Regional Network on AIDS, Livelihoods, and Food Security in Southern and Eastern Africa (RENEWAL). She has published widely on social protection and other issues related to poverty and development, including a new co-edited book, *Conditional Cash Transfers in Latin America*. Adato has a Ph.D. in Development Sociology from Cornell University and a Master of Public Administration from Harvard University.

Simona Bignami-Van Assche is Associate Professor of Social Statistics at the Université de Montréal. Her research on issues of data quality and validity of self-reported sexual behaviors, particularly in longitudinal studies, on the relationship of marriage and HIV, and examining questions on the role of poverty in HIV infection, has appeared in *AIDS, Demographic Research, Population Review*, and *Social Networks*, among other journals. She compiled a report for UNAIDS about orphans and vulnerable children in high HIV-prevalence countries in sub-Saharan Africa.

Agnes Binagwaho is the Minister of Health in Rwanda. She has served as Permanent Secretary of the Ministry of Health in Rwanda since October 2008. She is a specialist in emergency pediatrics, neonatology, and the treatment of HIV/AIDS, and she chairs the Rwandan Pediatric Society. From 1986 to 2002, she practiced medicine in public hospitals in Rwanda and several other countries before joining Rwanda's National AIDS Control Commission as Executive Secretary. She is a member of the editorial boards of the Public Library of Science, and the Harvard University Health and Human Rights Journal. Binagwaho also co-chaired the Millennium Development Goals Project Task Force on HIV/AIDS and Access to Essential Medicines for the Secretary-General of the United Nations under the leadership of Jeffrey Sachs, and was the global co-chair of the Joint Learning Initiative on Children and HIV/AIDS. In addition to her medical degree and a master's degree in pediatrics, she received an Honorary Doctorate of Sciences from Dartmouth College. Binagwaho serves as a visiting lecturer in the Department of Global Health and Social Medicine at Harvard Medical School.

Mark E. Boyes received his Ph.D. in psychology in 2010 from the University of Western Australia. His doctoral research focused on individual differences in stress reactivity and coping in the context of stressful situations. Boyes is a Postdoctoral Research Officer in the Department of Social Policy and Intervention at the University

of Oxford and is a Junior Research Fellow at Wolfson College. He is currently working on the Young Carers project (www.youngcarers.org.za), which is exploring the
impact of living in an AIDS-affected family on children's mental and physical health,
social development, and educational outcomes.

Kevin Clarke is a pediatrician with the South-to-South program who has worked in
child health and HIV/AIDS care in Zambia, Malawi, and South Africa. He graduated
from the University of Connecticut School of Medicine and trained in pediatrics at
the University of California, San Francisco. In 2007, he joined the Baylor International
Pediatric AIDS Initiative and was based at Zomba Central Hospital in Malawi's
Southern Region. During this time, he helped create the Malawi Pediatric HIV/AIDS
Treatment Support and Outreach mentorship program for building health care
worker capacity in pediatric HIV/AIDS care. He has served as Chairman of the
Tshwane Paediatric HIV Technical Working Group and is co-editor for the USAID-
funded publication, "Paediatric HIV Care and Treatment: A Toolkit for South
African Healthcare Workers."

Janine Clayton completed her training and qualified as a clinical psychologist at the
Child Guidance Clinic, University of Cape Town. She has extensive work experience
in the area of child and adolescent development within a psychodynamic framework, as well as in program development initiatives in southern Africa. Her most
recent work involves mainstreaming psychosocial support within HIV and AIDS
programs and organizations, focusing on the psychological well-being and protection of children.

Lucie D. Cluver is a lecturer at Oxford University, where she leads the Centre for
AIDS Interdisciplinary Research, and is an honorary lecturer at the University of
Cape Town. She trained as a social worker, and has practiced in South Africa and the
United Kingdom. Cluver works closely with the South African National Departments
of Social Development, Health, and Basic Education to develop policy-relevant
research on the impacts on children of AIDS-orphanhood and parental AIDS illness,
particularly related to mental health, physical health, and educational outcomes. She
has also acted as a scientific advisor to UNICEF, the World Health Organization, and
the South African National Action Committee for Children Affected by AIDS.

Mark Cotton is a Senior Specialist and Professor at the Department of Paediatrics
and Child Health, Stellenbosch University and Tygerberg Children's Hospital, as well
as Head of the Division of Pediatric Infectious Diseases. He serves as the Director of
the Children's Infectious Diseases Clinical Research Unit, and has published extensively in the field of pediatric HIV and immunology. He sits on the Provincial AIDS
Council, Western Cape, and the South African Antiretroviral Guidelines Committees;
is the International Vice-Chair of the Performance Evaluation Resource Committee
of the International Maternal Pediatric Adolescent AIDS Clinical Trials Group; and
is a technical advisor to the World Health Organization on pediatric classification of
HIV and antiretroviral therapy guidelines.

Hoosen M. Coovadia is the director of Maternal and Child Health at the University of
the Witwaterstrand, as well as an Emeritus Professor in Paediatrics and Child Health

and HIV/AIDS Research at the University of KwaZulu-Natal. He has been at the forefront of children's issues in developing countries for more than 40 years and has made significant contributions to the body of scientific evidence that guides the clinical management and public health control of the most common problems of poor South African children. His key publications have been in prevention of mother-to-child transmission of HIV-1, especially through breastfeeding; in infectious diseases, such as measles and hepatitis B; in protein-calorie and micronutrient malnutrition; and in renal disorders of black children. He has supervised numerous Ph.D. and master's degree theses, and provided mentorship and leadership to young researchers, many of whom currently hold leadership academic positions. Coovadia has also been involved in establishing and participating actively in antiapartheid organizations, helping shape health and development policy in an emerging democratic South Africa.

Chris Desmond is a research associate at the François-Xavier Bagnoud Centre for Health and Human Rights at Harvard University. He currently manages the "cost of inaction" research project at the François-Xavier Bagnoud Centre, which examines alternative approaches to evaluating the response to children affected by HIV/AIDS. Prior to moving to Harvard, Desmond was a research specialist at the Human Sciences Research Council in South Africa and a research fellow at the Health Economics and HIV/AIDS Research Division at the University of KwaZulu-Natal. Desmond's research has focused on issues relating to HIV and children, including those related to the costs of care, the appropriate targeting of responses, and policy development. His past work involved examining the possibilities for assessing country responses to HIV/AIDS, including investigating appropriate indicators of a successful response to children.

Angela Dramowski is currently a fellow in Paediatric Infectious Diseases at Tygerberg Hospital, Stellenbosch University, Cape Town, South Africa. She studied Medicine at the University of Cape Town and completed her residency at the University of the Witwatersrand. In 2009, she was awarded a Fogarty International Clinical Research Fellowship to study pediatric infectious diseases at the Children's Infectious Diseases Clinical Research Unit at Tygerberg Hospital under the supervision of Professor Mark Cotton. Her fields of interest include pediatric HIV and hospital-acquired infections.

Patrice L. Engle is a Professor of Psychology and Child Development at California Polytechnic State University. She has worked for the World Health Organization in developing models of combined health care and early stimulation, and for UNICEF in India and in New York as Global Early Child Development Advisor. She has developed guidelines for young children affected by HIV and AIDS for UNICEF in combination with the World Bank and analyzed early childhood in the National Plans of Action for orphans and vulnerable children in 17 high HIV/AIDS-prevalence countries for the Bernard van Leer Foundation. Engle is currently developing assessment tools for child development that can be used across countries, and has prepared an updated review on the effectiveness of programs to improve early child development in low- and middle-income countries, following on the 2007 *Lancet* Series on Child Development.

Geoff Foster is a specialist pediatrician with over 25 years of experience with the Ministry of Health in Mutare, Zimbabwe. He is a board member of the Firelight Foundation and co-founded and edits the international journal *Vulnerable Children and Youth Studies*. Foster is a leading expert on support for children affected by HIV/AIDS and has researched and consulted on issues of orphans and vulnerable children, faith-based organizations, and HIV/AIDS, with over 50 publications in peer-reviewed literature. In 1987, Foster founded Family AIDS Caring Trust, one of the first AIDS service organizations in Africa, and in 1993, he designed the FOCUS program, considered by UNICEF to be a model approach to community-based care for orphans and vulnerable children. In 2001, he was recognized by the Schwab Foundation as one of the world's outstanding social entrepreneurs and received the Order of the British Empire from Queen Elizabeth II for his contributions to HIV/AIDS research. Foster was one of the co-chairs of the multiagency Joint Learning Initiative on Children and HIV/AIDS (2006–2009).

Stefan E. Germann is the Director for External Partnerships, Research, and Learning for World Vision International's Health, HIV, and Nutrition team. For the past 18 years, Germann has been working in the field of HIV/AIDS and health and community care of children. His focus has been on orphans and children affected by AIDS in rural and urban communities. In 1998, he started the Masiye Camp program in Zimbabwe, which provides psychosocial support for children affected by AIDS, and in 2002 he co-founded REPSSI, which has the goal of scaling up psychosocial support for children affected by AIDS in Africa. He has published widely on children and youth affected by AIDS and is a member of the Firelight Foundation advisory council, a philanthropic organization supporting hundreds of community-based children and AIDS programs across Africa. In 2005, he started to work with World Vision International (WVI) in Asia as Director for program quality and accountability in the tsunami emergency response. In June 2006, he took up the position as WVI global Senior Orphans and Vulnerable Children's advisor, based in South Africa.

Yan Guo is a postdoctoral research fellow at the Pediatric Prevention Research Center, Wayne State University School of Medicine. She received her Ph.D. degree in sociology from Utah State University in 2009, specializing in demography and social change and development. She has been working on HIV/AIDS prevention projects in China funded by the U.S. National Institutes of Health (NIH), targeting most-at-risk populations, such as men who have sex with men. She has also worked on NIH-funded projects related to psychosocial well-being of children affected by HIV/AIDS in China.

Stuart Kean is Senior HIV and AIDS Policy Adviser with World Vision International. His work for the last 9 years has focused on policy and advocacy related to children affected by AIDS. This work includes advocating for the U.K. government, the European Union, and global institutions, especially the UN and G8/G20, to improve and implement their policy commitments for children affected by AIDS, as well as supervising research on progress toward achieving the UNGASS commitments for children, tracking resources allocated to OVC at the community level, and supporting World Vision to strengthen local advocacy capacity related to CABA. Kean is co-chair of the Children Affected by HIV & AIDS Working Group of the U.K. Consortium on AIDS and International Development and also co-chair of the Communities and Resources Working Group of the Inter Agency Task Team on Children and HIV & AIDS.

Malega Constance Kganakga is the Chief Director of the HIV/AIDS Division at South Africa's National Department of Social Development. She is a member of the South African National AIDS Council and led the development of two National Action Plans for OVC and families infected and affected by HIV and AIDS (2006–2008, 2009–2012). She has led many major policy and research programs, including a national surveillance system for orphaned children. Dr. Kganakga was previously the HIV/AIDS program manager for the Nelson Mandela Children's Foundation, and Head of Department and Associate Professor of Nursing at the Medical University of South Africa. Her Ph.D., earned in 2003, focused on home-based palliative care for people living with HIV and AIDS.

Xiaoming Li, Ph.D., is professor and director of the Pediatric Prevention Research Center at Wayne State University School of Medicine in Detroit, Michigan. Li's research interests include global health issues related to mental health and HIV/AIDS prevention. He has been funded by the World AIDS Foundation and NIH to conduct research in China since 2000. His recent work in China includes longitudinal psychosocial needs assessment among children affected by HIV/AIDS, culturally appropriate HIV behavioral intervention prevention among rural-to-urban migrant workers, and HIV and alcohol use risk reduction intervention among female sex workers and their clients. He has been also participating in HIV prevention research conducted in other international settings including Namibia, Vietnam, India, Mexico, and the Bahamas. He received his doctoral training at the University of Minnesota, in the areas of educational psychology and research methodology.

Vinod Mishra is currently Chief of the Population Policy Section of the United Nations Population Division. He was previously head of research at Measure DHS. He is interested in behavioral, social, and environmental aspects of health and population issues in developing countries. He has published hundreds of articles and reports on a wide range of topics, including obesity and associated health problems, reproductive and child health, fertility and family planning, effects of air pollution on health, and human impacts on land use and land cover. Before coming to the United States in 1990, he worked with the Institute of Economic Growth and the National Institute of Health and Family Welfare in India.

Happyson Musvosvi is a Clinical Advisor for Preventing Mother to Child Transmission with the South-to-South program. He graduated from the University of Zimbabwe Medical School in 1988, and then worked as a general practitioner for an urban faith-based hospital in Malawi and a rural district hospital in Botswana. He obtained a master's degree in public health at the University of California, Davis, in 2006, and then worked for the William J. Clinton Health Access Initiative as Clinical Mentor for the pediatric program in Ethiopia. He is deeply interested in global health issues and has a particular interest in scaling up quality HIV/AIDS care in limited resource settings.

Marie-Louise Newell is a Professor of Paediatric Epidemiology at University College London's Institute of Child Health, as well as Professor of Health and Population Studies at the University of KwaZulu-Natal. She is an international expert on mother-to-child transmission of HIV infection, with a career spanning about 25 years and more than 250 publications. From 1987 to 2006, she led the European Collaborative Study on HIV infection in pregnancy, and since 2006, she has been based in South Africa, where she is the Director of the Africa Centre for Health and Population Studies. Research at the Centre is focused on charting the HIV epidemic in rural KwaZulu-Natal, understanding the spread of the virus, and informing the pathogenesis of transmission. As Director, she has forged a strong partnership with the Department of Health in the delivery of the HIV Treatment and Care Programme in the Hlabisa subdistrict.

Nathan Nshakira is a medical doctor and public health specialist based in Kampala, Uganda. He is an independent consultant and associate lecturer in Public Health at Uganda Christian University, Mukono. Nshakira has worked in hospital-based and district health services in rural Uganda, and has also led NGO intervention programs on AIDS and poverty in Uganda and nine other African countries. He has provided consulting support to faith-based and donor-supported development programs across eastern and central Africa on HIV/AIDS, child health, and support to vulnerable children. He was a key researcher in the global Joint Learning Initiative on Children and AIDS in 2007–2009, focusing on external resource flows to support community-based responses to vulnerable children. He is currently providing long-term technical support to the Strengthening Decentralization for Sustainability Program, a 5-year USAID-supported initiative to enhance social service delivery in health, education, and social development through decentralized local governments in Uganda.

Mihyung Park is a Regional Program Development and Evaluation Officer for Asia and former Regional Program Development Officer for Africa at Samaritan's Purse, an international nongovernmental organization. She has been involved in HIV prevention programs, HIV testing programs, and OVC support programs in Ethiopia, Kenya, Mozambique, Liberia, and Uganda. Park holds a master's degrees from both the Harvard School of Public Health and the University of Oxford.

Linda Richter is a Distinguished Research Fellow at the Human Sciences Research Council in South Africa, an Honorary Professor in the Department of Paediatrics at the University of the Witwatersrand in South Africa, and an Honorary Fellow in the Department of Psychiatry at the University of Oxford in the United Kingdom. Currently, she is on contract from the Human Sciences Research Council to the Global Fund to Fight AIDS, Tuberculosis, and Malaria in Geneva as a Senior Specialist on Vulnerable Children. Richter has conducted both basic and policy research in child, youth, and family development as applied to health, education, welfare, and social development, and has published more than 200 papers and chapters in the fields of child, adolescent and family development, infant and child assessment, protein-energy malnutrition, street and working children, and the effects of HIV/AIDS on children and families, including HIV prevention among young people.

Marina Rifkin served as Program Monitoring Advisor with the South-to-South program from 2008 to 2010. She holds a master's degree in health science with a specialization in international health from the Johns Hopkins School of Public Health and has extensive experience in public health monitoring, evaluation, and surveillance. Prior to joining South-to-South, she served as an epidemiologist with the Institute for Global Health at the University of California, San Francisco, and as Research Associate with the International Vaccine Institute in Seoul, Korea.

Rachel Samuel is Director of Sustainable Health and Development Solutions, an international development organization based in the United Kingdom that addresses issues of health access and other key development challenges. Her work on HIV/AIDS began in 1998, at the University of Oxford, where her doctoral research included work on an HIV vaccine, developed in collaboration with the International AIDS Vaccine Initiative. During the past 10 years, Samuel has been actively engaged in HIV policy, advocacy, and research in the United Kingdom, Africa, and South Asia. Recently, as Policy Adviser to World Vision International on health and HIV/AIDS, she worked on global policy issues such as health care financing and integrating HIV and health. Her work has appeared in peer-reviewed journals and as resource materials for practitioners in India, Uganda, Kenya, and South Africa. She is currently working on health care financing for the rural and urban poor in India.

Annemadelein Scherer is an occupational therapist and currently appointed as the Neuro-Developmental Advisor at the South-to-South program. She previously worked in two military hospitals, where she was Head of the Paediatric Occupational Therapy Unit and Nodal Point for the Military HIV Prevention project. She joined the South-to-South team in December 2008, and is currently pursuing her master's degree in early childhood intervention at the University of Pretoria.

Amy Slogrove is a Paediatric Clinical Advisor with the South-to-South program. She completed her medical studies at the University of Natal, Durban, South Africa. She subsequently qualified as a specialist pediatrician at Tygerberg Children's Hospital and Stellenbosch University in 2009. Her master's thesis dealt with severe infections in HIV-exposed uninfected infants in South Africa, the determinants of which she is going to study further through a Ph.D.-level course at the University of British Columbia, Canada.

Liezl Smit is the Clinical Program Director of South-to-South, a USAID-supported program providing technical and system support for maternal and child public health programs related to HIV/AIDS. She is currently based at the University of Stellenbosch, Cape Town, South Africa. She completed her medical studies at the University of Stellenbosch, obtained a diploma in child health from the Royal College of Paediatrics and Child Health, London, and subsequently qualified as a pediatrician at Tygerberg Children's Hospital and Stellenbosch University in 2004. She obtained her master's degree in child health from Warwick University in 2008, and completed the Advanced Health Management Program at the Foundation for Professional Development at Yale University.

Nigel Taylor is Coordinator for the U.K. development agency Friends of Treatment Action and works in South Africa with the Treatment Action Campaign, a social movement dedicated to achieving decent health care for those living with HIV. Taylor has spent nearly 30 years working on poverty reduction in Africa. In addition to work in Gambia and the Sudan, Taylor worked for 14 years for Oxfam GB, including management positions in its Humanitarian Department responding to food crises and conflict in eastern and southern Africa, and as the Country Representative in South Africa. Living in South Africa from 1996 to 2003 was a formative period as the AIDS pandemic impacted on friends and work. From 2004 to 2010, he worked as a freelance consultant focusing on strengthening civil society and international donor responses to AIDS, with a particular interest in developing greater appreciation for the role of communities and faith organizations.

Douglas Webb is a social scientist currently based in Ethiopia with UNICEF. Most recently, he was the Chief of the Children and AIDS Section in the East and Southern Africa Regional Office of UNICEF in Kenya (2004–2008). Douglas obtained his Ph.D. from the University of London in 1995, which examined social responses to HIV and AIDS in South Africa and Namibia, in contexts of political transition. He worked as a research officer for UNICEF Zambia (1995–1997) and UNICEF Mozambique (1998), as well conducting research with the Southern African AIDS Dissemination Service (SAfAIDS) in 1997–1998. He was the HIV/AIDS Adviser for Save the Children UK (2000–2004) in London. While there, he was the vice chair of the U.K. Consortium on AIDS and International Development. More recently, he was a member of the Joint Learning Initiative on Children and AIDS (JLICA), 2006–2008. He has written over 30 articles and book chapters covering issues such as children affected by AIDS, adolescent sexual and reproductive health, and HIV and AIDS and development. He is the author of *HIV and AIDS in Africa* (Pluto Press, 1997) and co-editor of *Social Protection for Africa's Children* (Routledge, 2010).

Protecting Childhood in the
AIDS Pandemic

Meeting the Essential Needs of All Children

JODY HEYMANN, LORRAINE SHERR, AND RACHEL KIDMAN

As her adult daughter became desperately ill with AIDS, Nunuko Ndebele took leave from work to care for her. Nunuko had no brothers or sisters to turn to when Marie was dying. After the funeral, Nunuko shared the experience with no one in her community but her pastor. The ongoing stigma of HIV/AIDS and the fear of ostracism silenced her.

After her daughter's death, Nunuko became the primary guardian of her orphaned grandchildren, 11-year-old Mosadi and 6-year-old Kgomotso. It quickly became clear that Kgomotso was also sick with HIV. Nunuko described the fluctuations in Kgomotso's health:

> *At times, you think she's better and then she presents with symptoms . . . . Then we bring her to the hospital and she gets better, the next month it's like we never treated her in the first place.*

Nunuko focused all her energies on providing the best care she could for her children and grandchildren. Providing the care on her own for Kgomotso, however, was next to impossible on Nunuko's earnings. Kgomotso's frequent illnesses meant Nunuko often missed work and lost much-needed income.

> *Kgomotso needs love from me. Greater love. She is sick. We have been advised to provide her with a balanced diet . . . . When I have money, I buy a bag of oranges for the whole family. As the oranges are getting fewer, I tell the others that maybe we should leave these ones for the sick child.*

When Kgomotso was sick, Nunuko would keep her home from school to care for her, afraid not only that she might spread one of the opportunistic infections to others, but also that both she and her granddaughter would become stigmatized if people learned she was HIV infected.

Kasego Mpofu shared similar challenges, and profound worries, about raising her children. Although they were healthy, Kasego was not: She had tested positive for HIV. At the time of her diagnosis, Kasego worked cleaning other families' homes.

Poverty, exacerbated by her health costs and how HIV/AIDS affected Kasego's work, left a profound impact on the lives of her son and sister in the absence of better supports. She knew early learning was important and had wanted her son to attend preschool, but she had not been able to afford it. It was all she could do to keep her younger sister in school. Kasego's earnings went for her sister's education and saving for her son's future schooling, instead of for a bed, a table, or clothing. She lived in a one-room house with no furniture.

> *These problems, like the lack of food, have a particular effect on the children. I can see it in their end-of-term reports. The teachers write as comments that many times the children are just sleeping in class. At times, they are brought back from school, and it is reported that the children are crying they are so hungry. . . . They've all lost weight these days and I think it's because of starvation; they're not eating as they're supposed to be. . . . [T]o make matters worse, they go to school on bare feet. We can't afford shoes—if we buy them shoes, it means that we don't buy food.*

Kasego had hoped to return to school to get the skills to train for a better paid job. Once she found out that she was HIV positive, Kasego's dreams of returning to school diminished. Her focus turned to saving as much money as she could for her son and her younger sister, both dependent on her. Kasego was acutely aware that her death would leave them depending on each other and on whatever resources she had been able to save. But she could save little. After she had budgeted for health costs, rent, her sister's education and other essentials, Kasego only had 100 pula—US$19—left per month for her own food: "You can imagine the kind of food I can afford."

Far greater attention has been paid to addressing how HIV/AIDS affects individual adults than to addressing how it affects children and families. And far greater resources have been dedicated to medical care than to meeting other basic needs, from food to education. The experiences of Nunuko, Kasego, and their families illustrate the extent to which the needs of HIV-affected families go far beyond adults and medical care.

UNICEF and others have increasingly called for urgent efforts to meet the needs of children affected by AIDS. The goal of this edited volume is to provide recommendations from leaders around the world in the field about how we can move from research to action to address the critical needs of children in the era of AIDS—an issue long overdue.

THE NUMBERS AND NATURE OF CHILDREN TOUCHED BY AIDS

HIV has a ripple effect on children. The children affected include those whose lives have changed due to direct infection, through infection of family members, and through community ramifications in highly endemic environments. An estimated 17 million children have lost a parent to AIDS; another 2.5 million are currently living with the virus.[1] Many millions more are rendered vulnerable when AIDS affects their families and communities.

We are only now beginning to appreciate the myriad of ways in which AIDS has shaped children's lives. The initial focus on AIDS orphans—the most visible and easily quantifiable group of affected children—has given way to a broader view of vulnerability. AIDS can be a debilitating long-term illness, and children may feel its impacts and loss of parental time and ability to provide care before parents die. As the virus spreads in families, children can experience multiple sequential episodes of illness and death within their family. Mounting medical costs and lost income impoverish households, forcing some children to prematurely enter the labor market and others to become primary care providers. After parental death, children's lives may be further uprooted as they are absorbed into new families.

The burden of care due to HIV/AIDS is borne mainly by extended family: First, they care for the sick and dying relatives; then, they assume responsibility for the children left behind.[2] Today, the extended family cares for over 90% of double orphans.[3] Adults who take on these caregiving responsibilities often have less time for their own children, more demands on their financial resources, and greater difficulties meeting all basic needs. Children who have parents providing care to AIDS-sick relatives or who share scarce resources with foster children may also experience disadvantage. Moreover, in places with severe epidemics, entire social support systems may be eroded by the high burden of HIV/AIDS. Friends and neighbors, overwhelmed by their own AIDS-related caregiving, may no longer be able to lend assistance, leaving already vulnerable children in even more precarious situations. Finally, in communities severely affected by AIDS, traditional safety nets are often overwhelmed by cumulative mortality, teachers are absent from school because of their own illness or that of family members, and basic health facilities can be hamstrung by AIDS care—all of which leave children increasingly vulnerable. The impact is most severe in environments in which government- and state-level support is the weakest, where universal education, health care, and social welfare are either not available or only partially available.

Although an entire generation of children has grown up in the shadow of the AIDS crisis, the epidemic has recently begun to stabilize. In 33 countries, most in sub-Saharan Africa, HIV incidence fell between 2001 and 2009; in many other countries, the epidemic has slowed. AIDS-related deaths also peaked at 2.1 million in 2004, and have steadily declined since. This is largely due to the increasing availability of treatment: In 2009, 1.2 million people were newly enrolled in treatment, resulting in a 30% jump in the total number treated compared to the previous year.[4] Deaths among children have also declined, but at a slower pace than for adults, partially reflecting the slower rollout of pediatric treatment.

This encouraging news should not obscure the epidemic's immense scale or the devastating impact it continues to have on children. Thirty-three million people are infected with HIV, most of whom (23 million) are concentrated in sub-Saharan Africa. New infections remained exceptionally high at 2.6 million in 2009. Moreover, progress has not been universal: The epidemics in Eastern Europe and Central Asia are still growing. Treatment has greatly reduced AIDS mortality, but 10 million people eligible for treatment still do not have access to essential therapy. As a result, there were 1.8 million deaths from AIDS in 2009.[5]

The epidemic's incidence and impact among children continues to be severe. New HIV infections among children dropped more than 30% in the last half decade but remain at an inexcusable 370,000 a year, even though the means to prevent vertical transmission have been known, available, and well-documented since 1996. AIDS-related orphanhood has not yet begun to decline; in fact, it increased from 14.6 million orphans in 2005 to 16.6 in 2009. Orphaning—like the epidemic itself—is concentrated (90%) in sub-Saharan Africa, with six countries (Kenya, Nigeria, South Africa, Uganda, United Republic of Tanzania, and Zimbabwe) home to a combined 9 million AIDS orphans.[6] Reductions in HIV infection and AIDS mortality are desperately needed, but will not alone avert the impact on millions of children.

HOW CHILDREN'S LIVES ARE AFFECTED

Without adequate protections, children affected by AIDS are exposed to recurrent risks, often magnified by their cumulative nature. The immense range of physical health, mental health, and social problems has been catalogued.[7] Children affected by AIDS are more likely than other children to suffer from hunger and to be stunted, to lack access to medical services, to have developmental delay, to experience infection and injury, and to die. They also commonly experience disruption of normal childhood and adolescence, psychological challenges, lack of adult supervision and care, harassment, and heightened vulnerability to physical and sexual abuse. Encountering stigma and discrimination, and living in households impoverished by the epidemic, children face difficulties in accessing education and are more likely to prematurely enter the labor force. There is also growing evidence that youth affected by AIDS engage in riskier sexual behaviors and are more likely to contract HIV. Below, we delineate some of the challenges that AIDS-affected children and youth experience across their life course; these are all presented in more detail throughout the book.

Elevated Risk of Infection in Infancy

HIV is a threat to children's survival from the start if their parents are infected, as infants can acquire HIV prenatally, at birth, or while breastfeeding. As a result of pre-, peri-, and post-natal transmission, 370,000 infants became newly infected in 2009.[8] In high-income countries, proven prevention strategies have lowered mother-to-child transmission to only 2%. Unfortunately, most women elsewhere do not have access to the needed preventive therapy.

Moreover, HIV, often dormant for many years in adults, progresses rapidly in infants. Early pediatric treatment can keep children healthy, but this again is out of reach for most children in low- and middle-income countries, where fewer than 6% of newborns are even tested for the virus.[9] Two million children are living with the virus,[10] but pediatric ARV coverage lags behind adult coverage: 28% of HIV-positive children who need ARVs have access.[11] In the absence of universal treatment, a quarter of a million children die of AIDS annually, most before their second birthday. In the largest country epidemic, in South Africa, AIDS now accounts for 35% of deaths in children under 5.[12]

Challenges to Healthy Development in Preschoolers

Children infected with HIV demonstrate delays in cognitive and motor development, as well as higher levels of malnutrition, illness, and mortality.[13] Evidence is also emerging that children exposed but uninfected are demonstrating developmental delay and worsened mortality.[14]

Young children need adult supervision, yet children who live with a sick parent see the consistency of their care decline. When a parent dies, children experience both grief and the loss of their primary caregiver. Where high HIV/AIDS mortality has reduced the availability of caregivers, few close family members may be available to care for orphaned children. Those adults left behind struggle to balance competing child care and economic responsibilities. Barriers to meeting these conflicting demands can affect the lives of HIV-uninfected children as well as-infected, biological as well as those who have been brought into the home after they became orphans. Our previous research in Botswana, for example, found that parents caring for HIV-infected family members spent less time with their own preschool children and were almost twice as likely to leave these young children home alone, resulting in higher rates of injury.[15]

Young children are particularly susceptible to infectious disease; risk is amplified in children who are also malnourished. Yet, in AIDS-affected households, young children are often repeatedly and intimately exposed to infections, particularly when few healthy adult caregivers are available. Empirical studies examining orphans and children of chronically ill or HIV-infected parents have largely found that they are more likely to experience respiratory infections and diarrhea, and are also more likely to die.[16] Children living in households with other sick adults or experiencing recent adult deaths are likewise more prone to illness.[17] Not surprisingly, those children in the poorest households are at greatest risk.[18] Children living in families impoverished by AIDS lose access to necessities. They are more likely to be malnourished, which is an underlying factor behind half of all child deaths,[19] and more likely to miss preventive health care.

Limited Education in Childhood

Children's life chances are dramatically shaped by the extent to which they access education and succeed in school. Yet, children affected by AIDS are often held back by difficult circumstances. Children living with sick parents may drop out of school to act as caregivers. Orphans may be forced to adopt adult roles, such as caring for younger siblings or entering the paid labor force, that compete with their schooling. For both populations, stigma and isolation from their peers may further discourage attendance. AIDS-related impoverishment may also leave families without resources for school fees. Finally, all children in severely affected communities may experience high teacher mortality and worsening infrastructure, which further impede their access to quality education. Regardless of the reason, the outcome is clear: Amidst a high prevalence of both poverty and AIDS, only 76% of African children are enrolled in primary school.[20]

Disadvantage is concentrated among AIDS-affected children. For example, a study of 40 countries showed that orphans are 13% less likely to attend school, with double orphans the most disenfranchised.[21] However, the degree of disadvantage varies from country to country.[22] Orphan disparities widen with age[23] and extend to secondary school: A Ugandan study found 16% of youth aged 15–19 years lost school time and 29% dropped out of school following their parent's death.[24] Some studies report that maternal orphans living in poverty experience more educational deprivation than their paternal counterparts, whereas double orphaning has the most detrimental effects.[25] Finally, double orphans living with more distant relatives may be at greatest risk, as evidence suggests that these relatives are least likely to invest in their education.[26] Old problems, such as gender inequality, are exacerbated by HIV and AIDS, with a double jeopardy for young girls, who are more likely to be kept away from school, required to take over household care responsibilities, and diverted to support income-generation activities.

Similar to orphans, children who experience the death of any adult in a poor household—regardless of whether it is a parent—have worse education outcomes.[27] Children living with sick parents may have similar, or even greater, difficulties accessing and attending school.[28] For example, longitudinal studies have indicated that children's schooling is most affected while a parent is ill.[29] Clearly, AIDS is having a dramatic impact on children's human capital development, making it harder to escape the cycle of poverty.

Psychosocial Impact in Childhood

Children affected by AIDS experience a range of traumatic events, including parental illness and death, stigma, social isolation, and separation from siblings, all of which have profound impacts. Children with sick parents can suffer loss of support, anxiety and uncertainty about the future. They can be confronted with many additional demands as a result of HIV/AIDS—such as caregiving for sick relatives or younger siblings or premature entry into the labor force—that further disrupt normal childhood routines. The trauma of their parent's death, or that of another loved one, brings grief at the same time that their loss can uproot families, separate siblings, and isolate children from normal support networks. When families experience a death, they are four times more likely to dissolve,[30] disrupting care and social ties at a time when children are in particular need of support.[31]

The nature of the AIDS pandemic leads to repeated exposure to traumatic events that cumulatively wear down resilience and adaptation. Although far more research is needed, two reviews of existing studies suggest that children affected by AIDS are more likely to experience depression, anxiety, and post-traumatic stress disorders.[32] In the absence of effective interventions, these psychosocial problems worsen over time.[33]

During the middle years, children are normally developing social identities, and peer groups become increasingly important. Children are still very reliant on the adults around them, including extended family, teachers, and other community members who are intimately involved in their everyday lives. Rather than receiving support during this critical period, children affected by AIDS may become subjected to stigma, discrimination, and bullying[34] affecting self-esteem and coping abilities.[35]

HIV Risk and Resilience in Youth

Youth are often overlooked in the response to children affected by AIDS. They are caught between two groups: too old to be considered children, and too young to be considered adults. However, this age group faces unique vulnerabilities while adopting new social roles. A major concern for all youth is high-risk sexual activity: almost half (45%) of all new infections occur in youth between the ages of 15 and 24.[36] Most of these infections occur in sub-Saharan Africa, where girls of this age are two to five times more likely to contract HIV than are boys. Research has found heightened risk for orphaned youth;[37] in one South African study, orphans were 50% more likely to have had sex.[38] In Zimbabwe, female orphans likewise demonstrated greater rates of HIV infections, other sexually transmitted infections (STIs), and unwanted pregnancies.[39]

High rates of sexual violence, transactional sex, and a lack of information about how to protect oneself (e.g., only 19% of girls in developing countries have accurate knowledge about HIV transmission and prevention)[40] contribute to risky sexual behavior and heightened HIV transmission. These risk factors may be particularly prevalent among children affected by AIDS. For instance, many children affected by AIDS lack adequate adult supervision and protection,[41] and are more likely to be living in economically dire conditions with limited access to schooling and decent work opportunities.

The Erosion of Family and Community Resources

Families play a crucial role in the health, education, and welfare of most HIV-affected children. This fact goes almost without saying when it comes to HIV-infected and other vulnerable children living with their parents. However, it is equally true for most orphans, as over 90% of double orphans live with extended family members.[42] In sub-Saharan Africa, one in six households is now caring for at least one orphan.[43] Unfortunately, their ability to protect and care for these children is increasingly compromised by the HIV/AIDS pandemic. Research has documented that families affected by AIDS are particularly likely to lack both caregiving time and economic resources. They are also overlooked by service interventions. The need to care for sick and dying family members, orphans, and others drains time spent with healthy children. Illness and caregiving responsibilities also limit the hours adults in the family are able to work and thus reduce their ability to earn income;[44] medical costs further draw down limited financial resources.[45] This in turn exacerbates poverty,[46] reducing the economic resources available to meet children's nutritional requirements and access health care. A study in Botswana found that approximately half of all families caring for orphans reported financial difficulties as a result of the caregiving burden.[47] Many AIDS-affected households are unable to provide adequately for their children; a survey in Tanzania found that almost 40% of households could not cover basic expenses (such as education, food, medical care, and clothes) for orphans.[48] Several other studies have likewise demonstrated reduced access to food in families that foster orphans.[49] On the other hand, when given even the most meager resources in a variety of cash transfer programs (at times as little as US$7 a month), families respond with elevated input to children in the domains of education, health, and nutrition.[50]

AIDS is also shaping the demographic composition of households in ways that place children at greater risk. In places with severe epidemics, children are increasingly cared for by grandparents,[51] whose age and economic vulnerability may impede care. Fostering of unrelated orphans is also on the rise;[52] this shift in caretaking disadvantages orphans. Studies have shown that the further orphans are from their caregivers biologically, the less likely they are to be well cared for and have good educational outcomes.[53] In the most highly affected countries, children are also increasingly living without adult supervision, although child-headed households are still a relatively rare and usually transient occurrence.[54]

Vulnerable households have traditionally reached out to the community for assistance;[55] relatives, friends, and neighbors responded with substantial in-kind and monetary resources.[56] However, the AIDS epidemic is eroding this community safety net.[57] As the number of ill and orphaned increases, need rises at a time when friends and neighbors are no longer able to lend support.

Public programs, which form a final safety net for vulnerable households, are likewise being eroded by the epidemic. Teachers are absent from school because of their own illness or that of family members, basic health facilities are consumed by AIDS care, and social welfare programs face overwhelming caseloads[58]—all of which leave children increasingly vulnerable. Within these devastating conditions, families are demonstrating enormous resilience and ingenuity.

They are reforming and reconfiguring responsibilities to better meet children's needs, but they are nonetheless under extreme strain. This is most marked in environments in which state responsibility and provision is the most lacking. Indeed, large-scale generalized provision, such as universal education, pensions, and health care, can act as a buffer and protect children who would otherwise have little chance of a healthy development.

CURRENT NATIONAL AND GLOBAL EFFORTS

The global response, viewed from many perspectives, has shortchanged children. The political and strategic explanations are complex, but the ramifications are simple—initial neglect and delayed response. The first step is to prevent HIV infection in children. Effective interventions to reduce transmission were first published in 1994. A decade and a half later, rollout has only been step-wise. In 2005, only 15% of mothers in need of ARV treatment in low-income countries received ARVs; 53% did in 2009. This picture shows a marked rise, but equally large gaps remain. It means that 47% of known HIV-positive pregnant mothers are slipping through the net—a net which should be watertight. Moreover, it only represents those who are known to be HIV positive and is thus intimately linked to HIV testing rates—which are notoriously low. In 2009, UNICEF reported that only 29% of pregnant women in low- and middle-income countries received an HIV test—up from 7% in 2005, but far from universal.[59]

Treatment of HIV-infected children is the next stage in the response. Yet, rollout of treatment to children has been low and lagging behind that of adults. Current data suggest that 28% of children who are considered in need of treatment actually receive it.[60] The formulation of pediatric compounds lagged behind that of adult ones; for many years, doctors reported cutting adult pills for child doses, with the accompanying inaccuracy in doses that need to be modulated based on child size. This has begun to change as more pediatric formulations permeate the market. However, the costs of pediatric formulations remain higher than those of adult formulations. This has the effect of increasing the costs for child treatment and raising barriers to treatment at a time of constrained and restricted budgets. Additionally, treatment can only be considered when HIV status is known. Early infant testing is still lamentably low (under 6%).[61]

Developmental care has lagged even further behind medical care. Although health interventions are routinely informed by evidence-based practice, many of the social and community responses to children have been carried out with little evaluation, and thus the learning curve is interrupted.[62]

Moreover, funding has been at a fraction of the need. Although HIV/AIDS prevention and treatment have benefited from the Global Fund initiative, an examination of country bids reveals limited direct monies allocated to children. Although it may well be that children share some global categories (such as prevention or testing monies), prevention and treatment programs often focus on adults, and funding directed at orphans and vulnerable children (the one category separating out children) falls far below the need. Publically available data from countries that have submitted progress reports to the Joint United Nations Program on HIV and AIDS (UNAIDS) confirm this trend. In Africa, only Swaziland and Botswana allocate large shares of AIDS-related expenditures to orphans and vulnerable children (OVC), with 30% and 19% respectively;[63] OVC in other African countries receive small fractions of total expenditures: 10% in Burundi,[64] 7% in Mozambique,[65] 6% in Cameroon and Zambia,[66] 5% in Burkina Faso,[67] 4% in Niger,[68] 3% in Mali and Cote d'Ivoire,[69] 2% in Sierra Leone and Togo,[70] and 1% or less in Benin and Ghana.[71] Outside of Africa, the percentages are even smaller: around 1% in Thailand,[72] El Salvador,[73] and Nepal,[74] and less in every other reporting country, including large countries like Mexico and Indonesia.[75] Some countries, like Ghana or the Philippines, freely admit that they have no public programs for OVC,[76] whereas others, like Mozambique or Benin, explicitly acknowledge that the expenditures are low.[77] Countries like Thailand or Lesotho have seen the amounts spent on OVC decline over the last reporting period,[78] in Lesotho's case because of reliance on diminishing funds from external donors.[79]

TAKING ACTION IS ESSENTIAL TO GLOBAL GOALS

The important but too limited steps taken to date by countries and the global community have left children at the crux of our failure to adequately prevent and address the impact of HIV/AIDS. Both life stories and statistics make abundantly clear why anyone concerned about the impact of AIDS should be deeply committed to addressing its impact on children.

Yet, even those who are not focused on AIDS but are rather focused on major development goals need to understand what can be done to markedly improve the lives of children affected by AIDS. When world leaders came together in 2000, only one of the Millennium Development Goals (MDGs) explicitly focused on HIV. Within MDG 6, which targeted combating HIV/AIDS, malaria, and other diseases, little of the HIV emphasis was on children. Only one subtarget specified improving school attendance of orphans aged 10–14. Yet, the reality is that it will be difficult if not impossible to achieve many of the global community's goals in the hardest-hit countries without successfully meeting the needs of children affected by AIDS.

MDG 1 focuses on eradicating extreme poverty and hunger. A quick review of the countries with the worst poverty statistics includes many countries where individual, family, and national economic outcomes have been deeply affected by HIV/AIDS: Congo, Chad, the Central African Republic, Swaziland, Zambia, Nigeria, Malawi, Mozambique, Malawi, and Tanzania are among the top 20 countries in the world in both HIV prevalence and percentage of the population living on less than US$1.25 a day.[80] MDG 2 targets achieving universal primary education. As detailed above, children affected by AIDS are at heightened risk of not completing schooling. The countries in the world with the highest rate of out-of-school children include many of the countries with a high number of AIDS-affected children, including, among others, Nigeria, the Central African Republic, and Lesotho.[81] The same can be said for MDG 4, which focuses on child health: countries like Chad, the Central African Republic, Cameroon, Equatorial Guinea, Mozambique, Zambia, and Nigeria have high rates for both under-5 mortality and HIV prevalence. (These lists include countries that have the 20 highest prevalence rates in the world, according to UNAIDS in 2009, and at the same time perform poorly in MDGs 2 and 4, according to the UN organization charged with tracking progress toward these goals).[82]

Yet, at the same time, providing far greater hope, there are countries with high rates of HIV infection where children are nonetheless doing well in education and health. For example, Botswana and Namibia, which at 23.9% and 15.3% have the second and fifth highest adult HIV prevalence rates in the world, are outside of the top 50 in under-5 mortality; in a similar vein, Zambia, Tanzania, and Uganda, whose respective adult HIV prevalence rates are 15.2% (7th in the world), 6.2% (11th), and 5.4% (13th), have net primary school enrollment rates of 96.7%, 99.6%, and 97.2%, respectively. Clearly something can be done.

PROTECTING CHILDHOOD IN THE AIDS PANDEMIC: FINDING SOLUTIONS THAT WORK

Protecting Childhood in the AIDS Pandemic will bring together lessons from experts around the world on what has worked, and what needs to be done to transform the outcomes of children of all ages whose lives have been affected by HIV/AIDS.

Children's developmental needs change as they grow, and unique solutions are often required for each age group. Although the importance of a developmental approach to children's programs may seem straightforward, few global actors and countries have embraced one. Countries that have programs that specialize in the needs of one age group (e.g., prevention of mother-to-child HIV transmission in infancy) often simultaneously fail to address the related needs of another age group (e.g., prevention of sexually transmitted HIV in adolescence), just as programs that have successfully addressed medical needs have often failed to address psychosocial needs.

In research, although a great deal of needed work has been carried out on the problems children face, less has been done to systematically pull together the best evidence on solutions. Substantial empirical evidence is available to inform decisions. Each chapter tackles a critical policy or programming question. The chapters begin with an overview of the challenges, review the solutions that have been tried, and analyze evidence on program effectiveness to point readers toward interventions with the greatest potential. We hope that this will spur action among all engaged in meeting the needs of children affected by AIDS, from local programmers to national policy-makers to global donors.

Protecting Childhood in the AIDS Pandemic will begin with chapters that place children's lives in context. Programs that have targeted children's needs, without considering their sources of support in families and communities, have often both failed to meet children's needs adequately and been unsustainable. The first section of the book will focus on placing children affected by AIDS in the context of the families and communities in which they live.

The second section of the book is dedicated to examining what would work in meeting the full range of needs of children affected by AIDS—psychosocial, developmental, and educational—across the life course from infancy through preschool, middle childhood, and adolescence.

The third section of the book examines medical interventions for children affected by AIDS: from preventing transmission during pregnancy, birth, and breastfeeding to ameliorating prevention and medical services both to the child as he or she grows and to the adults around him or her.

The fourth section of the book provides insights from leaders who have worked in government, civil society, and academia at national and international levels on questions that cut across age groups and across the types of needs children have. Whose responsibility is it to provide services and support for children affected by AIDS? And who should programs target?

In addressing these issues, the book brings together people who have expertise on and have worked in sub-Saharan Africa, Europe, South Asia, East Asia, Australia, and Central and North America. The authors include leading members of government, international organizations, national research organizations and academia, and national and international nongovernmental organizations, as well as medical professionals and practitioners working in program implementation and delivery.

What we learned was clear. When we asked experts in HIV/AIDS around the world what needed to be done to better meet children's needs, they recommended solutions that would fundamentally strengthen health and social services for all poor and marginalized children and families—not just those affected directly by HIV/AIDS. In writing about preschool children, Engle highlights the need to ensure adequate infant and child nutrition, guarantee access to health care for all, and develop community childcare and early learning programs. Each of these recommendations matters for all children. At the same time, she also highlights some of the particular needs of children affected by AIDS, including ensuring that the best means of preventing mother-to-child transmission are followed and scaling up early testing of children. In describing how to best meet the needs of school-aged children, Li and Guo similarly focus on improving those programs that would meet the needs of all children living in poverty. When focusing on youth, Bignami-Van Assche and Mishra detail the health and education services and supports that all youth need access to in order to prevent becoming infected with HIV, as well as the services needed by youth who have become infected. In discussing meeting the needs of families of children affected by AIDS, Richter further emphasizes that the best solutions are those that would expand income support and health and education services for all those living in poverty, not solutions targeted to those with HIV only.

Although the authors more focused on medical intervention, including Coovadia and Newell, and Smit and colleagues, naturally focused recommendations on those most directly affected by AIDS, even these medical chapters make clear the large extent to which all health services need to be improved if the health care services for children affected by AIDS are to be effective. In short, when asked what the best ways to increase the chances of healthy development for all children affected by AIDS were, the majority of authors focused on the importance of improving services that would benefit all children living in poverty, even if they are disproportionately important to children affected by AIDS. When specifically asked to analyze all of the evidence on whether programs should be targeted at children affected by AIDS, Adato likewise makes a compelling and detailed case for why the target needs to be focused on all children living in poverty, with few exceptions. Addressing HIV/AIDS in this integrated manner would, for many countries and global funders, mean a substantial shift from the kind of vertical funding that was the primary approach as the dollars available for HIV/AIDS increased after the creation of the Global Fund in 2002.

We began this initiative with the knowledge that, in order to meet global goals to improve the health and education of all children and to lift children and adults alike out of poverty, we would have to do a better job at preventing HIV/AIDS and diminishing its impact on those infected and affected. By the end of developing this volume, it has become clear that, even if one only cares about children affected by HIV/AIDS, to meet their needs requires improving the educational and health care systems for all.

Developing programs and using resources to meet the needs of children affected by AIDS has at times been perceived to be in conflict with doing the same for other children living in poverty. If these programs are designed well, nothing should be further from the truth. The most effective programs for improving the lives of children affected by AIDS can and in fact must be successfully aligned with the most important programs addressing the needs of children and families living in poverty and otherwise marginalized. In this edited volume, our hope is to move these programs forward to meet the needs of all children at risk. The time is long overdue.

NOTES

1. UNAIDS. (2010). *UNAIDS report on the global AIDS epidemic 2010.* Geneva: UNAIDS.
2. UNICEF, UNAIDS, & USAID. (2004). *Children on the brink 2004: A joint report of new orphan estimates and a framework for action.* New York: UNICEF, UNAIDS, USAID; Madhavan, S. (2004). Fosterage patterns in the age of AIDS: Continuity and change. *Social Science and Medicine, 58*(7), 1443–1454.
3. Monasch, R., & Boerma, J. (2004). Orphanhood and childcare patterns in sub-Saharan Africa: An analysis of national surveys from 40 countries.*AIDS 18* (suppl. 2), S55–S65.
4. UNAIDS. (2010). *UNAIDS Report on the global AIDS epidemic 2010.*
5. Ibid.
6. Ibid.
7. Richter, L., Foster, G., & Sherr, L. (2006). *Where the heart is: Meeting the psychosocial needs of young children in the context of HIV/AIDS.* The Hague: Bernard van Leer Foundation.
8. UNAIDS. (2010). *UNAIDS Report on the global AIDS epidemic 2010.*
9. WHO, UNAIDS, & UNICEF. *Towards universal access: Scaling up priority HIV/AIDS interventions in the health sector: Progress report 2010.* Retrieved January 14, 2011, http://www.who.int/hiv/pub/2010progressreport/report/en/index.html

10. UNAIDS. (2010). *UNAIDS Report on the global AIDS epidemic 2010.*
11. Ibid.
12. WHO, UNAIDS, & UNICEF. (2010). *Towards universal access.*
13. Abubakar, A. et al. Paediatric HIV and neurodevelopment in sub-Saharan Africa: A systematic review. Tropical Medicine and International Health, 13(7), 880–887; Potterton, J. et al. (2009). Neurodevelopmental delay in children infected with human immunodeficiency virus in Soweto, South Africa. Vulnerable Children and Youth Studies, 4(1), 48–57; Newell, M. -L., Brahmbhatt, H., & Ghys, P. D. Child mortality and HIV infection in Africa: A review. AIDS, 18(suppl. 2), S27–S34.
14. Filteau, S. (2009). The HIV-exposed, uninfected African child. Tropical Medicine and International Health, 14(3), 176–187.
15. Heymann, J. (2006). *Forgotten families.* New York: Oxford University Press.
16. Watts, H. et al. (2007). Poorer health and nutritional outcomes in orphans and vulnerable young children not explained by greater exposure to extreme poverty in Zimbabwe. *Tropical Medicine and International Health, 12*(5), 584–593; Mishra, V. et al. Education and nutritional status of orphans and children of HIV-infected parents in Kenya. *AIDS Education and Prevention, 19*(5), 383–395; Zaba, B. et al. (2005). HIV and mortality of mothers and children: Evidence from cohort studies in Uganda, Tanzania, and Malawi. *Epidemiology, 16,* 275–280; Nakiyingi, J. et al. (2003). Child survival in relation to mother's HIV infection and survival: Evidence from a Ugandan cohort study. *AIDS, 17*(12), 1827–1834.
17. Gray, G. et al. (2006). The effects of adult morbidity and mortality on household welfare and the well-being of children in Soweto. *Vulnerable Children and Youth Studies, 1*(1), 15–28; Ainsworth, M., & Semali, I. (2000). *The impact of adult deaths on children's health in Northwestern Tanzania.* World Bank Policy Research Working Paper no. 2266. Washington, DC: World Bank; Kadiyala, S. et al. (2009). The impact of prime age adult mortality on child survival and growth in rural Ethiopia. *World Development, 37*(6), 1116–1128.
18. Ainsworth & Semali (2000). *The impact of adult deaths on children's health in Northwestern Tanzania.*
19. Bryce, J. et al. (2005). WHO estimates of the causes of death in children. *Lancet, 365*(9465), 1147–1152.
20. United Nations. (2010). *The millennium development goals report 2010.* New York: United Nations Department of Economic and Social Affairs.
21. Monasch & Boerma. (2004). Orphanhood and childcare patterns.
22. Ainsworth, M., & Filmer, D. (2006). Inequalities in children's schooling: AIDS, orphanhood, poverty, and gender. *World Development, 34*(6), 1099–1128.
23. Yamano, T., Shimamura, Y., & Sserunkuuma, D. (2006). Living arrangements and schooling of orphaned children and adolescents in Uganda. *Economic Development and Cultural Change, 54,* 833–856; Ueyama, M. (2007). *Mortality, mobility and schooling outcomes among orphans: Evidence from Malawi.* IFPRI discussion paper no. 00710. Washington, DC: International Food Policy Research Institute.
24. Sengendo, J., & Nambi, J. (1997). The psychological effect of orphanhood: A study of orphans in Raika district. *Health Transition Review, 7*(Suppl.), 105–124.
25. Ueyama. (2007). *Mortality, mobility and schooling outcomes among orphans;* Bicego, G., Rutstein, S., & Johnson, K. (2003). Dimensions of the emerging orphan crisis in sub-Saharan Africa. *Social Science and Medicine, 56,* 1235–1247.

26. Case, A., Paxson, C., & Ableidinger, J. (2004). Orphans in Africa: Parental death, poverty and school enrollment. *Demography, 41*(3), 483–508.

27. Yamano, T., & Jayne, T. (2005). Working-age adult mortality and primary school attendance in rural Kenya. *Economic Development and Cultural Change, 53*(3), 619–653; Ainsworth, M., Beegle, K., & Koda, G. (2005). The impact of adult mortality and parental deaths on primary schooling in north-western Tanzania. *Journal of Development Studies, 41*(3), 412–439.

28. Gray et al. (2006). The effects of adult morbidity and mortality on household welfare and the well-being of children in Soweto; Mishra et al. (2007). Education and nutritional status of orphans and children of HIV-infected parents in Kenya.

29. Ainsworth, Beegle, & Koda. (2005). The impact of adult mortality and parental deaths.

30. Hosegood, V. et al. (2004). The impact of adult mortality on household dissolution and migration in rural South Africa. *AIDS, 18*, 1585–1590.

31. Hosegood, V. (2009). The demographic impact of HIV and AIDS across the family and household life-cycle: Implications for efforts to strengthen families in sub-Saharan Africa. *AIDS Care, 21*(S1), 13–21.

32. Cluver, L., Gardner, F., & Operario, D. (2007). Psychological distress amongst AIDS-orphaned children in urban South Africa. *Journal of Child Psychology and Psychiatry, 48*(8), 755–763; Sherr, L., & Mueller, J. (2008). Where is the evidence base? Mental health issues surrounding bereavement and HIV in children. *Journal of Public Mental Health, 7*(4), 31–39; Gwandure, C. (2007). Sexual assault in childhood: Risk HIV and AIDS behaviours in adulthood. *AIDS Care, 19*(10), 1313–1315; Cluver, L., Fincham, D. S., & Seedat, S. (2009). Posttraumatic stress in AIDS-orphaned children exposed to high levels of trauma: The protective role of perceived social support. *Journal of Traumatic Stress, 22*(2), 106–112; Cluver, L., Gardner, F., & Operario, D. (2009). Poverty and psychological health among AIDS-orphaned children in Cape Town, South Africa. *AIDS Care, 21*(6), 732–741; Kaggwa, E. B., & Hindin, M. J. (2010). The psychological effect of orphanhood in a matured HIV epidemic: An analysis of young people in Mukono, Uganda. *Social Science and Medicine, 70*(7), 1002–1010.

33. Cluver, L., Kuo, C., & Kganakga, M. (2010, July 16–17). *Parenting, disability and HIV/AIDS: Understanding impacts on children in AIDS-affected families.* Paper presented at Children and HIV Family Support First conference, Vienna.

34. Foster, G. et al. (1997). Perceptions of children and community members concerning the circumstances of orphans in rural Zimbabwe. *AIDS Care, 9*(4), 391–405; Thurman, T. R. et al. (2006). Psychosocial support and marginalization of youth-headed households in Rwanda. *AIDS Care, 18*(3), 220–229; Cluver, L., Bowes, L., & Gardner, F. (2010). Risk and protective factors for bullying victimization among AIDS-affected and vulnerable children in South Africa. *Child Abuse and Neglect, 34*(10), 793–803.

35. Sarason, I. G., & Sarason, B. R. (1982). Concomitants of social support: Attitudes, personality characteristics, and life experiences. *Journal of Personality, 50*(3), 331–343.

36. UNAIDS. (2010). *UNAIDS Report on the global AIDS epidemic 2010.*

37. Thurman, T. et al. (2006). Sexual risk behavior among south African adolescents: Is orphan status a factor? *Aids Behavior, 10*, 627–635; Operario, D. et al. (2007). Prevalence of parental death among young people in South Africa and

risk for HIV Infection. *Journal of Acquired Immune Deficiency Syndromes, 44,* 93–98; Gregson, S. et al. (2005). HIV infection and reproductive health in teenage women orphaned and made vulnerable by AIDS in Zimbabwe. *AIDS Care, 17*(7), 785–794.

38. Thurman et al. (2006). Sexual risk behavior among south African adolescents.
39. Gregson, S. et al., HIV infection and reproductive health in teenage women orphaned, 2005.
40. UNICEF. (2010). *Progress for children: Achieving the MDGs with equity.* New York: UNICEF.
41. Heymann, J. (2006). *Forgotten families.* New York: Oxford University Press; Rajaraman, D., Earle, A., & Heymann, S. J. (2008). Working HIV care-givers in Botswana: Spill-over effects on work and family well-being. *Community, Work and Family, 11*(1), 1–17.
42. Monasch, R., & Boerma, J. (2004). Orphanhood and childcare patterns in sub-Saharan Africa: An analysis of national surveys from 40 countries.*AIDS 18*(suppl. 2), S55–S65.
43. UNAIDS. (2006). *UNAIDS report on the global AIDS epidemic 2006.* Geneva: UNAIDS.
44. Heymann. (2006). *Forgotten families;* Heymann, J. et al. (2007). Extended family caring for children orphaned by AIDS: Balancing essential work and caregiving in a high HIV prevalence nation. *AIDS Care, 19*(3), 337–345.
45. Palamuleni, M., Kambewa, P., & Kadzandira, J. (2003). *HIV/AIDS and food security in Malawi.* Zomba, Malawi: Chancellor College, University of Malawi.
46. Palamuleni, Kambewa, & Kadzandira. (2003). *HIV/AIDS and food security in Malawi;* Loewenson, R., & Whiteside, A. (2001). *HIV/AIDS: Implications for poverty reduction.* United Nations Development Programme Policy Paper. New York: UNDP; Bechu, N. (1996). The impact of AIDS on the economy of families in Côte d'Ivoire: Changes in consumption among AIDS-affected households. In M. Ainsworth, & O.M. Fransen (Eds.), *Confronting AIDS: Evidence from the developing world: Selected background papers for the World Bank policy research report.* United Kingdom: European Commission; Deininger, K., Garcia, M., & Subbarao, K. (2003). AIDS-induced orphanhood as a systemic shock: Magnitude, impact, and program interventions in Africa. *World Development, 31*(7), 1201–1220; Ainsworth, M., & Filmer, D. (2002). *Poverty, AIDS and children's schooling: A targeting dilemma.* Washington, DC: World Bank; Miller, C. et al. (2007). Emerging health disparities in Botswana: Examining the situation of orphans during the AIDS epidemic. *Social Science and Medicine, 64*(12), 2476–2486; Miller, C. et al. (2006). Orphan care in Botswana's working households: Growing responsibilities in the absence of adequate support. *American Journal of Public Health, 96*(8), 1429–1435.
47. Miller et al. (2006). Orphan care in Botswana's working households.
48. UNICEF (2003). *Africa's orphaned generations.* NY: UNICEF.
49. Miller et al. (2006). Orphan care in Botswana's working households; Rivers, J., Silvestre, E., & Mason, J. (2004). Nutritional and food security status of orphans and vulnerable children: Report of a research project supported by UNICEF, IFPRI, & WFP (Working Paper). New Orleans: Tulane University; Gillespie, S. (2008). Poverty, food insecurity, HIV vulnerability and the impacts of AIDS in sub-Saharan Africa. *IDS Bulletin, 39*(5), 10–18.

50. Adato, M., & Bassett, L. (2009). Social protection to support vulnerable children and families: The potential of cash transfers to protect education, health and nutrition. *AIDS Care, 21*(S1), 60–75.

51. Foster, G. (2000). The capacity of the extended family safety net for orphans in Africa. *Psychology, Health and Medicine, 5*(1), 55–62; Zimmer, Z., & Dayton, J. (2005). Older adults in sub-Saharan Africa living with children and grandchildren. *Population Studies, 59*(3), 295–312; Nyangara, F. (2004). *Sub-national distribution and situation of orphans: An analysis of the president's emergency plan for aids relief focus countries.* Washington, DC: USAID.

52. Nyangara. (2004). Sub-national distribution and situation of orphans.

53. Case, A., Hosegood, V., & Lund, F. (2005). The reach and impact of child support grants: Evidence from KwaZulu-Natal. *Development Southern Africa, 22*(4), 467–482; Nyangara, *Sub-national distribution and situation of orphans,* 2004.

54. Ayieko, A. (2000). *From single parents to child-headed households: The case of children orphaned by AIDS in Kisumu and Siaya districts.* New York: UNDP; Nyamukapa, C., Foster, G., & Gregson, S. (2003). Orphans' household circumstances and access to education in a maturing HIV epidemic in eastern Zimbabwe. *Journal of Social Development in Africa, 18*(2), 7–32; Richter, L., & Desmond, C. (2008). Targeting AIDS orphans and child-headed households? A perspective from national surveys in South Africa, 1995–2005. *AIDS Care, 20,* 1019–1028.

55. Foster, G. (2004). Safety nets for children affected by HIV/AIDS in southern Africa. In R. Pharoah (Ed.), *A generation at risk: HIV/AIDS, vulnerable children and security in Southern Africa.* Pretoria: ISS.

56. World Bank. (1997). Confronting AIDS: Public priorities in a global epidemic. New York: Oxford University Press; Mutangadura, G., & Makaudze, E. (2000). Urban vulnerability to income shocks and effectiveness of current social protection mechanisms: The case of Zimbabwe. Consultancy report submitted to the Ministry of Public Service, Labour and Social Welfare and the World Bank; Foster, G. (2005). Under the radar: Community safety nets for children affected by HIV/AIDS in poor households in sub-Saharan Africa. Harare, Zimbabwe: UNRISD.

57. Nyambedha, E., Wandibba, S., & Aagaard-Hansen, J. (2003). Changing patterns of orphan care due to the HIV epidemic in western Kenya. *Social Science and Medicine, 57,* 301–311; Mtika, M. (2001). The AIDS epidemic in Malawi and its threat to household food security. *Human Organization, 60*(2), 178–188.

58. Haacker, M. (2002). *The economic consequences of HIV/AIDS in Southern Africa.* Washington, DC: IMF; Cornia, G. (2002). Overview of the impact and best practice responses in favour of children in a world affected by AIDS. In G. Cornia (Ed.), *AIDS, public policy and child well-being.* Florence: UNICEF-IRC; Richter L., & Foster, G. (2005). *The role of the health sector in strengthening systems to support children's health development in communities affected by HIV/AIDS.* Geneva: CAH, WHO.

59. UNICEF. (2010). *Children and AIDS: Fifth stocktaking report.* New York: UNICEF.

60. Ibid.

61. Ibid.

62. King, E. et al. (2009). Interventions for improving the psychosocial well-being of children affected by HIV and AIDS. *Cochrane Database of Systematic Reviews, 2*, doi: 10.1002/14651858.CD006733.pub2

63. Botswana National AIDS Coordinating Agency & UNAIDS. (2007). *Botswana national AIDS spending assessment: 2003/2004 to 2005/2006.* Gaborone: Botswana NACA & UNAIDS; National Emergency Response Council on HIV & AIDS & UNAIDS. (2008). *The kingdom of Swaziland national AIDS spending assessment 2005/2006 and 2006/2007.* Swaziland: NERCHA & UNAIDS.

64. Ministere de la Lutte contre le SIDA. (2009). Estimation des flux de resources et de depenses nationales de lutte contre le VIH/SIDA et les IST, Burundi 2007–2008. Burundi: CNLS Burundi/ONUSIDA.

65. UNAIDS. (2007). Mozambique: National AIDS spending assessment (NASA) for the period 2004/2006. Mozambique: UNAIDS.

66. Comité National de Lutte contre le SIDA. (2009). Rapport de l'analyse des flux des ressources et des depenses nationales contre le SIDA (EF-REDES) au Cameroun en 2007. Cameroon: Comité National de Lutte contre le SIDA; National HIV & AIDS/STI/TB Council. (2008). *Zambia: National AIDS spending assessment for 2005 and 2006.* Zambia: Ministry of Health.

67. Conseil National de Lutte contre le SIDA et les Infections Sexuellement Transmissibles. (2009). *Estimations des flux de ressources et de depenses nationales de lutte contre le VIH/SIDA et les IST (EF-REDES), Burkina Faso.* Burkina Faso, Mali: Presidence du Faso, UNAIDS & UNDP.

68. Coordination Intersectorielle de Lutte contre le SIDA. (2009). *Estimation des flux de ressources et de depenses nationales contre le VIH/SIDA et les IST (REDES): Niger, 2007–2008.* Niger: Presidence de la Republique & UNAIDS.

69. Secretariat Executif du Haut Conseil National de Lutte contre le SIDA. (2009). *Estimation des flux de ressources et de depenses nationales de lutte contre le VIH et les IST (EF-REDES): Mali, 2007–2008.* Mali: Presidence de la Republique & ONUSIDA; Conseil National de Lutte contre le SIDA (2009). *Estimation des flux de ressources et de depenses nationales de lutte contre le SIDA (EF/ REDES):Côte d'Ivoire 2006, 2007 et 2008.* Cote d'Ivoire: Ministere de la Lutte contre le SIDA.

70. Republic of Sierra Leone. (2009). *National AIDS spending assessment (NASA) for the period 2006–2007.* Sierra Leone: National HIV/AIDS Secretariat & UNAIDS; Conseil National de Lutte contre le SIDA et les Infections Sexuellement Transmissibles. (2009). *Flux des financements et depenses consacrees a la reponse au VIH at au SIDA en 2006 et 2007 au Togo.* Lome, Togo: Presidence de la Republique & ONUSIDA.

71. Comite National de Lutte contre le SIDA. (2008). *Estimation des flux de ressources et de depenses nationales de lutte contre le VIH/SIDA et les IST (REDES): Bening, 2006–2007.* Benin, West Africa: Presidence de la Republique & UNAIDS; Asante, F. A., & Fenny, A. P. (2008). *National AIDS spending assessment 2007: Level and flow of resources and expenditures to confront HIV and AIDS.* Ghana: Institute of Statistical, Social & Economic Research, Ghana AIDS Commission & UNAIDS.

72. Tisayaticom, K. et al. (2009). *Thailand national AIDS spending assessment 2000–2004.* Thailand: International Health Policy Program & National Economics & Social Development Board.

73. Programa Nacional de ITS/VIH-SIDA. (2009). *Medición de gastos en SIDA.* El Salvador: Ministerio de Sanidad.
74. Sharma, M., & Nyanti, S. (2009). *Nepal: National AIDS spending report 2007.* Kathmandu: HIV/AIDS & STI Control Board, Government of Nepal, & UNAIDS.
75. Rivera Reyes, M. D. P., Barragan Robles, M., & Parra Bernal, L. D. (2008). *Medición del gasto en SIDA (MEGAS), México 2006–2007.* Mexico: CENSIDA & ONUSIDA; Nadjib, M., Megraini, A., & Darmawan, E. S. (2008). *Technical report: AIDS spending in Indonesia 2006–2007.* Indonesia: Center for Health Research, University of Indonesia.
76. Aranjuez, E. S. (2009). *Country report on national AIDS spending assessment (NASA): Year 2000–2004 in the Philippines.* Philippines: National Economic & Development Authority; Asante & Fenny. (2008). *National AIDS spending assessment 2007.*
77. Comite National de Lutte contre le SIDA. (2008). *Estimation des flux de ressources et de depenses nationales de lutte contre le VIH/SIDA et les IST (REDES): Bening, 2006–2007*; UNAIDS. (2007). *Mozambique: National AIDS Spending Assessment.*
78. Tisayaticom et al. (2009). *Thailand national AIDS spending assessment 2000–2004.*
79. Mokete, K. et al. (2009). *Lesotho: National AIDS spending assessment.* Lesotho, Africa: National AIDS Commission & UNAIDS.
80. UNAIDS. (2010). *UNAIDS Report on the global AIDS epidemic 2010*; World Bank. *World Development Indicators (WDI) and Global Development Finance (GDF)* database. Retrieved February 4, 2011, http://databank.worldbank.org/ddp/home.do?Step=12&id=4&CNO=2
81. UNAIDS. (2010). *UNAIDS Report on the global AIDS epidemic 2010*; UNESCO Institute of Statistics. *Data Centre* data base. Retrieved February 4, 2011, http://stats.uis.unesco.org/unesco/tableviewer/document.aspx?Report Id=143
82. UNAIDS. (2010). *UNAIDS Report on the global AIDS epidemic 2010*; United Nations Division of Statistics, *Millennium Development Goals Indicators* database. Retrieved February 4, 2011, http://mdgs.un.org/unsd/mdg/Data.aspx

PART ONE

The Critical Context
of Children's Lives

2

The Central Role of Families in the Lives of Children Affected by AIDS

LINDA M. RICHTER ■

Empirical studies of the impact of HIV and AIDS on families indicate both stress and coping.[1] However, unpublished programmatic literature, popular reports, and the media tend to portray families, especially families in sub-Saharan Africa, as being in crisis—nonexistent, broken, or disordered—having disintegrated under the strain of the dual impacts of longstanding poverty and increasing adult deaths due to AIDS. There are descriptions of whole villages without adults, of child-headed households coming into existence every few seconds,[2] and of millions of children without care.

The reality is quite different. In poor countries, many of which are characterized by postcolonial strife and ineffectual or corrupt governance, few social, health, and educational services function as safety nets. Under these circumstances, extended families, kin, and community provide what protection exists for vulnerable children. The vast majority of children affected by HIV and AIDS live with their families, and families remain the most important, and developmentally appropriate, form of support for all children—not only those in deep poverty or in areas affected by AIDS or other misfortunes. In addition, the erosion of rural lifestyles and the lack of employment in urban areas mean that many working-age adults continue to live with ageing parents and their children. But AIDS is depleting the capacities of families because it impoverishes households by draining income and destabilizing livelihoods and family structure, creates anxiety and grief among adults and children, and tears at community connectedness. Yet, very little effort and few resources are currently being directed to supporting families in their important functions of caring for and protecting children. This chapter argues for a reorientation from efforts by external agencies to provide assistance directly to individual children identified as orphans to systemic endeavors to protect families from destitution and to provide services to families, so that they can provide care for children now as well as in a sustainable way in the future.

The extreme perceptions of absent and failed families are fuelled by a number of factors. It is now recognized that the definition of an orphan in the HIV/AIDS litera-ture as a child who has lost one or both parents[3] inadvertently contributed to wide-spread misunderstanding of the issues affecting children. Adult deaths are used as a proxy for the social impact of the HIV and AIDS epidemics, especially on children. However, this definition of orphaned children misled donors and philanthropic organizations to try to "replace" lost parents and families by building orphanages, providing out-of-family care and support, providing psychosocial support directly to children, and supplementing parenting in other ways. In fact, though, epidemiologi-cal and demographic estimates indicate that more than 88% of children classified as orphans have a surviving parent,[4] most often their mother, and more than 90% of "orphans" live with close family.[5] Expanded access to treatment has slowed adult deaths, increased parental survival, and even led to improved conditions for chil-dren,[6] but much more needs to be done to bolster resources and support for families, including those coping with multiple members on long-term antiretroviral (ARV) medication.

Images of abandoned children without family control and parental guidance also prompted security fears that hordes of unsocialized children and youth would be forced to turn to crime or dragooned into rogue armies, thus contributing to unrest in already unstable regions of the world.[7] Ensuring orphaned children received moral direction and were under the control of responsible adults gave impetus to efforts to provide substitute family care, including by faith-based groups. But very few chil-dren affected by HIV and AIDS find themselves without any family support.[8] Unlike nuclear families in the West, families throughout the majority world are generally extensive, and socialization of children is seldom left solely to one or both biological parents. In Africa, for example, a parent's siblings are often referred to as *little mother* or *big father*, depending on whether they are younger or older than the child's parent.[9] Further, there is no evidence that children whose parents have died are unsocialized or aggressive; rather, they are more likely to be withdrawn and at risk of depression, both at the time of parental death and/or in the future.[10]

The idea of millions of bereft and orphaned children, abandoned and alone, while a distorted picture, has served the interests of advocates in their efforts to draw atten-tion to the severe difficulties faced by the many children and families affected by HIV/AIDS and poverty. Meintjes and Giese refer to the "spin" put on orphanhood, of which an unintended consequence has been to divert attention away from the context of longstanding poverty, as well as from families and children other than orphans who are also affected by HIV and AIDS.[11] The almost exclusive focus on orphans has individualized responses, predisposing local and international actors to individual case management and welfare approaches rather than to public health or social policy responses to affected children.[12] The latter is nevertheless more suited to the context, scale, and longstanding nature of the challenges facing children and families.

Most importantly, images of abandoned children, which are significant prompts for philanthropic behavior, have unfortunately drawn attention away from the importance of supporting families. In fact, they have unintentionally played into ten-dencies to blame families for the vulnerability of children, including for bringing HIV and AIDS into the household. However, families—vulnerable as they may be—are currently caring for affected children, even under worsening social and economic conditions. In contrast to services, programs and projects can help only intermittently and for short periods of time; only families can take responsibility for children on a day-to-day basis, as well as over their life course.

Despite the fact that families comprise the front-line response for children affected by HIV and AIDS, pitifully few resources and services are directed at bolstering and protecting vulnerable families. Fewer than 15% of families caring for orphans and vulnerable children in 2007 were estimated to have received any assistance from external agencies.[13] It has taken equally long to recognize the role that communities play in supporting vulnerable children and families and the importance of strengthening indigenous community systems of care.[14] Lack of appreciation of their roles has contributed to families and communities being passed over in HIV and AIDS funding, programming, and policy.[15]

THE IMPORTANCE OF FAMILIES IN THE LIVES OF CHILDREN AFFECTED BY HIV AND AIDS

Families were the first to respond to children affected by AIDS, both in the United States and in southern Africa,[16] and families have continued to be the vanguard of care and support for affected children. The same pattern of response is being seen in China, India, Eastern Europe, and other sites of concentrated AIDS epidemics.[17] When parents become ill or die, their spouses, siblings, parents, other family members, and neighbors help with or take on the care of affected children, as kith and kin have always had to do during times of calamity and misfortune.[18] Given the absence of government or civil society organizations and services, families remain the main sources of support for vulnerable people and groups in poor communities—whether by default or choice.[19] This inevitable mutuality does not romanticize families nor gloss over family schisms that can adversely affect children.[20]

Families are the social expression of a human life strategy for, among others, child survival and development. Whether constituted by biological or social ties, families provide for intensive support over the life course, as well as for the intergenerational transfer of social values, competencies, and assets.[21] In turn, families are embedded in wider networks of kin and are part of broader society.[22] Thus, family formation can be thought of as an expression of social "deep structure,"[23] comprising human motivational and behavioral dispositions to create (and recreate) social organization that provides not only for the nurture of an individual child in the immediate generation, but also secures accumulated knowledge, lineage, and the re-creation of family bonds in the future.[24] The implications of this deeply embedded pattern of affiliation to support and protect children are that both children and adults attempt to replicate parental and family arrangements of one kind or another when misfortune occurs, families are disrupted, or children abandoned. This is an expression of our desire, as human beings, for "family relatedness" to others and for stable bonds of mutual affection and predictable support, including under extremely difficult circumstances when the need for them and their salience is intensified.

Families are an inherent aspect of human social organization but, under social and individual stress, can become inadequate and even dysfunctional. There is a danger in romanticizing families, as occurred in the United States, where Goode referred to "the classical family of Western nostalgia."[25] Nonetheless, while families dissolve and change as part of the cycle of life and death, even in war, calamitous natural disasters, and genocide, family groups continue to be formed as the central pillar of social organization for human beings, and the critical foundation for ensuring the current and future well-being of children. In fact, one of the difficulties faced by children reared in orphanages—that is, outside of continuous intimate relationships with a shared or constructed history and future—is how their sense of self is diminished by the absence of a shared life story, an essential element to the establishment of one's own family.[26]

The Impact of HIV and AIDS on Families

Before the emergence of AIDS, major changes started to occur in families across the world, largely as a consequence of industrialization and ensuing social and geographic mobility. These include, for example, decreasing family size. Postindustrial family forms began to emerge that are being influenced by declining fertility, growing gender equality, and delays to and reductions in marriage. Goode speaks of the "desacralization" of marriage in the West, with legal, religious, psychological, and social distinctions between being married and not being married becoming increasingly blurred.[27] While traditional, extensive families remain predominant in the majority world, increasingly modern, or rather postmodern, families may consist of various mixes of biological, adoptive, and elected members, as occurs in reconstituted families following death or divorce and remarriage, with some blood relatives, partners and their families, and friends.[28] The specific impacts of HIV and AIDS are difficult to differentiate against these background trends.[29] Families dissolve throughout the life cycle as a result of births, deaths, and separations. These cannot be averted and, indeed, such dissolution may be adaptive. Even if families are under severe strain, the appropriate response is not to attempt to replace family in a child's life. Instead, families must be supported as they emerge, transform, and adapt in the face of the socioeconomic and psychosocial demands created by long-term deep poverty, stigmatization, and the effects of relentless AIDS epidemics.[30]

The first AIDS cases date back to the 1950s in Africa, with fairly rapid increases in HIV infection during the 1970s. At the time, however, AIDS was largely indistinguishable from deaths due to malnutrition, malaria, and diarrheal disease.[31] Heterosexual transmission and HIV infection in women was only recognized in the mid-1980s,[32] and vertical transmission some time later.[33] It was not until fairly recently that HIV/AIDS has been appreciated as a "family disease." That is, HIV and AIDS cluster in families because of the ways in which it is transmitted, its social impact on people in relation to one another, and the burden of care entailed by chronic illness and death.

The predominant route of HIV transmission in generalized epidemics is between long-term, often cohabiting partners who, in many cases, are husband and wife. For example, estimates from Rwanda and Zambia show that this form of horizontal transmission accounts for 60% to 95% of new infections.[34] Similarly, almost all infections in children are acquired vertically, from parent to child during pregnancy, delivery, and breastfeeding.[35] These patterns of infection cause HIV and AIDS to concentrate in families. Moreover, when an individual is affected by HIV/AIDS, those closest to them, the people they call family, are also affected.[36] All are exposed to infection, and they share apprehension about disclosure, stigmatization, ill-health and suffering, the costs and burdens of treatment, loss of income, and need for care and support. AIDS causes anxiety and stress throughout the family,[37] and the full impact of HIV and AIDS, including its social and economic effects, is only appreciated when not only the individual, but the family as a whole, is considered.[38]

Economic stress is among the first impacts of HIV at the household level. Affected individuals, often breadwinners, may stop working, and such income or produce is sorely missed. Available resources are used to access and purchase additional health services and care. As stresses increase, households sell assets, may become indebted, and inevitably reduce consumption. They buy less food and spend less on transport, school, and health care other than health expenses for those people who are acutely ill.[39] This chain of events occurs also in low-prevalence and concentrated epidemic settings.[40] Reduced household consumption affects children in particular. Parenting effort generally increases under conditions that threaten child well-being, but can decrease when parental health is threatened at the same time as prospects for survival, especially for very young children, decrease.[41] Children may experience hunger, withdrawal from school, increased work in the home and in livelihood activities, isolation due to stigma, neglect by withdrawn adult caregivers, anxiety over parental health, and fear for their own future security.

In generalized epidemics, large numbers of families are affected in these ways. An analysis at the district-level in southern Africa indicated that, whereas 32% of families had been directly affected by HIV and AIDS, another 29% (in total almost two-thirds of families) had experienced ripple effects, such as fostering affected children and assisting relatives with money for food and health care expenses.[42] The numbers of affected households (those estimated to have an adult member living with HIV or an adult member with AIDS, plus those that have experienced one or more deaths of adult members from AIDS) were calculated in 2003 to range from about 16% to 57% in 11 sub-Saharan African countries.[43]

INTERVENTIONS: FEASIBILITY AND EFFECTIVENESS

In high-prevalence settings, what are the most appropriate, feasible, and effective interventions for children, and to what degree are these interventions generalizable to low-prevalence environments and concentrated epidemics?

Desmond argues that, of the many serious consequences HIV and AIDS have for children, few are inevitable.[44] Rather, families with sufficient social and material resources, as well as access to needed services, can deflect or absorb the impacts of HIV/AIDS on children to personally manageable levels. For example, in the United States, as in other Western countries, a small proportion of children (3%–5%) experience parental death.[45] With sufficient ongoing support, the great majority of these children adjust to this experience and grow up to lead happy and productive lives. That is, it is not the experience itself that carries maximum threat, but the lack of stable and continuing assistance to help children manage their response to the loss. The greatest danger to children in high HIV prevalence settings is that the impacts of AIDS occur in the context of preexisting and pervasive poverty and lack of services, both of which debilitate the capacity of families to protect children through increased parenting and protection.

Under these circumstances, public health and policy responses are needed to achieve overall improvements in the conditions of all children and families, and such responses will tend to have the greatest benefits for the most vulnerable groups. Consider the curve in Figure 2.1, which describes the normal distribution of the health and well-being of children in any particular population. The right and left tails of the curve describe, respectively, children who are doing very much worse and very much better than average. Under conditions of general hardship and stress, the numbers of children doing poorly increases, making individual case-management approaches ineffective as the problems children experience cannot successfully be addressed one at a time. Instead, if the curve is shifted to the right—that is, if the circumstances of all children improve by virtue of one or more universal interventions—the numbers of children requiring individual assistance becomes smaller and more manageable through individually targeted interventions. This is the basis of public health, as compared to clinical medicine or case management.

In addition, not all children affected by HIV and AIDS need individual intervention by agencies external to the family. In Figure 2.2, a hierarchy of children's needs for psychosocial care, support, and intervention is depicted alongside recommended commensurate actions. All children need responsive care by their parents; a smaller number of children whose families are under stress may need additional stimulation, play, and routines, as may be provided in an early child development program or facility or through after-school care; a smaller number still may need supplementary community and social support to assist their families as they go through acute difficulties, as may be provided by support groups and home visiting programs; and only a small minority of children need individual-level intervention by trained paraprofessionals or professionals.

The Joint Learning Initiative on Children and HIV/AIDS (JLICA) made a strong recommendation with respect to strengthening families as a key public health intervention to protect children from the adverse effects of HIV and AIDS.[46] Strengthening families, from this point of view, involves four major sets of actions: first, recognizing

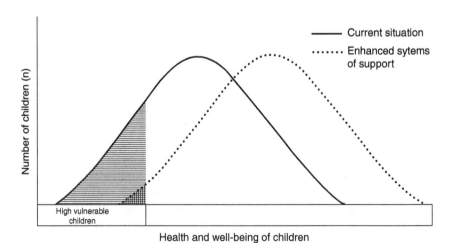

Figure 2.1 Universal curve shift to improve children's health and well-being.[47]

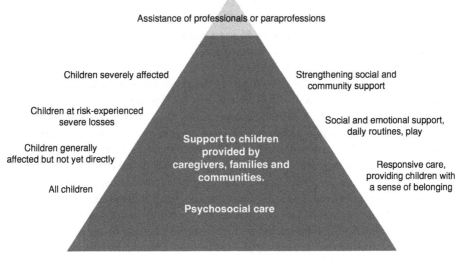

Figure 2.2 Hierarchy of children's needs for psychosocial care, support and intervention.[48]

and acknowledging the importance of families in the lives of children; second, ensuring that families have sufficient material resources to provide adequate care for children; third, assisting families in ways that enable children to thrive and have opportunities to realize their human potential; and, fourth, providing services in ways that sustain and reinforce family relationships and mutual commitments to build long-term, sustainable protection for children.[49]

Acknowledging the Central Role of Families in the Lives of Children

Services, programs, and projects set up to support and protect children do so effectively against the background of family care across the life course. Families are constant in the lives of children (and adults), whereas interventions and services are intermittent and generally short-lived. Two examples illustrate this point.

Unfortunately, far too many government programs and nongovernmental organizations (NGOs), that perceive the acute psychosocial needs of children affected by AIDS respond with attempts to provide "better parenting," substitute care, and psychosocial support directly to children. Committing children who have surviving parents and kin to orphanages, without first providing family support and counseling for unification, is an example of an attempt to provide "better parenting" than children are currently perceived to be receiving from their families. Attempts to "improve parenting" through substitute care were applied during colonial times in India, Australia, and the American West, among other places, principally to give local children what was thought to be a better chance in life than their indigenous families could provide,[50] in Eastern Europe to produce citizens and families in tune with state ideology,[51] and now in sub-Saharan Africa to save AIDS orphans.[52] Only a minority of children in orphanages are without parents; most are poor children.[53]

Nearly a century of research has established that orphanage and other forms of group residential care have adverse effects on the long-term psychological, social, and physical health of young children.[54] Despite the high cost of orphanages, estimated to be ten times or more than family care,[55] still not enough effort is being made in developing countries to provide assistance to families that have experienced bereavement, to undertake family reunification, or to support "kith-and-kin fostering" of separated and orphaned children.

The same observation applies to much of the provision of psychosocial care to affected children. Programs that distribute toys as comfort objects to bereaved children, for example, seldom hand the doll over to the mother or other primary caregiver to give to the child at an appropriate and meaningful time in the child's life, whether this is bedtime on that day, the child's birthday, or another special occasion. The latter approach supports and strengthens family bonds, enabling caregivers to respond to children's emotional needs, and it promotes love and appreciation from the child in return. Instead, when volunteers, often strangers in the community, hand dolls to children in contexts in which caregivers can barely manage to feed their families, families feel disempowered by their poverty and lack of agency, and children become confused. The same applies to feeding schemes in which volunteers hand out food for children while mothers sit helplessly by. In fact, many current child-focused interventions have the potential to strengthen the support system around a child by acknowledging and reinforcing the importance of parents, other intimate caregivers, and families in children's lives.

A strong conclusion from the available science on child development is to consider children inevitably as part of an ecology in which their parents, siblings, other intimate family, and kin provide the lifelong proximal material, social, and psychological environment for children's health and well-being.[56] Not all families are stable or able to provide fully for their children's needs. Such families require assistance to be able to protect and care for children. Two critical forms of help that families require are financial assistance to meet the basic needs of children, and family-centered services that build on and reinforce family members' mutual commitment to each other over the long term.

Ensuring the Economic Survival of Families

About 6 million young children in poor countries die each year from preventable conditions, principally undernutrition, diarrhea, malaria, measles, and pneumonia. Deaths from these causes are all associated with poverty, deprivation, and lack of accessible health services.[57] In the same vein, it is estimated that some 200 million children in resource-poor countries fail to reach their full human potential because of poor nutrition and deprivation.[58] Added to this is the burden on mortality, morbidity, and human development associated with HIV and AIDS.

Twenty percent of the world's population lives on less than US$1 a day, and half the world population (about 3 billion people) live on less than US$2 a day.[59] As indicated earlier, worsening socioeconomic conditions are an early impact of HIV and AIDS on families. Poor families have little food security and few, if any, assets and savings. They thus have no cushion to absorb lost income and livelihoods and the increased health care costs associated with HIV/AIDS.[60] Desperate poverty saps children's development, mental health and social adjustment, work and school performance, and family capital.[61] Eventually, it recycles vulnerability to HIV infection and intergenerational poverty.[62]

Increasing poverty and its knock-on effects on children and families suggest as an urgent first step a social security, rather than a social welfare, approach to assisting the neediest families. There is a continuum of social security or social protection strategies that range from income transfers to microlending to public works to skill training and employment. Access to water, sanitation, education, and health services are also provisions that significantly benefit the poorest communities affected by HIV and AIDS.[63]

However, the degree of incapacity of the worst-hit and poorest families affected by HIV and AIDS means they cannot benefit from upstream developmental approaches. Older women caring for grandchildren, for example, may not be physically able to work even if offered the opportunity, nor do most have the capacity to generate income to repay a small loan. For this reason, direct income transfers are most appropriate for highly vulnerable, work-constrained families. They are less labor intensive, require less administration than in-kind benefits, and they maximize the choices of poor families. Items from food parcels, for example, are often sold to enable a family to buy soap or pay for transport to a health facility. Income transfers can also be implemented immediately in collaboration with local civic organizations and scaled up as capacity and funds allow. Whether conditional on accessing services of benefit to children and families or not, they provide a rights-based approach to providing immediate relief. At the same time, they promote human and social capital, thus building capacity to fight HIV/AIDS and recover from its impacts.[64]

Income transfer programs can take many forms, including old-age pensions and child grants. The amounts involved in providing small income transfers are low relative to total foreign aid. As an example, if a recent Zambian pilot project that provides US$15 per month to each of the poorest 10% of households was implemented in all low-income countries in sub-Saharan Africa, it would cost only 3% of the aid to Africa agreed upon at Gleneagles.[65] A comprehensive review of the effectiveness of income transfers concluded that there is sufficient evidence that they offer the most feasible and effective strategy for scaling up to a national system of social protection for children affected by HIV and AIDS.[66]

Several universal social security income transfer programs are in place in southern Africa. South Africa, for example, has a very large rights-based transfer scheme for the elderly, people with disabilities, and children in poor households. Botswana, Lesotho, Mauritius, and Namibia also pay universal pensions to older persons, transfers with considerable benefit for children, as pension money is generally spent on food and education.[67] Evaluations have demonstrated that children in recipient households have more food, and exhibit better growth and higher school enrollment.[68] Strong arguments have been made for social security to be targeted toward the poorest members of society rather than specifically toward AIDS-affected individuals and households.[69] Orphan targeting, for example, tends to reach fewer vulnerable poor children than does a program with a focus on child poverty.[70] Pilot programs likely to be scaled up significantly over the next few years are under way in Malawi and Kenya. As these programs have been set up to be rigorously evaluated, very useful research results will shortly become available.

Box 2.1

MALAWI'S CASH TRANSFER PROGRAM: FROM PILOT TO NATIONAL SOCIAL PROTECTION SYSTEM[71]

Nearly 3 years ago, with support from UNICEF, the Government of Malawi launched a pilot program called Social Cash Transfer (SCT) in the Mchinji District as a means to tackle poverty. To qualify, families must be labor-constrained and meet the criteria for being at the extreme poverty line, such as an inability to have more than one meal each day or to purchase essential nonfood items like soap, clothing, and school supplies. The Mchinji District Secretariat identified four intervention and four comparison villages, each containing about 1,000 households, of whom about 100 families (10%) received cash transfers.

The extent of need in the area is illustrated by baseline findings that indicate that, of 3,331 people in 881 households, 44% of all adults were 65 years and older, 27% had a chronic illness, and 20% reported some type of disability. The transfers received vary by household size and the number of school-going children in the households, with an average of US$14 per month per household and an overhead cost of about 13%.

The program has been expanded and, as of 2009, is reaching some 28,000 households with approximately 106,000 beneficiaries, 65% of whom are children. It is estimated that some 70% of beneficiary households are affected by HIV/AIDS. An external evaluation has been undertaken by Boston University and the University of Malawi, and significant positive impacts of the cash transfer have been found in the areas of adult and child health status and health-seeking behaviors; consumption and diversification of foodstuffs and food security; child enrollment and retention in school; household productive assets; and child labor.

The Malawian government is currently designing a National Social Protection Programme with the aim of addressing all vulnerable categories of the population. The program is being scaled up nationwide to reach approximately 300,000 households. In addition, increased efforts are being made to link social protection with additional social services to provide a more comprehensive response to the needs of families affected by HIV and AIDS.

Assisting Families to Promote Children's Development

As previously indicated, the focus on orphaned children has framed mitigation for children affected by HIV and AIDS as an individual, rather than a social and national problem. Public health, policy, and systemic approaches to children aim to dramatically reduce the total number of children in need of individual interventions. These can be effected by, among others, social protection, state-supported preschool programs, free education and health care, school feeding, removing barriers to access, and improving the care children receive at home and in their community.

In a comprehensive review commissioned by the JLICA, Chandan and Richter examined well-evaluated programs to improve family care environments.[72] These included home visiting, parent education and parent behavioral skills training, early child development and youth development programs, and two-generational interventions aimed at improving children's development, as well as parental employment and well-being.

Parenting and family programs generally include a package of services and support that is specifically tailored to the needs of particular families. Nonetheless, they usually comprise one or more of the following components: parenting education, parent skill building, home visiting, social support, counseling and case management services, health care provision, early childhood education, adult education and job training, financial assistance, and advocacy.[73]

Home visiting programs, in particular, seek to improve outcomes for children by targeting parenting knowledge, beliefs, and practices, and by providing social support and practical assistance. In the main, they are prevention programs, seeking to avert future problems by working with parents when children are young.[74] Early childhood development programs are generally targeted toward vulnerable children and families, such as those living in poverty, and are intended to counteract the factors that place low-income children at risk of poor outcomes. Two-generation programs and "combination programs" offer early childhood programs in combination with parenting education as well as adult education, literacy, or job skills and training.[75]

In examining the evidence on family strengthening from high-income contexts and considering the applicability of approaches to high-prevalence, resource-constrained settings, two key areas—home health visiting for pregnant mothers and young children, and early childhood development programs, whether as individual or combined home-, center-, or community-based—emerge as areas of feasible, effective, and promising interventions. Home health visiting programs could build upon existing structures of home-based care and community health worker programs in sub-Saharan Africa (see Box 2.2). These programs have become an established intervention strategy for meeting the health care needs of people living with HIV and AIDS.[76]

Box 2.2

COMMUNITY-BASED HOME VISITING: ISIBINDI IN SOUTH AFRICA

Isibindi (Courage) is an initiative of the National Association of Child Care Workers in South Africa (NACCW) that provides accredited training in child and youth care. *Isibindi* is a community-based program that trains unemployed community members in an accredited child and youth care course to provide integrated child and youth care services to vulnerable families. Each *Isibindi* project is managed through a partnership between NACCW and an implementing agency. The U.S. President's Emergency Plan to Fund AIDS Relief (PEPFAR) is funding the NACCW to replicate the *Isibindi* model nationally, in partnership with the national Department of Social Development.

Isibindi home-based care workers live in the vicinity of the families they support and visit the affected households allocated to them every day. They cook food, help to clean the house, dress children, wash clothes, supervise homework, and in many small ways are integrated into the household and assist the family to remain functional and supportive despite a desperately ill or recently deceased parent. They provide counseling and psychosocial assistance as part of their routine activities with families, or in the "life space" of children. Care workers are supervised through a mentorship hierarchy and training is ongoing.

Isibindi workers also facilitate the family's access to social grants, education, health and available social services, and accompany family members to services when needed. The goal of the program is to maximize benefits to children, families, youth, and communities. In the process of assisting children and families, local organizations are assisted to grow and access further resources through their association with NACCW; communities are strengthened through the injection of young people's skills and resources; and child and youth care workers are set on a career path in a recognized profession. Since 2004, PEPFAR has supported 56 of NACCW's 63 *Isibindi* projects, providing direct services to over 48,000 orphans and vulnerable children, and training 1,000 child and youth care workers.

However, some important caveats are in order. While it is useful to learn from successful and effective programs in the North, interventions tested and refined in resource-rich countries are not easily implemented, given the huge gap in what is feasible in poor countries. Well-trained professional staff, high-quality and high-fidelity programs, high-density or dose-of-program elements, long duration, and integration with other services have all been identified as essential to program successes.[77] It is clear that the implementation of family strengthening activities, such as home visiting and early child development programs, must unfold alongside and build upon efforts to economically strengthen families.

Providing Family-centered Services for Children Affected by HIV and AIDS

Family-centered services are premised on the fact that the family is the basic unit of care for children, a group with the primary motivation and responsibility for ensuring that children survive and thrive. In addition, families have the greatest influence on children's health and well-being prior to, during, and following interventions by health and social welfare professionals.[78]

But a family perspective has been slow to emerge from the individualistic focus in the United States, with which the response to HIV/AIDS began.[79] The impact of AIDS on families and the potential of families to be at the forefront of prevention, treatment, and care has not been fully appreciated, partly because people in high-risk groups (such as men who have sex with men, commercial sex workers, and injecting drug users) are inaccurately assumed to be isolated from family life.[80] In fact, though, substantial numbers of individuals in these groups live with family, including their parents and children. The rationale and evidence for family-centered services for children affected by HIV and AIDS is only starting to be assembled.[81]

From the perspective of family-centered services, families are defined inclusively as individuals who, by birth, adoption, marriage, or declared commitment, share deep, personal connections and who expect to receive and are obligated to provide support to each other, especially in times of need.[82] In fact, HIV and AIDS have contributed to this broader, evolving, postmodern view of family, challenging traditional concepts of kin.[83]

Adopting a family lens entails also subscribing to a life cycle and life course perspective of children affected by HIV/AIDS. This is illustrated by what are called the four pillars of prevention of vertical transmission—the prevention of HIV infection among young men and women of reproductive age, the prevention of unintended pregnancies, the prevention of transmission from mother to child (PMTCT), and the ongoing care of children and their families. Running through these three areas of prevention are care and support for women and children affected by HIV and AIDS. Such a life course understanding is important to devising feasible and effective programs. For example, Hladik et al. developed a model based on Ugandan data that demonstrated that expanded family planning had the potential to avert more child infections than ARV-PMTCT.[84] A piecemeal approach to individuals that ignores their most fundamental social context across time is akin to tackling only one aspect of a complex multifaceted problem. The danger with this is that early successes may be reversed because later-stage factors were not considered. For example, eliminating HIV transmission to children is critical, but it does not address known risks to the mortality, morbidity, and development of exposed but uninfected children.[85]

While there are several definitions of family-centered services, all are based on a bio-psychosocial systems approach, in which the primary focus for care is the individual in the context of his or her family.[86] With respect to HIV and AIDS, this entails recognizing that HIV affects everyone in the family; that members of the family are invaluable to prevention, treatment, and care; and that services for one individual provide an ideal entry point to others also at risk. Services provided to a person infected with HIV need to be extended to those in his or her intimate circle, including partners and members of his or her family. In fact, recognition of infection in one person in a family is a way of reaching many others who may not otherwise be detected. For example, home-based voluntary counseling and testing approaches have demonstrated the existence of a large undiagnosed and untreated population of children.[87]

A recent systematic review illustrates the benefits of a family-centered approach to ARV treatment for children.[88] Adherence rates are excellent, some even "near perfect," when parents and children are treated together.[89] Attendance at scheduled clinic visits is also very high, family-care patients have been found to be more likely to comply with return visits, and their loss to follow-up is low.[90] Survival 1 year into highly active antiretroviral therapy (HAART) is reported to be between 90% and 98%.[91] A 3-year retrospective study of children receiving routine pediatric ART in Malawi found that children receiving family-centered services had better outcomes than did controls on a number of measures: survival, retention in care, continuing ART, and transfer to other ART sites.[92] Family-centered services do, however, face a number of challenges, including making contact with and recruiting family members, especially those dispersed by migrant labor, which includes men.[93]

GAPS IN IMPLEMENTATION

The evidence is clear, demonstrating the clustering of HIV in families, the adverse social and material impacts on families and households when one member is infected with HIV, and the extensive and robust role played by families in care. What are less clear are the nature and determinants of intrafamily variations in response and how these can be addressed by feasible and effective interventions. More also needs to be known about individual psychosocial services required for the children and families who demonstrate persistent emotional and behavioral problems and how these need to be linked into broader social welfare, psychological, and psychiatric services. There are also large gaps in evidence with regard to the effectiveness of interventions at scale and over time, and relative costs and benefits of alternative interventions, and there is little science to guide implementation and expansion of programs.

Intrafamily Variations in Response to Children

It is clear that not all families, at all times, have the capacity to be supportive when someone in their midst is infected, when a relative's household needs financial assistance, or when a child needs to be cared for in the kin network. In fact, there is ample evidence that some families stigmatize, isolate, and mistreat infected and affected relations, including children. Orphaned children fostered in kin households have been reported to be less likely to be enrolled in school, receive less food, and do more work than other children.[94] Little is known about the extent of such prejudice in family fostering or the degree to which orphaned children—as a result of their grief, pessimism, and depression—perceive they are mistreated compared to their peers, rather than actually experience callousness and deprivation at the hands of extended kin.[95]

The notion of *parental solicitude*, based on a proposed evolutionary predilection to favor consanguinity or people related by blood, contends that parents give preference to biological children.[96] Analyses have been conducted indicating that, in South Africa, for example, biological versus stepmothers spend more money on food.[97] However, this hypothesis is not likely to account in any substantial way for the nonresponsiveness of some families toward the children of kin. First, the biological argument, as applied to complex social groups, includes extended kin in the circle of so-called *nepotistic benevolence*.[98] In addition, social and cultural definitions of family, kin, and clan, as well as norms governing obligations within those groups (as exist among most people in sub-Saharan Africa),[99] modify basic biological predispositions. Although much is written in general about family conflict arising from contravention of norms and personal friction, little is known about how such events and histories affect family generosity with respect to care for kin children, or what feasible and effective interventions could be put in place for family conflict resolution for the benefit of children's care.

Several studies indicate that paternal orphans are highly likely to remain living with their mothers, whereas maternal orphans are less likely to remain living with their fathers, suggesting that the presence of an engaged and involved father influences family responses to children affected by AIDS.[100] However, these proportions vary significantly across countries according to base rates of marriage and cohabitation, the mortality rates of men and women, and the proportion of nonorphaned children who live with one or both parents.[101] For example, Hosegood et al. found that a large proportion of children in Malawi and Tanzania continued to live with their father if he was the surviving parent,[102] but this figure was much lower in

South Africa, where low marriage rates and high adult labor migration cause many nonorphaned children to live apart from one or both parents.[103] In fact, the most recent estimates of living arrangements of orphans in South Africa indicate that, while an average of 70% of paternal orphans live with their mothers, only about 25% of maternal orphans live with their fathers.[104] There are indications that maternal orphans are worse off than paternal orphans on follow-up, with significant decrements in attained height and schooling.[105]

The majority of children affected by HIV and AIDS who do not live with one of their parents tend to live with grandparents,[106] although frequently other young adults are present in the household. Grandparents throughout the world are playing an increasing and important role in the care of children, especially with the rise of women in the labor market.[107] Although grandparents in developing countries are often younger than in the global North, hard lives and disability may make it difficult for them to care for young children, especially without any predictable or sustainable income. Although this issue is of great concern, there is, in fact, very little published literature on the profile, circumstances, and needs of grandparent caregivers, or on how they may best be assisted.

Box 2.3

Psychosocial and Income Support to Aged Caregivers and Very Vulnerable Families in Tanzania[108]

The KwaWazee project was started at the end of 2003 in the Kagera region of north-western Tanzania, an area severely affected by HIV and AIDS. Its aim was to provide poor and vulnerable people over the age of 60, including those caring for children without parents, with a regular cash income in the form of a pension and a child benefit. By the end of 2007, nearly 600 older people were receiving a regular monthly pension of Tsh. 6,000 (US$5). Additionally, those who were primary caregivers received child benefits of Tsh. 3,000 (about US$2.50) for each grandchild.

An evaluation of the project indicated that the assistance significantly improved the psychological well-being and food security of children and their older caregivers. Improvements included a reduction in the need to beg for food among pension recipients, less reported illness among older caregivers, an ability to save some money for "rainy days," and better nutrition and hygiene for children in beneficiary households, as well as fewer absences from school among children in households that received cash transfers.

An interesting feature of the evaluation is that it explored the social, interpersonal, and emotional consequences of material support. Pensioners experienced greater reciprocity with family and neighbors as a result of their less precarious financial situation. They were also more likely to get credit from shops, traders, and neighbors because of their enhanced capacity to pay back, and intergenerational relationships improved with the reduced dependency of older caregivers.

Older people who received a pension were significantly less anxious about the future, less stressed, less lonely, and had fewer difficulties with sleeping. At the same time, they felt more confident about how they were coping with the challenges of

their lives. Older people who looked after grandchildren were significantly less wor-
ried about meeting the children's needs. Importantly, children felt more loved as a
consequence of their grandmothers' ability to meet their material needs.

By far, poverty is the most significant determinant of family capacity to care for
children affected by HIV and AIDS. Lack of resources to take on additional dependents without dangerously compromising the consumption of existing family members, many of whom are already living in destitution, is a critical determinant of the
quality of care of children.[109] Several studies in Africa and in China, for example,
have found that families are willing to care for relatives' children and that they see
care of children as a family responsibility, but are anxious and fearful about their
ability to cope with additional costs.[110] Moreover, a number of studies indicate that
destitution, hunger, lack of clothes and shelter, and inability to go to school are a
significant cause of psychosocial distress among children who have lost parents.[111]
Cluver and Orkin, for example, estimate that, in their sample of over 1,000 adolescents, poverty (as well as stigma) raised the likelihood of a child manifesting psychological distress from less than 20% to over 80%.[112] Much more needs to be known
about effective interventions that can feasibly be implemented at scale to address
poverty in ways that ameliorate child and caregiver distress associated with hardship
and want.

Psychosocial and Other Specialized Services
for Children and Families

Most large-scale (national or cross-national) studies find inconsistent and sometimes
even statistically insignificant differences in nutritional and educational outcomes of
children orphaned, presumptively, by AIDS.[113] This is partly because the majority of
children in sub-Saharan Africa live in very poor conditions, so their health and
development are already severely constrained; orphanhood is frequently only one of
a number of severe stresses and deprivations experienced by children. It is also partly
because orphaned children may be variously fostered into poorer or better-off kin
households, living arrangements that substantially affect child outcomes for better or
worse. A recent UNICEF analysis of national data from 38 countries between 2003
and 2006 found that poverty, rather than orphan status, predicted poorer outcomes
among children, assessed in terms of wasting, school enrollment, and age of sexual
debut.[114]

Nonetheless, several in-depth studies report poorer psychosocial adjustment
among orphans than among nonorphans in a variety of high-prevalence and concentrated epidemic settings, with orphans found to report more distress, anxiety, and
depression.[115] Many of the studies are limited by small samples, selection bias, lack of
suitable control and comparison groups, short follow-up periods, and measurement
challenges associated with adapting constructs across social and cultural settings.
Nonetheless, the consistency of findings and data from at least one longer-term study
calls for better understanding of the duration and clinical significance of children's

distress, and for the most cost-effective approaches to address psychosocial difficulties in these settings.

At least one study has reported long-term differences in the adult outcomes of orphans as compared to nonorphans. Beegle et al. followed-up on 781 children who had lost a mother before the age of 15 years and found that orphans had attained significantly lower adult height and fewer years of schooling than nonorphaned children from the same site in Tanzania.[116] On the basis of these findings, the authors argue that circumstances resulting from maternal death cause children's poor development and reduce opportunity over the long-term. Several papers speculate that paternal death is associated with a drop in economic security, and maternal death with psychosocial difficulties as well as socioeconomic disadvantage;[117] Cluver et al. found that socioeconomic problems and stigma associated with HIV and AIDS account for a significant proportion of children's distress.[118]

Studies in the West have confirmed that children who experience parental death have elevated risk for negative outcomes, but the majority of children do not experience serious problems or what has been called *problematic grief*.[119] Although there are reports of effective bereavement programs for children,[120] in the field as a whole, it has been difficult to demonstrate the long-term positive effects of interventions, mainly because most individuals in control groups tend to improve with time. Viewed from the perspective of maximizing resilience, efforts should be made to minimize hardships for bereaved children and to maintain their social connections and routine. For example, children who have "natural mentors" in their lives show significantly less distress,[121] and a recent review of evidence-based practices stresses the importance of parental support, arguing that "positive parenting by the surviving parent is the single most consistently supported malleable mediator of the adjustment of parentally bereaved children,"[122] and that "providers (of educational, health, and social services for children) should be educated regarding the importance of positive parenting."[123]

Far too little is known about effective and feasible interventions for bereaved children in the context of HIV/AIDS. We need tools to distinguish not merely whether children experience distress—which they surely do—but whether children have sufficient supports, particularly love and affection from their surviving parent and positive family interactions,[124] as well as material and social support, to stand a good chance of pulling through. Certainly enough is known to design interventions based on experience and knowledge gained over decades of research on the issues faced by children of dying parents.

Implementation of Effective and Sustainable Interventions at Scale

There is growing concern about the narrow targeting, short reach, impracticality, and undocumented effectiveness of current approaches to support children and families affected by HIV and AIDS. For example, Schenk and Michaelis found that the quality of evidence for community-based care and support programs for children was weak.[125] In 2000, John Williamson observed that:

Developing programs that significantly improve the lives of individual children and families affected by HIV/AIDS is relatively easy with enough resources, organizational capacity, and compassion. Vulnerable individuals and house-holds can be identified, health services can be provided, school expenses of orphans can be paid, food can be distributed, and supportive counseling can be provided. Such interventions meet real needs, but the overwhelming majority of agencies and donors that have responded so far have paid too little attention to the massive scale of the problems that continue to increase with no end in sight. As programs to date have reached only a small fraction of the most vul-nerable children in the countries hardest hit by AIDS, the fundamental chal-lenge is to develop interventions that make a difference over the long haul in the lives of the children and families affected by HIV/AIDS at a scale that approaches the magnitude of their needs.[126]

And, indeed, to date, few interventions for children have been formulated, resourced, or implemented on a scale commensurate with the impact of the epi-demic. Based on the few reports from countries available in 2007, it is estimated that fewer than 15% of households supporting children orphaned or made vulnerable by HIV and AIDS are reached by either community-based or public sector support programs.[127] This figure is barely up from the 5% estimated 8 years earlier, in 1999.[128] The latter figure was derived from Uganda, where a massive community response was mounted to support children affected by HIV/AIDS. However, the authors estimate that only 5% of orphans were reached by the combined efforts of NGOs, government, and other donors, and that community-based organizations reached only 0.4% of orphans.[129]

It is clear that families and communities are at the heart of the response to children affected by HIV and AIDS, and that, although they can provide support and protec-tion at a local level for individual children, effective mechanisms for organizing and realizing this potential have yet to be developed. Many civil society organizations (CSOs) have unique identities based on founder ideals and commitments. Those that see themselves as watchdogs of human rights resist notions of service provision on behalf of government, whose methods and bona fides they frequently question. They prize their independence and autonomy, including from other organizations, and chafe under donor requirements when these are perceived to be at odds with com-munity needs. Yet CSOs are frequently partial, servicing only some sections of a community, either by geographical or social demarcation, and they have struggled to produce evidence of their effectiveness in the area of care and support for children affected by HIV and AIDS.

Considering that joint efforts by CSOs and governments are required to provide for children and families at scale, Richter and Desmond propose that each brings a comparative advantage.[130] The state's key advantages are its size and coverage. The advantage of national reach is important in contexts of poverty and high HIV preva-lence. The state also has continuity and longevity, and can use redistributive taxes to fund programs. The state also has authority. It has the ability to implement legisla-tion, enforce compliance, and create and change policy conditions. Unfortunately, to some extent, the state's advantages are also its weaknesses. As a result of their size, governments are slow-moving and lack flexibility. When considering all possible variations in the design of responses, it is difficult to adapt to specific local contexts. It is in these situations that the comparative advantages of CSOs become clearer.

The state has the reach to address national problems, whereas CSOs have the capacity to reach individuals.

Box 2.4

EXAMPLE OF GOVERNMENT ACTION TO PROVIDE SUPPORT TO CHILDREN
THROUGH POLICY AND FUNDING INVOLVING CLEAR CRITERIA FOR ACTION,
STANDARDIZATION, AND ENTITLEMENT[131]

A policy developed in China's Henan Province is family-centered and attempts to provide support to children through families, community structures, and services, including financial aid, although at a very low level.

The Henan Province, consisting of close to 100 million people, is a predominantly grain farming area located in eastern central China. It is one of the most severely HIV and AIDS affected areas in China, with some 20,000 people infected. Illegal blood collection is the primary source of infection. In the early 1990s, many poor farmers from Henan and other similar provinces were infected when they sold their blood plasma to unauthorized collectors. The virus then spread to families, affecting women and children.

Henan Province's six-point program includes assistance for children orphaned by AIDS. Orphans are placed with other families and adopted. They receive free compulsory education, with a monthly allowance of RMB 130, and RMB 30[132] for adoption (about US$20 and US$5, respectively). The government is committed to build one road, one school, one standardized clinic, one orphanage, and one education room at villages hard hit by HIV/AIDS.

In addition, the province attempts to standardize assistance to widows and orphans affected by AIDS. Orphans raised by their relatives attend primary and junior middle school free of charge and receive financial support to attend institutions of higher learning. Until 18 years of age, each child receives an annual allocation of RMB 180 for medical care. Orphans adopted by relatives receive RMB 130 a month through the local civil affairs department for 3 years from the date of fostering or adoption.

Civil society organizations, free of the bureaucracy, responsibility, and size of the state, can be far more flexible. They can see a problem and adapt their services promptly. Not only can they be flexible, but they can also be creative. Seeing the possibility that something might work, they have the freedom to try it and find out. Civil society organizations can develop services and responses that are only relevant in one particular context and adapt them for another. They do not have the same pressure to provide uniform services or basic services to everyone in their catchment areas. Civil society organizations can respond to individual distress on a case-by-case basis, which is often difficult and inefficient for the state to do.

As governments move toward more systemic responses, CSOs can adopt a variety of roles, including providing services on commission to the state, facilitating families' receipt of and benefit from state services, helping to link families to different state services and to civil society and community-based agencies, and conducting well-evaluated demonstration projects, as well as pursuing activism and empowerment. Unfortunately, there are many instances in which services that are state responsibilities are either absent or inadequate. Notable examples include failure to provide health care, preschool care, or education for all children. The void has often been filled by CSOs and, in particular, by faith-based organizations (FBOs). The manner in which CSOs step in to provide what should be state services has long-term implications, especially if pressure is being put on the state to expand its provision. Civil society organizations' services need to be provided in such a way that they can coordinate with, link into, or even be taken over by state services. This has often been the case with hospitals and schools established by FBOs. The FBO might establish a hospital or school to fulfill a need, but as state capacity improves, the FBO might withdraw, sometimes financially, sometimes administratively, and at times completely.

Box 2.5

COLLABORATIONS BETWEEN CIVIL SOCIETY ORGANIZATIONS AND THE
STATE TO PROVIDE SERVICES FOR VULNERABLE FAMILIES: SUPPORTING
HIV-AFFECTED FAMILIES IN THE UKRAINE THROUGH LEGAL AND
OTHER SERVICES[133]

The All-Ukrainian Network of People Living with HIV (AUKN) and their partners provide a continuum of support for HIV-infected and/or -affected children to keep them from being placed in institutions or becoming street children due to the breakdown of their family. Ukraine is a country "in transition," with one of the most severe AIDS epidemics in Europe, principally as a result of drug use. It is estimated that about 50,000 families in Ukraine are affected by HIV and AIDS, most with little income, and drug and alcohol abuse is common. Parents sometimes resort to sex work to obtain money. Although Ukraine has a well-developed social and health care system, corruption and discrimination are significant barriers to access for very vulnerable families and children.

The project has agreements with national and local government to provide services and to encourage collaboration between relevant departments and civil society organizations.

Each family goes through a needs assessment with a social worker and psychologist and is provided with an individually tailored comprehensive package of care. The number and frequency of services depend on family's needs, but can include all or some of the following: individual and family counseling; parenting and family support; referrals to the other agencies, including social services and educational and recreational activities for children at a day care facility.

Legal help is essential as sex workers, drug users, men who have sex with men, and people living with HIV and AIDS are persecuted by the militia, including falsification of criminal cases in order for the militia to meet its quota of arrests. Assistance is also needed to overcome refusal for hospital admission and provision of medical care. Property rights are also a major problem for many families, and many cases are undertaken to restore or enforce property rights and prevent eviction.

The amounts of money involved in all aspects of the response to HIV and AIDS have increased substantially in recent years, especially with the contributions of the Global Fund to Fight AIDS, Tuberculosis and Malaria, and the U.S. President's Emergency Plan to Fund AIDS Relief (PEPFAR). While lagging behind other responses, the money directed toward children has also increased. With increasing funds comes increasing pressure to show impact. Excessive monitoring and evaluation can become counterproductive, but it does draw attention to impact. While small programs focused on specific aspects of children's needs may work in a particular area, larger amounts of money increase the pressure to show broader, more substantial and sustainable impacts. It is clear that to have the required greater impact requires larger and more systemic responses.

CONCLUSION

This chapter argues that families, rather than individual children, need to be the target for assistance in efforts to mitigate the effects of HIV and AIDS on children. The reasons are that, first, families in all their diversity have evolved for the care and protection of children, and children grow and develop optimally in supportive family environments; and second, HIV and AIDS affect families specifically and severely challenge their capacity. To date, though, efforts to assist children affected by HIV/AIDS have tended to be individualistic, focusing on orphaned children and using a case management and social welfare approach.

However, the scale of the HIV and AIDS epidemic, particularly when considered against the backdrop of widespread poverty, calls for large scale responses that bolster and strengthen families as well as community-based organizations. The strengthening and expansion of health and education services to children is an obvious area for increased state action. Cash transfers provide another avenue for the state to support children via their families. These systemic responses can be designed to improve the well-being of all children while simultaneously providing additional support to those most vulnerable as a result of HIV/AIDS, poverty, or a combination of both. In many contexts, the most vulnerable children are actually in the majority, because such a high percentage of children in low- and middle-income countries live in poverty.

The key principle guiding interventions should be to amplify benefits to families, who, in turn, should be assisted to protect and support children through greater access to better-quality health, education, and social services, together with social protection and family-centered services. As Rutayuga recommended, we must build on existing strengths—extended families, kinship systems, and community structures—not bypass them in our efforts to serve children.[134] This is best achieved through partnerships between affected groups, CSOs, and all levels of government. Greater state involvement through systemic expansion of services to families in no way implies a reduced or diminished role for advocates and community-based organizations. Even in the richest countries with the highest levels of services, CSOs monitor government services, exert pressure on governments to expand and improve services, and themselves render services under conditions in which it is not feasible for the state to do so, or to do so at the required level of quality.

Provisions that directly assist families, such as cash transfers, early child development services, after-school care, and home-based support need to be expanded beyond the levels of projects and programs, to become entitlements of all families in their efforts to care for children.[135] Such rights-based approaches, based on collaborations between funders, governments, and civil society, have made the expansion of HIV prevention and AIDS treatment services possible. Mitigation, especially through care and support of vulnerable children and their families, needs to be taken along the same path.

NOTES

1. For example, see Caldwell, J. et al. (1993). African families and AIDS: Context, reactions and potential interventions. *Health Transition Review, 3* (Suppl.), 1–16, or Hosegood, V. et al. (2007). Revealing the full extent of households' experiences of HIV and AIDS in rural South Africa. *Social Science & Medicine, 65*(6), 1249–1259.

2. Lloyd, M. (2008). *AIDS orphans rising: What you should know and what you can do to help them succeed.* Ann Arbor, MI: Loving Healing Press.

3. UNAIDS. (2008). *Report on the global AIDS epidemic.* Geneva: UNAIDS.

4. Richter, L., & Desmond, C. (2008). Targeting AIDS orphans and child-headed households? A perspective from national surveys in South Africa, 1995–2005. *AIDS Care: Psychological and Socio-medical Aspects of AIDS/HIV, 20*(9), 1019–1028.

5. Heymann, J. et al. (2007). Extended family caring for children orphaned by AIDS: Balancing essential work and caregiving in high HIV prevalence nations. *AIDS Care, 19*(3), 337–345; Phiri, S., & Tolfree, D. (2005). Family- and community-based care for children affected by HIV/AIDS: Strengthening the front line response. In G. Foster, C. Levine, & J. Williamson (Eds.), *A generation at risk: The global impact of HIV/AIDS on orphans and vulnerable children* (pp. 11–36). Cambridge, UK: Cambridge University Press.

6. Zivin, J., Thirumurthy, H., & Goldstein, M. (2009). AIDS treatment and intra-household resource allocation: Children's nutrition and schooling in Kenya. *Journal of Public Economics, 93*(7–8), 1008–1015.

7. Singer, P. (2002). AIDS and international security. *Survival, 44*, 145–158.

8. Foster, G. (2004). Safety nets for children affected by HIV/AIDS in Southern Africa. In R. Pharoah (Ed.), *A generation at risk? HIV/AIDS, vulnerable children and security in Southern Africa* pp. 65–92. Pretoria, Cape Town: Institute of Security Studies.

9. Chirwa, W. (2002). Social exclusion and inclusion: Challenges to orphan care in Malawi. *Nordic Journal of African Studies, 11*(1), 93–113; Verhoef, H. (2005). A child has many mothers: Views of child fostering in Northwestern Cameroon. *Childhood, 12*(3), 369–390.

10. Bray, R. (2003). Predicting the social consequences of orphanhood in South Africa. *African Journal of AIDS Research, 2*(1), 39–55; Cluver, L., & Gardner, F. (2006). The psychological well-being of children orphaned by AIDS in Cape Town, South Africa. *Annals of General Psychiatry, 5*(1), 8; Richter, L. (2004). The impact of HIV/AIDS on the development of children. In R. Pharoah (Ed.), *A generation at risk: HIV/AIDS, vulnerable children and security in Southern Africa* (pp. 9–32). Pretoria, Cape Town: Institute of Security Studies.

11. Meintjes, H., & Giese, S. (2006). Spinning the epidemic: The making of mythologies of orphanhood in the context of AIDS. *Childhood, 13*(3), 407–430.

12. Richter & Desmond. (2008). Targeting AIDS orphans and child-headed households?.

13. United Nations Secretary General. (2006). *Declaration of commitment on HIV/AIDS. Five years later.* New York: UN Secretary General.

14. Foster, G. (2002). Supporting community efforts to assist orphans in Africa. *New England Journal of Medicine, 346*(24), 1907–1910.

15. Desmond, C. (2009). Consequences of HIV for children: Avoidable or inevitable? *AIDS Care: Psychological and Socio-medical Aspects of AIDS/HIV, 21*(1), 98–104.

16. Frierson, R., Lippmann, S., & Johnson, J. (1998). AIDS: Psychological stresses on the family. *Psychosomatics, 28*(2), 65–68; Beer, A., Rose, A., & Tout, K. (1988). AIDS: The grandmother's burden. In A Fleming et al. (Eds.), *The global impact of AIDS* (pp. 171–174). New York: Alan R. Liss Inc.

17. Bharat, S. (1999). Facing the challenge: Household responses to HIV/AIDS in Mumbai, India. *AIDS Care: Psychological and Socio-medical Aspects of AIDS/HIV, 11*(1), 31–44; Franco, L. et al. (2009). Evidence base for children affected by HIV and AIDS in low prevalence and concentrated epidemic countries: Applicability to programming guidance from high prevalence countries. *AIDS Care: Psychological and Socio-medical Aspects of AIDS/HIV, 21*(1), 49–59; Li, L. et al. (2008). Impacts of HIV/AIDS stigma on family identity and interactions in China. *Families, Systems, & Health, 26*(4), 431–442.

18. Rutayuga, J. (1992). Assistance to AIDS orphans within the family/kinship system and local institutions: A program for East Africa. *AIDS Education and Prevention,* Fall Supplement, 57–68.

19. Iliffe, J. (1986). *The African poor: A history.* Cambridge, UK: Cambridge University Press.

20. Bahre, E. (2007). Reluctant solidarity: Death, urban poverty and neighbourly assistance in South Africa. *Ethnography, 8*(1), 33–59.

21. Belsky, J. (1997). Attachment, mating, and parenting. *Human Nature, 8*(4), 361–381; Geary, D., & Flinn, M. (2001). Evolution of human parental behavior and the human family. *Parenting: Science and Practice, 1*(1), 5–61.

22. Taylor, S. et al. (2000). Biobehavioral responses to stress in females: Tend-and-befriend, not fight-or-flight. *Psychological Review, 107*(3), 411–429.

23. Bugental, D. (2000). Acquisition of the algorithms of social life: A domain-based approach. *Psychological Bulletin, 126*(2), 187–219.

24. Foley, R., & Lee, P. (1989). Finite social space, evolutionary pathways, and reconstructing hominid behavior. *Science, 243*(4893), 901–906.

25. Goode, W. (1963). *World revolution and family patterns.* New York: Free Press (p. 3).

26. Murray, S., Malone, J., & Glare, J. (2008). Building a life story: Providing records and support to former residents of children's homes. *Australian Social Work, 61*(3), 239–255.

27. Goode, W. (1993). *World changes in divorce patterns.* New Haven, CT: Yale University Press.

28. Levine, C. (1990). AIDS and changing concepts of family. *The Milbank Quarterly, 68*, 33–58.

29. Hosegood, V. (2009). The demographic impact of HIV and AIDS across the family and household life-cycle: Implications for efforts to strengthen families in sub-Saharan Africa. *AIDS Care: Psychological and Socio-medical Aspects of AIDS/HIV, 21*(1), 13–21.

30. Mathambo, V., & Gibbs, A. (2009). Extended family childcare arrangements in a context of AIDS: Collapse or adaptation? *AIDS Care, 21*(S1), 22–27.

31. Piot, P. et al. (1988). AIDS: An international perspective. *Science, 239*(4840), 573–579.

32. Centres for Disease Control. (1983). Immunodeficiency among female sexual partners of males with acquired immune deficiency syndrome (AIDS). *Morbidity and Mortality Weekly Report, 33*, 661–664.

33. Mundy, D. et al. (1987). Human immunodeficiency virus isolated from amniotic fluid. *The Lancet, 330*(8556), 459–460.

34. Dunkle, K. et al. (2008). New heterosexually transmitted HIV infections in married or cohabiting couples in urban Zambia and Rwanda: An analysis of survey and clinical data. *The Lancet, 371*(9631), 2183–2191.

35. De Cock, K. et al. (2000). Prevention of mother-to-child HIV transmission in resource-poor countries. *JAMA: The Journal of the American Medical Association, 283*(9), 1175–1182.

36. Shang, X. (2000). Supporting HIV/AIDS Affected families and children: The case of four Chinese counties. *International Journal of Social Welfare, 18*(2), 202–212; Schuster, M. et al. (2000). HIV-infected parents and their children in the United States. *American Journal of Public Health, 90*(7), 1074–1081.

37. Li. (2008). Impacts of HIV/AIDS stigma on family identity.

38. Bonuck, K. (1993). AIDS and families: Cultural, psychosocial, and functional impacts. *Social Work in Health Care, 18*(2), 75–89.

39. Richter, L. et al. (2009). Strengthening families to support children affected by HIV and AIDS. *AIDS Care: Psychological and Socio-medical Aspects of AIDS/HIV, 21*(1), 3–12.

40. Franco et al. (2009). Evidence base for children affected by HIV and AIDS in low prevalence and concentrated epidemic countries.

41. Quinlan, R. (2007). Human parental effort and environmental risk. *Proceedings of the Royal Society B: Biological Sciences, 274*(1606), 121–125.

42. Cornia, G. (2007). Overview of the impact and best practice responses in favour of children in a world affected by HIV and AIDS. In G. Cornia (Ed.), *AIDS, public policy and child well-being* (2nd ed., pp. 1–30). Florence: UNICEF Innocenti Research Centre.

43. Besley, M. (2005). *AIDS and the family: Policy options for a crisis in family capital.* New York: United Nations Department of Economic and Social Affairs.

44. Desmond. (2009). Consequences of HIV for children.

45. Rogers, R., Hummer, R., & Nam, C. (2000). *Living and dying in the USA: Behavioral, health and social differentials of adult mortality.* San Diego: Academic Press.

46. Richter et al. (2009). Strengthening families to support children; Richter, L., & Sherr, L. (2009). Strengthening families: A key recommendation of the joint learning initiative on children and AIDS (JLICA). *AIDS Care, 21*, 1–2.

47. Richter, L., Foster, G., & Sherr, L. (2006). *Where the heart is: Meeting the psychosocial needs of young children in the context of HIV/AIDS.* The Hague: Bernard van Leer Foundation.

48. Ibid.
49. Richter, L. (2010). An introduction to family-centred services for children affected by HIV and AIDS. *Journal of the International AIDS Society, 13*(suppl. 2), S1.
50. Jacobs, M. (2005). Maternal colonialism: White women and indigenous child removal in the American West and Australia, 1880–1940. *The Western Historical Quarterly, 36*(4), 453–476; Sen, S. (2007). The orphaned colony: Orphanage, child and authority in British India. *Indian Economic & Social History Review, 44*(4), 463–488.
51. Leon, J. (2009). The shift towards family reunification in Romanian child welfare policy: An analysis of changing forms of governmental intervention in Romania. *Children & Society, 25*, 228–238.
52. Bhargava, A., & Bigombe, B. (2003). Public policies and the orphans of AIDS in Africa. *British Medical Journal, 326*(7403), 1387–1389.
53. Tolfree, D. (1995). *Roofs and roots: The care of separated children in the developing world.* Aldershot, UK: Arena.
54. Frank, D., & Klass, P. (1996). Infants and young children in orphanages: One view from pediatrics and child psychiatry. *Pediatrics, 97*(4), 569; Judge, S. (2003). Developmental recovery and deficit in children adopted from Eastern European orphanages. *Child Psychiatry and Human Development, 34*(1), 49–62.
55. Desmond, C., & Gow, J. (2001). *The cost-effectiveness of six models of care for orphan and vulnerable children in South Africa.* Pretoria: UNICEF.
56. Bronfenbrenner, U. (1986). Ecology of the family as a context for human development: Research perspectives. *Developmental Psychology, 22*(6), 723–742.
57. Jones, G. et al. (2003). How many child deaths can we prevent this year? *The Lancet, 362*(9377), 65–71.
58. Grantham-McGregor, S. et al. (2007). Developmental potential in the first 5 years for children in developing countries. *The Lancet, 369*(9555), 60–70.
59. UNDP. (2007). *Human development report 2007/2008. Fighting climate change: Human solidarity in a divided world.* New York: UNDP.
60. Richter et al. (2009). Strengthening families to support children.
61. Besley. (2005). *AIDS and the family.*
62. Bell, C., Devarajan, S., & Gersbach, H. (2006). The long-run economic costs of aids: A model with an application to South Africa. *The World Bank Economic Review, 20*(1), 55–89; Earls, F., Raviola, G., & Carlson, M. (2008). Promoting child and adolescent mental health in the context of the HIV/AIDS pandemic with a focus on sub-Saharan Africa. *Journal of Child Psychology and Psychiatry, 49*(3), 295–312.
63. Desmond. (2009). Consequences of HIV for children.
64. Adato, M., & Bassett, L. (2009). Social protection to support vulnerable children and families: The potential of cash transfers to protect education, health and nutrition. *AIDS Care: Psychological and Socio-medical Aspects of AIDS/HIV, 21*(1), 60–75; World Bank. (2008). *Conditional cash transfers: Reducing present and future poverty. World Bank policy research report.* Washington, DC: World Bank.
65. Department for International Development (2005). *Can low-income countries in Africa afford social transfers?* Social Protection Briefing Note Series, No 2. London: Department for International Development.
66. Adato & Bassett. (2009). Social protection to support vulnerable children and families.

67. Samson, M., & Kaniki, S. (2008). Social pensions as developmental social security in Africa. In D. Failu, & F. Veras (Eds.), *Poverty in focus: Cash transfers: Lessons from Africa and Latin America* (15th ed., pp. 22–23). Brasilia: International Poverty Centre.

68. Case, A., Lin, I., & McLanahan, S. (2000). How hungry is the selfish gene? *The Economic Journal, 110*(466), 781–804; Duflo, E. (2003). Grandmothers and granddaughters: Old age pensions and intrahousehold allocation in South Africa. *The World Bank Economic Review, 17*(1), 1–25.

69. Richter, L. (2010). Social cash transfers to support children and families affected by HIV/AIDS. *Vulnerable Children and Youth Studies: An International Interdisciplinary Journal for Research, Policy and Care, 5*(2), 81–91.

70. Handa, S. (2008). The orphan targeting dilemma in Eastern and Southern Africa. In D. Hailu, & F. Soares (Eds.), *Cash transfers: Lessons from Africa and Latin America* (pp. 18–19). Brasilia: International Poverty Centre.

71. See Miller, C., Tsoka, M., & Reichert, K. (2010). Targeting cash to Malawi's ultra-poor: A mixed methods evaluation. *Development Policy Review, 28*(4), 481–502; Kulumeka, H. (2010). *Targeting households to reach vulnerable groups: Lessons learned from the Malawi social cash transfer programme.* Paper presented at the CCABA symposium, XVIIIth International AIDS Conference, Vienna.

72. Chandan, U., & Richter, L. (2009). Strengthening families through early intervention in high HIV prevalence countries. *AIDS Care: Psychological and Socio-medical Aspects of AIDS/HIV, 21*(1), 76–82.

73. Comer, E., & Fraser, M. (1998). Evaluation of six family-support programs: Are they effective? *Families in Society, 79*(2), 134; Layzer, J. et al. (2001). National evaluation of family support programs. Final report Vol. A. The meta-analysis. Cambridge, MA: ABT Associates.

74. Gomby, D., Culross, P., & Behrman, R. (1999). Home visiting: Recent program evaluations: Analysis and recommendations. *The Future of Children, 9*(1), 4–26; Olds, D. et al. (2000). Update on home visiting for pregnant women and parents of young children. *Current Problems in Pediatrics, 30*(4), 109–141.

75. Karoly, L., Kilburn, R., & Cannon, J. (2005). *Early childhood interventions: proven results, future promises.* Santa Monica: Rand Corporation.

76. World Health Organization. (2000). *Home-based long-term care. Report of a WHO study group.* Geneva: WHO; Campbell, S. (2004). Care of HIV/AIDS patients in developing countries. *Primary Health Care, 14*(8), 22–26.

77. Brookes, S. et al. (2006). Building successful home visitor-mother relationships and reaching program goals in two early Head Start programs: A qualitative look at contributing factors. *Early Childhood Research Quarterly, 21*(1), 25–45.

78. Richter. (2010). An introduction to family-centred services.

79. Rotheram-Borus, M. et al. (2005). Families living with HIV. *AIDS Care, 17,* 8, 978–987.

80. Levine, C. (1990). AIDS and changing concepts of family.

81. Richter. (2010). An introduction to family-centred services.

82. Levine. (1990). AIDS and changing concepts of family.

83. Bonuck, K. (1993). AIDS and families.

84. Hladik, W. et al. (2009). The contribution of family planning towards the prevention of vertical HIV transmission in Uganda. *PLoS ONE, 4,* 11, e76–91.

85. Filteau, S. (2009). The HIV-exposed, uninfected African child. *Tropical Medicine & International Health, 14*, 3, 276–287; Isanaka, S., Duggan, C., & Fawzi, W. (2009). Patterns of postnatal growth in HIV-infected and HIV-exposed children. *Nutrition Reviews, 67*, 6, 343–359.

86. Shelton, T., Jeppson, E., & Johnson, B. (1987). *Family-centred care for children with special health needs.* Washington, DC: Association for the Care of Children's Health.

87. Were, W. et al. (2006). Undiagnosed HIV infection and couple HIV discordance among household members of HIV-infected people receiving antiretroviral therapy in Uganda. *JAIDS Journal of Acquired Immune Deficiency Syndromes, 43*, 1, 91–95.

88. Leeper S., et al. (2010). Lessons learned from family-centred models of treatment for children living with HIV: Current approaches and future directions, *Journal of the International AIDS Society, 13*, Suppl 2, S3.

89. Byakika-Tusiime, J. et al. (2009). Longitudinal antiretroviral adherence in HIV+ Ugandan parents and their children initiating HAART in the MTCT-plus family treatment model: Role of depression in declining adherence over time. *AIDS and Behavior, 13*, 82–91.

90. Sendzik, D., & Thompson, K. (2006). HIV family-centred care: Supporting quality care for HIV-positive caregivers, *Proceedings of the XVI International AIDS Conference,* Toronto, Canada; Sendzik, D., & Thompson, K. (2006). Family-centred approach improves adherence to care, *Proceedings of the XVI International AIDS Conference,* Toronto, Canada.

91. Griensven, J. et al. (2008). Success with antiretroviral treatment for children in Kigali, Rwanda: Experience with health center/nurse-based care. *BMC Pediatrics, 8*, 1, 39; Van Winghem, J. et al. (2008). Implementation of a comprehensive program including psycho-social and treatment literacy activities to improve adherence to HIV care and treatment for a pediatric population in Kenya. *BMC Pediatrics, 8*, 1, 52.

92. Midturi, J. et al. (2008). A retrospective case-controlled analysis of children enrolled in a family-centred care clinic at Baylor College of Medicine-Abbot fund children's clinical centre of excellence (COE). *Proceedings of the XVII International AIDS Conference,* Mexico City, Mexico.

93. Tonwe-Gold, B. et al. (2009). Implementing family-focused HIV care and treatment: The first two years' experience of the mother-to-child transmission-plus program in Abidjan, Cote D'Ivoire. *Tropical Medicine & International Health, 14*, 2, 204–212.

94. Makame, V., & Grantham-Mcgregor, S. (2002). Psychological well-being of orphans in Dar El Salaam, Tanzania. *Acta Paediatrica, 91*, 4, 459–465.

95. Atwine, B., Cantor-Graae, E., & Bajunirwe, F. (2005). Psychological distress among AIDS orphans in rural Uganda. *Social Science & Medicine, 61*, 3, 555–564.

96. Daly, M., & Wilson, M. (1980). Discriminative parental solicitude: A biological perspective. *Journal of Marriage and Family, 42*, 2, 277–288.

97. Case, Lin, & McLanahan (2000). How hungry is the selfish gene?

98. Kurland, J. (1979). Paternity, mother's brother, and human sociality. In N. Chagnon & W. Irons (Eds.), *Evolutionary biology and human social behavior: An anthropological perspective* (pp. 145–180). North Scituate, MA: Duxbury Press.

99. Chirwa, W. (2002). Social exclusion and inclusion.
100. Denis, P., & Ntsimane, R. (2006). Absent fathers: Why do men not feature in stories of families affected by HIV/AIDS in KwaZulu-Natal? In L. Richter & R. Morrell (Eds.), *Baba: Men and fatherhood in South Africa.* (pp. 226–236). Cape Town: HSRC Press.
101. Monasch, R., & Boerma, J. (2004). Orphanhood and childcare patterns in sub-Saharan Africa: An analysis of national surveys from 40 countries. *AIDS, 18,* S55–S65.
102. Hosegood V., et al. (2007). The effects of high HIV prevalence on orphanhood and living arrangements of children in Malawi, Tanzania, and South Africa. *Population Studies: A Journal of Demography, 61,* 3, 327–336.
103. Preston-Whyte, E. (1993). Women who are not married: Fertility, 'illegitimacy,' and the nature of households and domestic groups among single African women in Durban. *South African Journal of Sociology, 24,* 3, 63–71.
104. Kibel, M. et al. (2010). *South African child gauge 2009/2010.* Cape Town: Children's Institute, University of Cape Town.
105. Beegle, K., De Weerdt, J. & Dercon, S. (2009). The intergenerational impact of the African orphans crisis: A cohort study from an HIV/AIDS affected area. *International Journal of Epidemiology, 38,* 2, 561–568.
106. Urassa, M. et al. (1997). Orphanhood, child fostering and the AIDS epidemic in rural Tanzania. *Health Transition Review, 7,* 141–153.
107. Gray, A. (2005). The changing availability of grandparents as carers and its implications for childcare policy in the UK. *Journal of Social Policy, 34,* 4, 557–577.
108. See Hoffman, S., Heslop, M., Clacherty, G., & Kessy, F. (2008). *Salt, soap and schools for school: Evaluation summary. The impact of pensions on the lives of older people and grandchildren in the KwaWazee project in Tanzania's Kagera region.* London: HelpAge International and REPSSI.
109. Deininger, K., Garcia, M., & Subbarao, K. (2003). AIDS-induced orphanhood as a systemic shock: Magnitude, impact, and program interventions in Africa. *World Development, 31,* 7, 1201–1220.
110. Madhavan, S. (2004). Fosterage patterns in the age of AIDS: Continuity and change. *Social Science & Medicine, 58,* 7, 1443–1454.
111. Zhao G. et al. (2007). Care arrangements, grief and psychological problems among children orphaned by AIDS in China. *AIDS Care: Psychological and Socio-medical Aspects of AIDS/HIV, 19,* 9, 1075–1082.
112. Cluver, L., & Orkin, M. (2009). Cumulative risk and AIDS-orphanhood: Interactions of stigma, bullying and poverty on child mental health in South Africa. *Social Science & Medicine, 69,* 8, 1186–1193.
113. Monasch & Boerma. (2004). Orphanhood and childcare patterns in sub-Saharan Africa; Birdthistle, I. (2003). *Understanding the needs of orphans and other children affected by HIV and AIDS in Africa: State of the science. Working Draft.* Washington D.C, USAID.
114. Akwara, P. et al. (2010). Who is the vulnerable child? Using survey data to identify children at risk in the era of HIV and AIDS. *AIDS Care: Psychological and Socio-medical Aspects of AIDS/HIV, 22,* 9, 1066–1085.
115. Cluver, L., Gardner, F., & Operario, D. (2007). Psychological distress amongst AIDS-orphaned children in urban South Africa. *Journal of Child Psychology and Psychiatry, 48,* 8, 755–763; Fang, X. et al. (2009). Parental HIV/AIDS and psychosocial adjustment among rural Chinese children. *Journal of Pediatric*

Psychology, 34, 10, 1053–1062; Nyamukapa, C. et al. (2008). HIV-associated orphanhood and children's psychosocial distress: Theoretical framework tested with data from Zimbabwe. *American Journal of Public Health, 98,* 1, 133–141.

116. Beegle, De Weerdt, & Dercon. (2009). The intergenerational impact of the African orphans crisis.

117. Birdthistle. (2003). *Understanding the needs of orphans and other children affected by HIV and AIDS in Africa.*

118. Cluver & Orkin. (2009). Cumulative risk and AIDS-orphanhood.

119. Worden, J., & Silverman, P. (1996). Parental death and the adjustment of school-age children. *Omega: Journal of Death and Dying, 29,* 219–230.

120. Sandler, I. et al. (2010). Long-term effects of the family bereavement program on multiple indicators of grief in parentally bereaved children and adolescents. *Journal of Consulting and Clinical Psychology, 78,* 2, 131–143.

121. Onuoha, F., & Munakata, T. (2010). Inverse association of natural mentoring relationship with distress mental health in children orphaned by AIDS. *BMC Psychiatry, 10,* 1, 6.

122. Haine, R. et al. (2008). Evidence-based practices for parentally bereaved children and their families, *Professional Psychology: Research and Practice, 39,* 2, 116.

123. Ibid., p. 119.

124. Ibid., pp. 113–121.

125. Schenk, K., & Michaelis, A. (2010). Community interventions supporting children affected by HIV in sub-Saharan Africa: A review to derive evidence-based principles for programming. *Vulnerable Children and Youth Studies: An International Interdisciplinary Journal for Research, Policy and Care, 5,* 2(Supp 1), 40–54.

126. Williamson, J. (2000). *Finding the way forward: Principles and strategies to reduce the impacts of AIDS on children and families.* New York, USAID.

127. United Nations Secretary General. (2006). *Declaration of commitment on HIV/AIDS.*

128. Deininger, Garcia, & Subbarao. (2003). AIDS-induced orphanhood as a systemic shock.

129. Ibid.

130. Richter, L., & Desmond, C. (2007). *Children in communities affected by HIV/AIDS: Emerging issues.* The Hague: Bernard van Leer Foundation.

131. See UNICEF (2006, March 22–24). *The situation of children and HIV/AIDS in China.* A background paper for East Asia and Pacific regional consultation on HIV/AIDS and children, Hanoi, Viet Nam. New York: UNICEF.

132. One U.S. dollar equals roughly 6.8 Chinese yuan.

133. See White, T., Dudina, O., & Aslett, A. (2009). *Children plus: Working with marginalized families living with HIV in Ukraine.* Paper presented at the Road to Vienna symposium: Family-centred services for children and families affected by HIV/AIDS, Geneva.

134. Rutayuga. (1992). Assistance to AIDS orphans within the family/kinship system and local institutions.

135. Richter. (2010). Social cash transfers to support children.

3

Strength Under Duress

Community Responses to Children's Needs

GEOFF FOSTER, NATHAN NSHAKIRA, AND NIGEL TAYLOR ∎

Children bear the brunt of many disasters, and the AIDS catastrophe is no exception. Many people living in the midst of the epidemic see its impact on children as the most serious consequence.[1] In contrast, many external responses to HIV and AIDS are adult-focused and do not consider the special needs of children living with, exposed to, or affected by the virus. Yet, while families and communities continue to shoulder the burden of supporting vulnerable children, the significance of these home-grown responses remains largely unrecognized by policy-makers, donors, and others.[2]

Treatment responses for children affected by HIV and AIDS have lagged behind those for their adult counterparts. Globally, children living with HIV and AIDS constitute 6% of people living with HIV infections, yet account for 14% of all AIDS-related deaths; and mortality rates in children with HIV are more than twice the rate in their adult counterparts.[3] These extreme differences are largely accounted for by high mortality rates in HIV-infected infants. Most infants living with HIV/AIDS do not receive recommended appropriate care—they fail to receive early diagnosis, are not started on efficacious cotrimoxazole prophylaxis, and do not obtain lifesaving antiretroviral treatment (ART) (Box 3.1). As a consequence, up to 40% of infants living with HIV/AIDS die before their first birthday.[4]

Efforts to prevent the spread of HIV to exposed children through vertical transmission have also been inadequate. Effective prevention technologies for children have been available for over a decade in developed countries and have drastically reduced mother-to-child transmission rates to less than 2%. Yet, these interventions still do not reach a good proportion of affected mother-and-infant pairs in low-income countries. As a consequence, large numbers of infants continue to acquire this deadly infection.

While global initiatives are being rolled out to meet the needs of children living with and exposed to HIV infection, systematic responses for the largest group of children affected by HIV/AIDS—orphans and vulnerable children (OVC)—have been slow to emerge. Only 12% of HIV-affected children in sub-Saharan countries received any support from external sources beyond their own families and communities (Figure 3.1).[5] Increasing engagement by political leaders has accompanied the development of national plans of action for orphans and vulnerable children in

Box 3.1

Children Affected by HIV/AIDS in Developing Countries[6]

Proportion of children living with HIV/AIDS in developing
  countries: 95%
Number of children who have lost one or both parents
  due to AIDS in Africa: 14.9 million
Orphan-to-nonorphan school attendance ratio in Africa[†]:   0.93
Orphans and vulnerable children in households receiving
  any external support[†‡]:   12%
HIV-positive pregnant women receiving antiretroviral therapy
  for prevention of mother-to-child transmission in low- and
  middle-income countries[†*]:   53%
Infants born to HIV-positive pregnant women started on
  cotrimoxazole prophylaxis in low- and middle-income
  countries: 14%
Antiretroviral therapy coverage in children in low- and
  middle-income countries[†*]:   38%

[†] United Nations General Assembly Special Session (UNGASS) core indicator; [‡] Average for 18 countries in sub-Saharan Africa; [*] Multi-country data is not available for (a) prevention of mother-to-child transmission (PMTCT) using more efficacious regimes; (b) early infant diagnosis rate of HIV-infected infants or (c) proportion of HIV-infected infants started on antiretroviral therapy (ART).

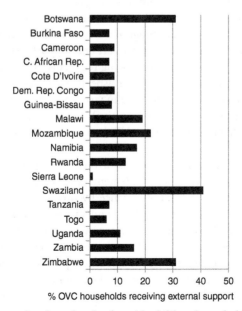

% OVC households receiving external support

Figure 3.1 Percentage of orphaned and vulnerable children households receiving any free external support.[6]

many affected countries. However, lack of resources for their implementation, and failure to incorporate these plans into national developmental frameworks mean their effectiveness has been limited.[7] Consequently, families, together with communities, have of necessity responded to the impacts of HIV and AIDS on vulnerable children, and bear some 90% of the financial costs of the woefully inadequate response.[8]

To the extent to which they are capable, communities have been energetic, creative, and generous in addressing the predicament of orphans and vulnerable children. Communities provide far more services and direct support for children affected by HIV and AIDS than do government ministries, donors, and international non-governmental organizations (NGOs) combined.[9] Systematic responses by those living outside affected communities, such as the provision of resources to support communities and the implementation of supportive national plans of action, are poorly developed. Although community engagement in HIV/AIDS programs increases their sustainability and likelihood of success,[10] most responses initiated by affected communities are inadequate and small-scale since they are self-resourced. Not surprisingly, most remain unnoticed outside their own neighborhoods. This chapter argues for stronger national and international responses to mitigate the impacts of HIV and AIDS on children by complementing and strengthening community OVC responses.

THE SCOPE OF COMMUNITY PROGRAMS FOR ORPHANS AND VULNERABLE CHILDREN

Communities play critical roles in providing material and psychosocial support, social and economic safety nets, and enhanced access to basic services that assist families in caring for children affected by HIV and AIDS.[11] Community OVC programs may be defined as interventions supporting the care of children within their own neighborhood that involve community engagement, commitment, and initiative in program implementation and involve community leaders in overseeing child care and well-being.[12] Community programs seek to build the capacity of caregivers and communities by enhancing traditional care and support systems based on family, kinship, or community ties.[13] As well as being recipients of assistance, children play active roles as care providers and in other aspects of the response. Their contributions are often not recognized or analyzed in terms of their significance, impacts on child development (both positive and negative), and the ways in which they can be harnessed and directed in, for example, skills building for personal coping and future income generation.[14]

Community OVC programs encompass a variety of approaches. Some address household food insecurity through supplementary feeding, nutrition, or agriculture programs. Others support school attendance by providing uniforms and fees, or strengthen primary health care for childhood diseases through school-based or facility-based interventions.[15] Many community-led initiatives involve volunteers who provide regular visits to affected households, and some programs involve specific components of psychosocial support,[16] address poverty through income-generating activities,[17] foster positive prevention behaviors to mitigate future impacts of HIV,[18] or plan for children's future fostering and prevent land-grabbing through will-writing.[19]

CLASSIFICATION OF COMMUNITY RESPONSES

Lack of understanding is widespread surrounding the nature of community responses for vulnerable children. Part of this confusion is caused by difficulties in terminology. It may help to describe the role of organizations as being either "community-based" or "community-oriented," depending on whether a program is implemented by an organization based within or outside an affected community. Further refinement of terminology may be necessary when community groups participate in external agency initiatives, depending on the degree to which community groups own and manage initiatives.

Terms describing local structures are sometimes used inappropriately, further contributing to poor understanding in this area. The term "*community*" is often taken to imply a discrete grouping of people who interact socially on a continuous basis.[20] But some groups, confusingly, use "community" interchangeably with "civil society" or "nongovernmental organization." The term "community-based organization" (CBO) is frequently mentioned in discussions of responses for vulnerable children. But the term is used inconsistently to refer to a variety of entities. Some use "CBO" as an across-the-board term to describe all types of civil society organizations, including large NGOs.[21] Some donors and intermediary organizations that partner national, provincial, and district-level NGOs refer to these as CBOs, in order to imply to their supporters, rightly or wrongly, that they are really "reaching the community." Others use "CBO" to refer to loose entities operating locally or to better-established organizations operating across broader areas. Greater precision in defining what exactly is meant by these terms would aid understanding in this important area of development and contribute to the framing of supportive responses.

A classification system consisting of four types of community-based structures for responding to vulnerable children has been proposed recently: *community initiative, community-based organization, community service organization* (CSO), and *community coordinating committee.*[22]

Community initiatives are composed of local community members who come together out of concern for vulnerable children. Priority activities are visiting vulnerable households, practical care for vulnerable children, and providing material and psychosocial support for affected households. Key outcomes are to enable vulnerable children to continue with schooling, and to provide them with basic physical, psychosocial, and spiritual care, building upon a cultural tradition of providing assistance within the community at times of need.[23]

Community initiatives rarely have any formal institutional arrangement, and they operate more on a verbal, rather than a written, basis. Typically, these groups are based within and are accountable to their local community. Distinctive characteristics include consensus-based decision-making, self-reliance, local leadership, voluntarism, and innovation.[24] Most have no organizational budget, staff, or facilities, and any external funding is used to provide inputs for vulnerable children and their caregivers. The very nature of community initiatives—their informality, rootedness within the community, and small-scale—has meant that they have rarely connected with external initiatives. They remain "under the radar" of many key stakeholders and have not been a traditional entity for donors to support.[25]

Community-based organizations often develop out of community initiatives: The two types of organization may be considered to lie on a continuum of volunteer-driven responses for vulnerable children. Community-based organizations are more likely to have established governance and supervisory structures, documentation, and linkage to external agencies. Many have developed plans with budgets and utilize paid or unpaid staff and volunteers to provide a range of services for their community. They tend to grow where resources are more accessible, for example in district centers and cities, and where they are led by better educated, well-connected leaders. Many CBOs have buy-in and credibility from their surrounding community and are appreciated by community members and funders for their provision of services at relatively low cost. Their accountability draws upon the motivation and insights of local people. Essentially, they combine the strengths of community initiatives with the advantages that come from formal institutionalization.

Community service organizations, although similar in many respects to CBOs, may be distinguished by their strong upward, rather than downward, accountability.[26] Some organizations based within communities may not have a continuous presence in the local community, are not accountable to local community structures, and are viewed as "outsiders" by community members. In some cases, CBOs have developed into community service organizations that deliver services under the direction of external organizations. The availability of funding for HIV and AIDS has transformed organizations into focusing their energies on delivering programs that are designed and monitored by external organizations.[27] Although CSOs may not have strong links to the communities they serve, they nevertheless perform important functions by providing services to marginalized community members in the absence of an effective public sector.

Community coordination committees are another type of organization that exists in many countries. These are instituted by governments and have the function of mobilizing, coordinating, and supporting other community-based responses. In some cases, committees have a mandate relating to child protection. They tend not to be implementers, or conduits for funding, as these functions potentially conflict with their coordination role. Examples of coordination committees include Most Vulnerable Children Committees at district, ward, and village levels in Tanzania; Community AIDS Committees, part of the formal structure of response to HIV and AIDS in Malawi; and Children's Coordinating Committees at district, sector, and cell levels in Rwanda.[28]

DEVELOPMENT OF COMMUNITY RESPONSES

Community action for children affected by HIV and AIDS is typically channeled through local organizations such as churches, schools, and associations. In Africa, community initiatives for children affected by HIV and AIDS preceded programs established by NGOs, international agencies, and governments (Figure 3.2).[29] By 1987, CBOs in Tanzania were providing educational assistance, food, and clothing to children orphaned by AIDS.[30] Over 20 years later, similar responses continue to proliferate, the majority being established by faith-based organisations (FBOs).[31]

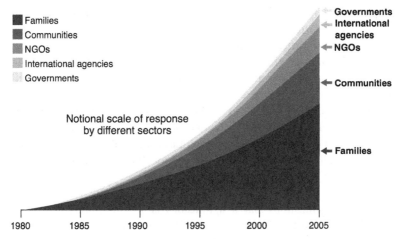

Figure 3.2 Notional onset and scale of responses to children affected by HIV/AIDS in sub-Saharan Africa by sector.[32]

Recent studies have documented the extent of community responses for children affected by HIV and AIDS:

- All entities delivering health, education, and other development services in four regions in Zambia were comprehensively mapped. Of the 265 entities identified, 73% provided HIV/AIDS-related services, nearly two-thirds of which were

---

Box 3.2

Faith-based Responses for Children Affected by HIV/AIDS

Nearly all the Christian congregations surveyed in Namibia had HIV/AIDS responses, whereas one-third implemented responses for children affected by HIV and AIDS.[33] Respondents valued the compassion and commitment of people of faith and their capacity to deliver spiritual and psychosocial support in addition to medical care. When asked to identify the most valued attribute of religious health services, respondents in Zambia and Lesotho ranked the intangible contributions of spiritual encouragement and compassionate care above more visible services of material support and curative care.[34]

One faith-based initiative was established with four volunteers identifying 187 orphans. Three years later, it involved 30 volunteers supporting 467 vulnerable children. As initiatives become better established, they often move beyond an initial "relief" focus on food and education and develop longer-term development foci including psychosocial support, economic empowerment, and HIV prevention.[35]

---

implemented by FBOs. Almost all FBOs delivered HIV/AIDS services, with around one-quarter supporting orphans and vulnerable children.[36]

- A study in four districts of Uganda identified 108 initiatives responding to vulnerable children. This represented one response per 1,300 people which, if extrapolated, would indicate some 25,000 OVC initiatives throughout the country.[37]
- Over three-quarters of children in Malawi lived in households that received transfers of cash or in-kind gifts from relatives, friends, and neighbors. Some 40% of children lived in communities with local support groups for the chronically ill offering counselling, support for vulnerable children, food or other in-kind gifts, and medical care.[38]

Faith-based organizations play a significant role in community-level responses to vulnerable children (see Boxes 3.2 and 3.3).[39] As well as establishing initiatives, religious bodies are able to connect these through extensive, well-organized networks.[40] A six-country study of 651 faith-based responses for vulnerable children found these involved over 9,000 volunteers supporting a cumulative total of some 150,000 OVC. Initiatives provided children affected by HIV and AIDS with a wide range of services, including provision of food and clothing, assistance with the costs of health care and education, psychosocial and spiritual support, and HIV prevention activities (Figure 3.3).[41]

Box 3.3

ZIMBABWE ORPHANS THROUGH EXTENDED HANDS (ZOE)

Since 1993, the Zimbabwe Orphans Through Extended Hands (ZOE) program has worked closely with all denominations, especially Pentecostal, Baptist, and independent church groups, to provide services to all vulnerable children, regardless of their religious affiliation. Volunteers from the various religious groups work together to provide children and their caregivers with assistance such as regular home visits; food and clothing; social, emotional, and spiritual support; and income-generating activities. Although external funding is also needed, all of the projects are funded largely through congregational collections. Between 2001 and 2005, ZOE's network grew from 19 initiatives involving 109 churches to 60 initiatives involving 600 churches. This included an increase from 247 volunteers supporting some 3,500 children to 2,000 volunteers supporting over 60,000 vulnerable children.[42]

THE IMPACT OF COMMUNITY RESPONSES

Community responses for vulnerable children are widespread, but few have ever been evaluated. An extensive literature review identified only 21 published evaluations of OVC interventions, with the large majority being reviews of programs implemented by international NGOs. Only two interventions were administered by local CBOs, an indication of the limited resources devoted to evaluation of smaller

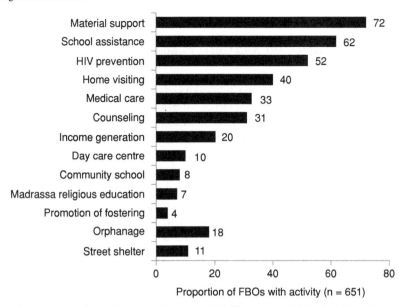

Figure 3.3 Services for orphans and vulnerable children provided by faith-based organizations.[43]

organizations' responses. The study concluded that "considering the widespread experience in implementing programs for orphans and vulnerable children represented by spending to date, the evidence base guiding resource allocation is disappointingly limited."[44]

However, the evidence that does exist, from these and other sources, suggests that community-based responses for vulnerable children have innate strengths:

- Volunteers from community initiatives effectively identify vulnerable children, provide psychosocial support, and supply labor assistance to affected households.[45]
- Community initiatives are sustainable and are good at getting material resources through to the most vulnerable children and their caregivers. This is what they have done since the onset of the AIDS pandemic, largely from their own resources.[46]
- Community groups ensure that those most in need are the first to benefit from any assistance, psychosocial support, or protection interventions, and provide clear criteria to decide who are the most vulnerable needing immediate assistance and who can wait.[47]
- The proximity of community groups to those they serve allows them to recognize, adapt, and respond quickly to changing needs and priorities.[48]
- Initiatives established by those directly affected, especially if they involve children and youth, are more likely to address important psychosocial dimensions of impact[49] (see Box 3.4).

Box 3.4

NGWANGWA ORPHAN CARE AND CHITUKUKO GROUP, BALAKA, MALAWI

The Ngwangwa Orphan Care and Chitukuko Group, in Balaka, Malawi, was started by a group of parents who had either lost children to HIV/AIDS or had taken orphans into their homes. They conducted a needs assessment of 32 villages that identified over 3,000 orphans in their region. In response, they initiated several activities, including village-based daycare centers, communal gardens to benefit vulnerable children, and an education committee to keep children in schools. Ngwangwa also offers caregivers counseling and training in child development. Daycare centers are run by volunteers in their own homes, with the support and oversight of village HIV/AIDS committees. Ngwangwa supports the centers by providing training and play materials. One meal is provided to children each day. The centers are open for at least 4 hours daily, allowing caregivers to work.[50]

Taylor has summarized the comparative advantages and shortcomings of community structures (Table 3.1). Each of the different structures has strengths and weaknesses in terms of their capacity, reach, and functioning in various areas. It is important that external agencies involved in implementing and partnering these structures appreciate these differences.

THE ROLE OF EXTERNAL AGENCIES IN SUPPORTING COMMUNITY RESPONSES

In recent years, significant increases in external funding to support HIV and AIDS responses have occurred. As a result, many local organizations involved in supporting AIDS-affected children and their families are interacting with external agencies—donors, national and international NGOs, and governments. When provided in the right way—for example, to assist community efforts to support vulnerable children—external resources in the form of money, material support, or technical assistance can provide a critical boost.

One study conducted under the Joint Learning Initiative on Children and HIV/AIDS (JLICA) examined the relationship between external organizations and community responses in Uganda. Most (61%) of the 108 OVC initiatives identified were local, founded and led by people within the community or based in institutions such as churches and schools. The remainder were externally based, implemented by Ugandan or international NGOs and FBOs. Sixty percent of local initiatives received support in the form of materials (81% of initiatives), finances (75%) or technical assistance (31%) from international donors and government.[51] The high rate of external support was testimony to the government of Uganda's commitment to promoting community responses. One objective of the JLICA was to clarify the most appropriate roles for external organizations in supporting community responses for affected children and researchers made a number of critical observations about the role of external agencies in supporting community OVC responses:[52]

Table 3.1 STRENGTHS AND WEAKNESSES OF DIFFERENT COMMUNITY STRUCTURES[53]

	Community Initiatives	Community-based Organizations	Community Service Organizations	Community Coordinating Committees
Strengths	• Commitment, motivation, and compassion • Rootedness • Reach: identify the most vulnerable • Accountability and ownership within local community • Innovation and flexibility to respond to changing context • Locally resourced • Sustainable	• Some commitment, motivation, and compassion • Some rootedness and reach • Varying degrees of accountability and ownership • May scale up and draw in large numbers of volunteers	• Provision of defined services • Ability to provide remuneration to volunteers • External linkages assist capacity development • May provide services to large numbers	• Inherent authority • Connect to structures within community • Often have defined roles • Accountability within community
Weaknesses	• Small-scale • Low level of training • Potential for dominant leadership • Partiality	• Potential for dominant leadership • Potential for partiality and abuse of resources • Dependence on external resources with sustainability concerns • Some not locally rooted and accountable	• May not respond to community concerns or may respond inflexibly • Dependence on external resources with sustainability concerns • Often not locally rooted and accountable	• Potential for dominant leadership • Potential for partiality

• *Community-led initiatives frequently fail to access external support.* Communities are frequently overlooked in the distribution of available international and local funds for scaling up OVC responses, despite their commitment and the magnitude of responsibilities they take on. Many community organizations struggle to resource their work and are unsuccessful in making applications to receive external support to expand their initiatives, even after considerable effort.[54] The criteria determining which applicants should receive support favor those with connections, writing skills, and adaptability to donor requirements. Community members involved in activities supporting children were dissatisfied with disbursement delays, unrealistically tight time frames, inflexibility, and lack of dependability and trustworthiness of intermediaries.[55]

• *Many vulnerable children are excluded from external support.* Many external support initiatives target assistance toward individual children using narrow criteria that do not coincide with community perceptions of vulnerability. This limits the effectiveness of communities to provide appropriate support to those with greatest need. Conditions may be applied to who may be supported— orphans only or children of certain ages, for example—and support may be restricted to certain needs, such as the payment of school fees.[56] In Uganda, only 36% (594/1,631) of needy children accessed assistance. Although the proportion of boys and girls receiving help was similar, only 18% of children under 6 were assisted, compared to 44% of older children, largely because of the emphasis of programs on educational support.[57] Although 59% of external support was targeted exclusively at individual children, only 8% was directed specifically toward strengthening households containing vulnerable children, raising concerns about equity since non-targeted children living in the same household might fail to benefit from external support.

• *External monitoring frameworks impose unrealistic burdens on local organizations.* Community groups indicate dissatisfaction about the functioning of monitoring systems imposed by external partners as conditions for funding. Groups in Mozambique complained that each donor required a different dataset, using different reporting tools and schedules. Time spent in fulfilling donor requirements was incompatible with their goal of assisting vulnerable children, to the point that some CBOs complained they were being transformed into service delivery agents for donors and intermediary NGOs. Monitoring indicators lacked relevance, with data collection focused on counting children and activities rather than on monitoring children's well-being. Local use of data by community implementers for decision-making, planning, and advocacy for better services was minimal.[58]

• *External funding initiatives benefit intermediaries more than beneficiaries.* Considerably more time and money has been invested by donors and their partners in monitoring recipient OVC activities than on assessing the impact and effectiveness of aid delivery. It is difficult to determine overall amounts of funding being provided at international and national levels for the support of vulnerable children, and there is little information available on how much support actually reaches beneficiaries.[59] Although few studies have been published assessing cost effectiveness, current large-scale funding initiatives appear to benefit intermediaries more than intended households and communities, and eat up external resources before they reach affected children (Box 3.5). There is scope for further study of community responses, given the limited evidence base on the effectiveness of external resources.

Box 3.5

Cost Effectiveness of Large-scale International Nongovernmental Organization-led Orphan and Vulnerable Children Programs

Funding to support international nongovernmental organizations (NGOs) administering large-scale orphans and vulnerable children (OVC) programs has increased significantly during the past decade, and several have been evaluated.[60] Important questions about these programs include: How effective are large international NGO OVC programs in delivering support to vulnerable children? And, what proportion of donated funds benefit vulnerable children? Catholic Relief Services (CRS) is an international faith-based organization that operates extensive HIV/AIDS programs, with OVC programs in Botswana, Haiti, Kenya, Rwanda, Tanzania, and Zambia. It received US$103 million, from the U.S. President's Emergency Plan for AIDS Relief (PEPFAR) for HIV/AIDS activities in 2007, the second highest amount of funding of any organization.[61] The CRS implemented the US$5 million 5-year STRIVE (Support to Replicable, Innovative Village/Community Level Efforts) program for vulnerable children in Zimbabwe starting in 2001, funded by the U.S. Agency for International Development (USAID).

One of the aims of STRIVE was to test "innovative interventions that allow resources to reach children at risk quickly and efficiently" and specifically collect data on operational costs. The CRS initially provided subgrants of between US$147,000 and US$196,000 to "eight local community and faith-based organizations" that supported between 2,800 and 8,000 vulnerable children. Another eight local and international NGOs received subgrants of between US$46,000 and US$649,000. Costs per child reached during the first phase of STRIVE varied from US$4 to US$65 per child per year; 14 local "community-based organizations" had annual costs of between US$4 and US$20 per child, whereas two international NGOs had costs of around US$65 per child. The two international NGOs were subsequently dropped from the second phase of STRIVE because their service delivery costs were considered too high.[62]

The USAID increased its grant provision on two occasions and provided nearly two-thirds of the US$11 million total cost of STRIVE. The final evaluation found that the approach of making subgrants through a U.S. private voluntary organization was costly, with few resources reaching communities and children. The CRS/STRIVE employed 20 staff members, and the administrative cost of the USAID grant was estimated at between US$3.24 and US$3.59 million (45%–50% of the total USAID contribution). Only half the grant was available for program activities, such as on-granting to subgrantees, operations research, and technical assistance. The CRS used $2.8 million of the total USAID grant for subgrants to partners that received grants in both phases. The average subgrant to these partners was US$257,000, around US$50,000 per year. The CRS required that each subgrantee employ at least three officers. Partners also incurred other operational costs, thus "diminishing the resources available for community activities." One partner allocated 63% of the STRIVE grant to salaries and 23% to other administrative costs, leaving only 14% for program activities. The consequence of this funding approach was that most of the subgrants were used for operating expenses—"an inverted pyramid where resources seemed to dissolve at successive levels, leaving little for actual on-the-ground activities." The evaluation concluded that "community interventions were very small—even tiny."[63] Although this program was specifically established to conduct operational research on cost effectiveness, there is a lack of corresponding data on the effectiveness of OVC programs implemented by other organizations.

THE ROLE OF GOVERNMENT IN COORDINATING COMMUNITY ORPHANS AND VULNERABLE CHILDREN RESPONSES

National responses to the crisis of increasing numbers of vulnerable children in Africa have been slow to emerge. National strategic HIV/AIDS plans have generally overlooked the care of orphans and vulnerable children.[64] Although in many countries ART rollout and prevention of mother-to-child transmission responses have been supervised and coordinated by ministries of health for some years, significant government responses to the crisis of increasing numbers of vulnerable children have only occurred recently, and their scale has been limited.[65]

In 2007, UNICEF's East and Southern African Regional Office (ESARO) commissioned a nine-country study to map the involvement of civil society in national responses for children affected by HIV/AIDS. The study reviewed the responses of different sectors, noting that these involved a few well-resourced international organizations, many local NGOs, and innumerable community-level initiatives. The study focused on *alignment*, a process in which external agencies and civil society engage with government and align their activities with the vision, principles, and strategies contained in national plans of action. The study identified important principles underlying OVC responses and suggested ways in which community responses may be better funded, coordinated, and monitored, summarized below:[66]

> • *Funding is strongly linked to alignment.* The recent, welcome expansion of external funding of OVC activities is being accompanied by increasing calls for greater involvement of communities in decision-making and alignment through coordinated national responses. Many civil society OVC responses are aligned more closely with donors than with national coordination structures. The sheer number of international contributions to OVC responses strains the capacity of national coordinating bodies. Decisions concerning which OVC services to provide and where to situate them are often made by Western donors and international NGOs. Donors have been slow to collaborate with one another and with national responses, while competitive funding processes have led to unwillingness by organizations to collaborate with one another. Alignment is more likely to be achieved as national coordination structures develop operational OVC policies, establish coordination structures and monitoring

mechanisms, and engage with funders through collaborative arrangements such as pooled donor funds.[67]

• *Coordination structures should be strengthened.* Coordination of OVC responses takes place through both government structures and civil society networks that, in many countries, are weak and fragmented. The lack of coordinated civil society responses has led to their limited involvement in national decision-making. Even when one or two international or national NGOs do become involved, the organizations frequently lack a mandate to represent nationwide civil society OVC responses.[68] The lack of local networks linked to national structures has encouraged the establishment of small, geographically diverse donor-linked networks. Government leadership is critical for ensuring coordination among stakeholders at national, district, and local levels. Government-facilitated networks can strengthen community-level initiatives, enable them to align with national plans, policies, and programs, and ensure community voice in decision-making.

• *Reporting systems should be standardized.* Diverse reporting systems have proliferated, with data delivered by NGOs and CBOs to funders and intermediaries often bypassing government structures. National OVC monitoring systems were functional in only one-third of the countries in the ESARO study.[69] Even if donor monitoring data were provided to governments, lack of uniformity would make it difficult for governments to utilize data and evaluate the effectiveness of OVC responses. One solution might be to establish standardized national OVC monitoring systems containing a small number of essential indicators supplemented by other context-specific monitoring data to meet the needs of funders. Although uniformity of reporting systems is desirable, "alignment up," whereby civil society modify their activities to fit with national plans of action, should be accompanied by "alignment down," whereby governments ensure that OVC monitoring systems meet the needs of implementers at community level.

RECOMMENDATIONS TO STRENGTHEN COMMUNITY RESPONSES FOR VULNERABLE CHILDREN

Governments are becoming more involved in responses to children affected by HIV/AIDS through situation assessments, national plans of action, and the establishment of coordinating structures and national monitoring systems. But national OVC scenarios have been characterized by "alignment anarchy," in which government coordination on OVC issues has been weak.[70] Enhanced and supportive government OVC coordination would have many advantages, such as increased protection and services, decreased gaps and duplication, coordinated access to external resources, improved national information systems, sharing of good practices, and increased cost efficiency. Governments might lead efforts to coordinate and strengthen community initiatives and ensure that actions by external agencies are appropriate and do not damage or undermine community responses. Recommendations have been proposed to assist national OVC responses and strengthen the responses of communities[71]:

• *Communities should have a determining voice in how resources for affected children are allocated and used in their local settings.* The views of children should, whenever possible, be taken into account in decision-making processes. Donors and implementing agencies must create mechanisms for regular, substantive community consultation and involvement in the design, implementation, monitoring, and evaluation of externally funded programs (including cash transfer schemes) that support children affected by HIV and AIDS.

• *Community initiatives must be strengthened, so that they can sustain and expand the scale and scope of their activities.* Donors and their NGO partners should be dissuaded from presenting their programs as directly benefitting vulnerable children and terming them "community-based" when they involve little community involvement in decision-making and so little funding actually directly benefits and reaches affected households and children. Access to external resources and technical support provision by community-level responses are key, but in delivering external resources, the context, needs, and capacities of communities have to be considered.

• *Government-led coordination structures should develop charters of best practice.* These charters would guide international development partners, governments, and local civil society in supporting children and families affected by HIV and AIDS. In addition, working groups involving both government and civil society should be convened to make recommendations on how to ensure that external resources intended for children are effectively utilized, and to engage communities in designing and using monitoring systems.

CONCLUSION

Even though income transfer programs targeting vulnerable households are becoming established, for the foreseeable future, extended family and community groups will remain the most important sources of support to households containing orphans and vulnerable children.[72] But community responses are no panacea – they may be poorly conceived and at odds with national and international best practice guidelines or they may overlook extremely vulnerable households due to stigmatisation. Not enough is known about the characteristics of communities, for example, how stronger leadership or level of preexisting organization may influence outcomes. Further research on these and other questions could help maximize the effectiveness of community-driven OVC initiatives.

In recent years, HIV/AIDS responses for vulnerable children have been increasingly driven by international NGOs and donors, with issues framed from external perspectives. External aid for vulnerable children can be more efficiently utilized by local communities if provided in appropriate amounts, through suitable mechanisms. There has been insufficient involvement of governments and community-level actors in decision-making. The effectiveness of externally driven programs to support vulnerable children would be enhanced if governments and affected communities were involved in their design. Governments have a role to play in ensuring that programs benefit their populations by providing appropriate resources and support to affected communities, households, and children.

Millions of children whose lives are blighted by the impacts of HIV and AIDS face problems that are largely invisible to outside agencies. Despite their scale and scope, community contributions remain "under the radar"—taken for granted, unac-knowledged, and under-supported by many governments, donors, and international agencies. Because community-based responses are barely seen, appropriate responses such as the provision of resources and the establishment of comprehensive national and international strategies have also been overlooked. Heightened visibility of the situation of people living with HIV contributed to the expansion of counseling, test-ing, and ART programs through expanded health sector responses in the last decade. It is our hope that raising awareness of the plight of affected children and the signifi-cance of community initiatives will be key to persuading governments and donors to increase the proportion of their funding and the quality of their support that reaches the grassroots level to assist effective and appropriate community OVC responses.

NOTES

1. Bolton, P., & Wilk, C. M. (2004). How do Africans view the impact of HIV? *AIDS Care, 16*, 123–128.

2. Foster, G., Laugharn, P., & Wilkinson-Maphosa, S. (2010). Editorial: Out of sight, out of mind? Children affected by HIV/AIDS and community responses. *Firelight Supplementary Issue: Community Action: Supporting Children and Families Affected by HIV/AIDS and Poverty in Sub-Saharan Africa, Vulnerable Children and Youth Studies, 5*(S1), 1–6; Gosling, L. (2005). *Study on civil society involvement in rapid assessment, analysis, and action planning (RAAAP) for orphans and vulnerable children.* London: UK Consortium on AIDS and International Development.

3. Joint United Nations Programme on HIV/AIDS (UNAIDS). (2009). *AIDS epidemic update.* Geneva: UNAIDS.

4. Newell, M. L., Coovadia, H., Cortina-Borja, M., Rollins, N., Gaillard, P., & Dabis, F. (2004). Mortality of infected and uninfected infants born to HIV-infected mothers in Africa: a pooled analysis. *Lancet, 364*(9441), 1236–1243.

5. UNICEF. (2009). *Children and AIDS: Fourth stocktaking report.* New York: UNICEF.

6. Data from Joint United Nations Programme on HIV/AIDS (UNAIDS). (2008). *Report on the global AIDS epidemic.* Geneva, Switzerland: UNAIDS; UNAIDS (2009) *AIDS epidemic update*; UNICEF (2009). *Children and AIDS: Fourth Stocktaking Report.* UNICEF (2010). *Children and AIDS: Fifth Stocktaking Report.* New York: UNICEF.

7. Webb, D., Gulaid, L., Ngalazu-Phiri, S., & Rejbrand, M. (2006). Supporting and sustaining national responses to children orphaned and made vulnerable by HIV and AIDS: Experience from the RAAAP exercise in sub-Saharan Africa. *Vulnerable Children and Youth Studies, 1*(2), 170–179.

8. Richter, L. (2008, August 3–8). No small issue: Children and families. Presented at the XVIIth International AIDS Conference, Universal Action Now, Mexico City, Mexico.

9. Gosling. (2005). *Study on civil society involvement in rapid assessment.*

10. Campbell, C., Nair, Y., & Maimane, S. (2007). Building contexts that support effective community responses to HIV/AIDS: A South African case study. *American Journal of Community Psychology, 39*, 347–363.

11. Foster, G., Deshmukh, M., & Adams, A. M. (2008). *Inside-out? Strengthening community responses to children affected by HIV/AIDS.* Boston/Geneva: JLICA

Learning Group 2, Community Action. Retrieved June 6, 2009, http://www.jlica.org/userfiles/file/JLICA_LG2_FINAL%281%29.pdf?PHPSESSID=63b2584f6b5d5ac5e1f344d46cc8d4cb

12. Schenk, K. (2008). *What have we learnt? A review of evaluation evidence on community interventions providing care and support to children who have been orphaned and rendered vulnerable.* Boston/Geneva: (JLICA), Learning group 2 on community action. Retrieved June 6, 2009, http://www.jlica.org/userfiles/file/JLICA%20paper%20Schenk%2023Sept%20%281%29.pdf?PHPSESSID=63b2584f6b5d5ac5e1f344d46cc8d4cb; Thurman, T. R., et al. (2006). Sexual risk behavior among South African adolescents: Is orphan status a factor? *AIDS and Behavior, 10*(6), 627–635.

13. Phiri, S. N., Foster, G., & Nzima, M. (2001). *Expanding and strengthening community action: A study to explore ways to scale-up effective, sustainable community mobilization interventions to mitigate the impact of HIV/AIDS on children and families.* Unpublished draft, USAID Displaced Children and Orphans Fund.

14. Akintola, O. (2004). *A gendered analysis of the burden of care on family and volunteer caregivers in Uganda and South Africa.* Durban: HEARD/UKZN and USAID.

15. Subbarao, K., Coury, D., & World Bank. (2004). *Reaching out to Africa's orphans: A framework for public action.* Washington, DC: World Bank.

16. Foster, G., et al. (1996). Supporting children in need through a community-based orphan visiting programme. *AIDS Care, 8*(4), 389–403; Gilborn, L. Z., Apicella, L., Brakarsh, J., Dube, L., Jemison, K., Kluckow, M., et al. (2006). *Orphans and vulnerable youth in Bulawayo, Zimbabwe: An exploratory study of psychosocial well-being and psychosocial support programs.* Washington, DC: Population Council - Horizons Program.

17. Donahue, J., & Williamson, J. (1998). *Community mobilization to address the impacts of AIDS: A review of the COPE II program in Malawi.* Washington, DC: USAID.

18. Gachuhi, D. (1999). *The impact of HIV/AIDS on education systems in the eastern and southern Africa region and the response of education systems to HIV/AIDS: Life skills programmes.* New York: UNICEF. Retrieved September 27, 2010,http://hivaidsclearinghouse.unesco.org/search/resources/HIV%20AIDS%20199.pdf

19. Horizons, Makerere University, & Plan/Uganda. (2004). *Succession planning in Uganda: Early outreach for AIDS-affected children and their families.* Washington, DC: Population Council.

20. Foster, G. (2005). Under the radar: Community safety nets for children affected by HIV/AIDS in extremely poor households in sub-Saharan Africa. Geneva: United Nations Research Institute for Social Development. Retrieved June 6, 2009, http://www.sarpn.org.za/documents/d0001830/Unrisd_children-hiv_Jan2005.pdf

21. Wikipedia. Non-governmental organization. Retrieved September 27, 2010, http://en.wikipedia.org/wiki/Non-governmental_organization; Depp, R. M., Marunda, S., & Yates, E. (2006). *Final assessment: USAID/Zimbabwe assistance to orphans and vulnerable children through Catholic Relief Services STRIVE program.* Washington, DC: Global Health Technical Assistance Project. Retrieved September 27, 2010, http://pdf.usaid.gov/pdf_docs/PDACI766.pdf; Catholic Relief Services (CRS). (2004). *Turning the tide: Lessons learned, sound practice*

and corrective action in OVC programming: STRIVE Phase 1 Summary Report. Harare: Catholic Relief Services.

22. Taylor, N. (2010). The different forms of structures involved in the community response for vulnerable children, and what are they best placed to do. *Firelight Supplementary Issue: Community Action: Supporting Children and Families Affected by HIV/AIDS and Poverty in Sub-Saharan Africa. Vulnerable Children and Youth Studies, 5*(S1), 7–18.

23. Luzze, F. (2002). Survival in child-headed households: A study on the impact of World Vision support on coping strategies in child-headed households in Kakuuto county, Rakai district, Uganda. MA thesis, Oxford Center for Mission Studies.

24. Foster, G. (2002). *Understanding community responses to the situation of children affected by AIDS- Lessons for external agencies.* Geneva: United Nations Research Institute for Social Development. Retrieved September 27, 2010, http://www.unrisd.org/80256B3C005BCCF9/httpNetITFramePDF?ReadForm &parentunid=DB1400AC67D49680C1256BB8004E0C3D&parentdoctype=pa per&netitpath=80256B3C005BCCF9/%28httpAuxPages%29/DB1400AC67D4 9680C1256BB8004E0C3D/$file/foster.pdf

25. Tembo, F., & Wells, A. (2007). *Multi-donor support to civil society and engaging with 'nontraditional' civil society. A light-touch review of DFID's portfolio.* London: Overseas Development Institute. Retrieved November 20, 2009, http:// www.odi.org.uk/RAPID/Publications/Documents/Multidonor_Support.pdf; Foster, G. (2005). Under the radar.

26. Kelly, K., & Birdsall, K. (2007). *Pioneers, partners, providers: The dynamics of civil society and AIDS funding in southern Africa.* Johannesburg: CADRE/OSISA.

27. J. Williamson (2007, September 24), Three Approaches to Working in Communities: Roles, Responsibilities, Resources. Presentation at JLICA Symposium, Meeting Children's Needs in a World with HIV/AIDS: An International Symposium. Harvard Medical School, Boston.

28. Donahue, J., & Mwewa, L. (2006). *Community action and the test of time: Learning from community experiences and perceptions: Case studies of mobilization and capacity building to benefit vulnerable children in Malawi and Zambia.* Washington, DC: USAID Displaced Children and Orphans Fund; Government of Rwanda. (2006). *Strategic plan of action for orphans and other vulnerable children, 2007–2011.* Kigali: MIGEPROF; Taylor, N. (2008). *Watering the banana trees: The role of international donors in supporting community responses to vulnerable children in countries severely affected by HIV and AIDS.* Unpublished draft produced for IATT on AIDS and Children.

29. Foster, G. (2006). Future imperfect? Charting a roadmap for children living in communities affected by HIV and AIDS. *Children First, 64.* Retrieved June 6, 2009, http://childrenfirst.org.za/shownews?mode=content&id=27131& refto=4922

30. World Bank & University of Dar es Salaam. (1992, September 16–20). *The economic impact of fatal adult illness in sub-Saharan Africa.* Report of a workshop held in Bukoba, Tanzania.

31. African Religious Health Assets Program (ARHAP). (2006). *Appreciating assets: The contribution of religion to universal access in Africa.* Report for the World Health Organization. Cape Town: ARHAP. Retrieved June 6, 2009 http://www. arhap.uct.ac.za/downloads/ARHAPWHO_entire.pdf

32. Foster, G. (2006). Future imperfect?
33. Yates, D. (2003). *Situational analysis of the church response to HIV/AIDS in Namibia: Final Report.* Windhoek, Namibia: Pan African Christian AIDS Network.
34. ARHAP. (2006). *Appreciating assets.*
35. Foster. (2005). *Religion and responses to orphans in Africa.* In G. Foster, C. Levine, & J. Williamson (Eds.), *A generation at risk: The global impact of HIV/AIDS on orphans and vulnerable children* (pp. 159–180). New York: Cambridge University Press.
36. African Religious Health Assets Program (ARHAP). (2006). *Appreciating assets.*
37. Nshakira, N., & Taylor, N. (2010). External resources for vulnerable children flowing through community-level initiatives: The experiences, concerns and suggestions of initiative leaders and caregivers in Uganda. *Firelight Supplementary Issue: Community Action: Supporting Children and Families Affected by HIV/AIDS and Poverty in Sub-Saharan Africa. Vulnerable Children and Youth Studies,* 5(S1), 71–80; Foster, Deshmukh, & Adams. (2008). *Inside-out?*
38. Kidman, R., & Heymann, S. J. (2009). The extent of community and public support available to families caring for orphans in Malawi. *AIDS Care, 21*(4), 439–447; Malawi National Statistics Office. (2005). *Malawi second integrated household survey (IHS2) 2004–2005: Basic information document.* Zomba, Malawi: Malawi National Statistics Office; Malawi National Statistics Office. (2005). *Integrated household survey, 2004–2005: Volume I Household socio-economic characteristics.* Zomba, Malawi: Malawi National Statistics Office.
39. Foster, Deshmukh, & Adams. (2008). *Inside-out?*
40. Foster, G. (2005). Religion and responses to orphans in Africa.
41. Foster, G. (2004). *Study of the response by faith-based organisations to orphans and vulnerable children.* New York: World Conference of Religions for Peace and UNICEF. Retrieved September 7, 2008, http://www.wcrp.org/files/RPT-ovc.pdf
42. Olson, K., Sibanda, Z., & Foster, G. (2006). *From faith to action.* Santa Cruz, CA: Firelight Foundation.
43. Foster (2004). *Study of the response by faith-based organizations.*
44. Schenk, K. (2008). *What have we learnt?*
45. Blackett-Dibinga, K., & Sussman, L. (2008). *Strengthening the response for children affected by HIV and AIDS through community-based management information systems.* Washington, DC: Save the Children (US) and (JLICA), Learning Group 2 on Community Action. Retrieved from http://www.jlica.org/userfiles/file/Body%20of%20Document.pdf?PHPSESSID=34902c401d45246478014602d64f489a; Family AIDS Caring Trust and The International HIV/AIDS Alliance. (2001). *Expanding community-based support for orphans and vulnerable children.* United Kingdom: International HIV/AIDS Alliance; Loewenson, R., Mpofu, A., James, V., Chikumbrike, T., Marunda, S., Dhlomo, S., et al. (2008). *Review of links between external, formal support and community, household support to orphans and vulnerable children in Zimbabwe.* Zimbabwe: TARSC/National AIDS Council and JLICA, Learning Group 2 on Community Action; Nshakira, N., & Taylor, N. (2008). *Strengthening mechanisms for channeling resources to child protection and support initiatives: Learning from communities supporting vulnerable children in Uganda.* Kampala: FARST Africa; Foster, Deshmukh, & Adams. (2008). *Inside-out?*
46. Taylor, N. (2010). The different forms of structures.

47. Donahue, J., & Mwewa, L. (2006). *Community action and the test of time.*
48. Loewenson et al. (2008). *Review of links.*
49. Ibid.
50. Olson, Sibanda, & Foster. (2006). *From faith to action.*
51. Nshakira & Taylor. (2008). *Strengthening mechanisms for channeling.*
52. Foster, Deshmukh, & Adams. (2008). *Inside-out?*
53. Based on Taylor. (2010). *The different forms of structures.*
54. Birdsall, N. (2005). *Faith-based responses to HIV/AIDS in South Africa: An analysis of the activities of faith-based organisations in the National HIV/AIDS Database.* Johannesburg: Centre for AIDS Development, Research and Evaluation; Taylor, N. (2005). *The warriors and the faithful: The World Bank MAP and local faith-based initiatives in the fight against HIV and AIDS.* HIV/AIDS Briefing Paper no. 5. Teddington, UK: Tearfund; Taylor, N. (2005). *Many clouds, little rain? The global fund and local faith-based responses to HIV and AIDS.* HIV/AIDS Briefing Paper no. 4. Teddington, UK: Tearfund; Taylor, N. (2006). *Working together? Challenges and opportunities for international development agencies and the church in the response to AIDS in Africa.* HIV/AIDS Briefing Paper no. 7. Teddington, UK: Tearfund.
55. Nshakira & Taylor. (2008). *Strengthening mechanisms for channeling resources.*
56. Aniyom, I., Obono, O., Oyene, U., Laniyan, C., & Adebayo, B. (2008). *Strengthening community and civil society response to orphans and vulnerable children in Cross River State, Nigeria.* JLICA Technical Report: Learning Group 2 on Community Action. Cross River State, Nigeria: State Agency for the Control of AIDS; Loewenson, et al. (2008). Review of links.
57. Nshakira & Taylor. (2008). *Strengthening mechanisms for channeling resources.*
58. Blackett-Dibinga & Sussman. (2008). *Strengthening the response for children.*
59. Foster, G. (2005). *Bottlenecks and dripfeeds: Channelling resources to communities responding to orphans and vulnerable children in Southern Africa.* London: Save the Children (UK). Retrieved June 6, 2009 http://www.savethechildren.org.uk/scuk/jsp/resources/details.jsp?id=2985&group=resources&section=publication&subsection=details; Garmaise, D. (2006). *The Aidspan guide to developing global fund proposals to benefit children affected by HIV/AIDS.* New York: Aidspan. Retrieved June 6, 2009 http://www.globalaidsalliance.org/page/PDFs/Aidspan_Global_Fund_Pediatric_Guidelines.pdf
60. Schenk. (2008). *What have we learnt?*; Schenk, K. (2009). Community-based interventions providing care and support to orphans and vulnerable children: A review of evaluation evidence. *AIDS Care, 21,* 918–942; Schenk & Michaelis. (2010). Community interventions supporting children.
61. AVERT. PEPFAR Funding: How is the money spent? Retrieved October 28, 2010, http://www.avert.org/pepfar-funding.htm
62. Catholic Relief Services (CRS). (2003). *Report on the mid-term review of the STRIVE project.* Harare, Zimbabwe: Catholic Relief Services. Retrieved October 28, 2010, http://sara.aed.org/tech_areas/ovc/strive-report.pdf; Catholic Relief Services (CRS). (2004). *Turning the tide.*
63. Depp, Marunda, & Yates. (2006). *Final assessment.*
64. Tarantola, D., & Gruskin, S. (2009). Universal access: Are national strategic plans sensitive to human rights. In R. C. Marlink, & S. J. Teitelman (Eds.), *From the ground up: Laying a strong foundation.* Washington, DC: Elizabeth Glaser Pediatric AIDS Foundation.

65. Webb, D., Gulaid, L., Ngalazu-Phiri, S., & Rejbrand, M. (2006). Supporting and sustaining national responses to children orphaned and made vulnerable by HIV and AIDS.

66. Foster, G. (2008). *Getting in line: coordinating responses of donors, civil society and government for children affected by HIV and AIDS.* Nairobi: UNICEF ESARO. Retrieved June 6, 2009 http://www.aidsportal.org/repos/CSO%20Alig nment%20with%20National%20Responses_ESAR_09_20081.pdf.

67. Lewnes, A., & Monasch, R. (2008). *A partnership making a difference: Zimbabwe's programme of support to the national action plan for orphans and other vulner-able children.* Zimbabwe: Ministry of Public Service, Labour, and Social Welfare and UNICEF.

68. Gosling, L. (2005). *Study on civil society involvement in rapid assessment.*

69. Foster. (2008). *Getting in line.*

70. Ibid.

71. Foster, Deshmukh, & Adams. (2008). *Inside-out?*; Foster. (2008). *Getting in line.*

72. L. Richter, "Social cash transfers to support children and families affected by HIV/AIDS," *Firelight Supplementary Issue: Community Action: Supporting Children and Families Affected by HIV/AIDS and Poverty in Sub-Saharan Africa, Vulnerable Children and Youth Studies* 5, No. S1 (2010): 81–91.

PART TWO

Challenges to Child Development

4

Early Childhood

The Building Base for the Future

PATRICE L. ENGLE ■

As children move from early infancy through adolescence, both the impact of HIV/AIDS and the interventions needed to ensure that each child can survive and thrive change in accordance with the child's developmental trajectory. The period below age 5 has received far too little specific attention in interventions for orphans and vulnerable children (OVC). Yet, this is the critical period of high risk and high opportunity for growth and development. It should be the highest priority for programming.

It has been estimated that over 200 million young children in the developing world do not fulfill their potential for development. With estimates of a loss of up to 20% of gross domestic product (GDP) a year due to this lost potential, many countries are beginning to look at this missed opportunity.[1]

Richter et al. have eloquently argued that all children need three things: a special relationship with at least one caregiver, social and economic support for the dyad, and being part of a larger social system.[2] This chapter attempts to specify what these three levels entail for young children who are vulnerable because of HIV/AIDS or are affected by HIV/AIDS.

To achieve these three conditions, some supports are well recognized, but others are just beginning to be understood. It is well recognized that caregivers of young children need access to food and health care services, and children need to be registered at birth. But caregivers also need knowledge and skills, as well as motivation and energy to meet the multiple needs of young children. For example, caregivers need to know how to talk to young children about difficult issues and to understand age-appropriate psychosocial support, since children who are living with HIV have unique age-related care and emotional support needs. As this chapter will show, strategies are beginning to be developed that are particularly appropriate for children aged 0–5 who are affected by HIV and AIDS.

Whereas programs and policies for OVC have increased in recent years, most attention has been given to school-aged children. Assessment of research and practice in four areas carried out by the Joint Learning Initiative on Children and HIV/AIDS (JLICA) provides useful conclusions about the current state of programs. The JLICA Learning Group 2 report, which examined community responses to young children, identifies the lack of attention to programs for young children as a critical unmet need, particularly given their long-term importance when instituted during a child's early years.[3]

This chapter begins with a description of children's developmental trajectory in the period from birth through the beginning of school (age 5–6 in most countries). Second, it describes how this trajectory is influenced by the specific challenges posed by living with HIV or being vulnerable to the effects of HIV and AIDS. Third, it outlines interventions that have been developed for this age group, including evidence for effectiveness and the plans and policies that are put in place to help these children. Finally, it discusses recommendations for what can be done to improve the well-being of children affected by HIV and AIDS in this age group.

WHAT IS CHILD DEVELOPMENT, AND HOW DOES IT CHANGE IN THIS AGE RANGE?

Child development refers to the ordered emergence of interdependent skills of sensory-motor, cognitive-language, and social-emotional functioning. A child's development is strongly affected by her health and nutritional status, as well as by learning opportunities in her environment. A child continues to develop into adulthood, and every stage is important, but the early phase (prenatal through age 5) is particularly critical for later development. This is the period during which the brain develops most rapidly, cognitive and language skills grow, social and emotional patterns are formed, and both risk and opportunity for change are largest. It is also a period during which there are no recognized social investments (e.g., school) other than initial contact with health services; thus, variations in family well-being and economic level play a substantial role.

Brain architecture, or the structure and function of the brain, plays a major role in a child's eventual functioning. Both brain architecture and developing abilities are built "from the bottom up," with simple circuits and skills providing the scaffolding for more advanced circuits and skills over time. Brain architecture is built over a succession of *sensitive periods*, each of which is associated with the formation of specific circuits that are associated with specific abilities. The development of increasingly complex skills and their underlying circuits builds on the circuits and skills that were formed earlier. Through this process, early experiences create a foundation for lifelong learning, behavior, and physical and mental health.[4]

Improving early child development may be the most effective strategy for developing human capital and reducing poverty and inequalities. Increased productivity is an important component of most poverty reduction strategies, but often primary schooling does not help to reduce disparities and to begin to break the cycle of poverty. Poorer and stunted children often enter school later, are more likely to repeat or drop out, and perform worse than better off children. Early childhood is a unique period during which to help children initiate schooling on a more equal level and begin to move forward.

Children's readiness to learn at school entry is a significant component in determining their progress in school. In minority populations in the United States, the poorer the child's environment, the greater the impact of the early environment, and the less likely the child will be to improve in school relative to age mates.[5] Heckman analyzed a large number of interventions to improve poor children's well-being prior to school, during school, and in adolescence in the United States, and found that the only cost-effective ones were those in early childhood that targeted the most disadvantaged.[6] In the absence of interventions for young disadvantaged children, social class divisions between children at school entry continue and often widen through the school years. School readiness is influenced by cognitive ability, social-emotional competence (e.g., the ability to function in groups of other children and communicate with strange adults), effective approaches to learning (e.g., openness to learning, curiosity, and interest), and sensory-motor development (e.g., critical skills, such as writing).

These domains of development have been shown to be improved by parenting styles, quality of the home environment, and early child development programs. For example, the amount of language exposure a child experiences, particularly language used in a meaningful context such as a conversation with the child (rather than on TV), is strongly associated with later language development, which in turn helps school performance in later years.[7] The quality of the home environment, including having learning materials that provide children with opportunities for touching, manipulation, problem-solving, and responsive play and care with adults and older siblings, contributes to child development in many cultures.[8] Children who do not have these learning opportunities are at risk for not developing their potential.

Developing an early emotional and trusting connection to a caregiver is critical for an infant's well-being.[9] Emotional security develops through a child's attachment or unique bond with at least one consistent caregiver who responds to the child's physical and emotional needs soon after they are expressed. The lack of attachment with at least one consistent caregiver can affect a child's brain development and overall functioning.[10] When these emotional deficits are severe, as in cases of early exposure to systematic abuse or poor-quality nonparental care, children may fail to grow and can have impaired cognitive function through biological effects on brain structure.[11] As they get older, these children are more at risk of problem behaviors.[12]

Poverty and social context increase young children's exposure to biological and psychosocial risks; these in turn affect development through changes in brain structure and function and in behavior.[13] Major well-documented risks include stunting (often associated with low birth weight and lack of exclusive breastfeeding), iron deficiency anemia, iodine deficiency, and lack of stimulation in the environment. Additional potential risk factors include exposure to violence, maternal depression, parental loss, and environmental toxins.[14] Concurrent risks, which are very common, have a much greater impact on child development than do single risks.

Because the factors influencing a child's early development are biological, psychological, and social, supporting a child's right to development requires a holistic and intersectoral approach to the early years (conception to school entry), and should include protection from various forms of risk. This approach should include enabling policies, accessible quality basic services, and appropriate family and community care.

EARLY CHILD DEVELOPMENT AND HIV/AIDS

Living in the context of high HIV/AIDS prevalence results in a lower chance of optimal development and an increased likelihood of risks during this critical period, both for children who are HIV positive and for those affected by HIV and AIDS.

This section first defines the number of children infected and affected by HIV and AIDS, and then examines evidence of the effects of the pandemic on their nutrition and development.

YOUNG CHILDREN LIVING WITH HIV (HIV-POSITIVE)

In 2007, an estimated 370,000 (330,000–410,000) children younger than 15 years became infected with HIV. Globally, the number of children younger than 15 years living with HIV increased from 1.6 million (1.4 million–2.1 million) in 2001 to 2.0 million (1.9 million–2.3 million) in 2007. Almost 90% live in sub-Saharan Africa.[15] Probably 90% of these children acquired the virus in utero, during birth, or through breastfeeding, with a much smaller number becoming infected as young adolescents.[16]

These children are likely to die at a young age, since, without treatment, the virus is aggressive in children and progresses quickly.[17] In highly infected areas, HIV is an underlying cause of over a third of all child deaths before age 5.[18] Untreated, most children born with HIV die before their 10th birthday, and many die earlier. In fact, recent data suggest that the peak of infant mortality in young HIV-infected children may be in the first 2–3 months of life.[19]

Figure 4.1 from the 2008 Joint United Nations Program on HIV and AIDS (UNAIDS) report illustrates that the number of children infected with HIV is increasing over time. However, even though the total number is growing, the rate of increase is slowing; Figure 4.2 shows that the number of new infections appears be shrinking.[20] In part, this is due to smaller numbers of new infections as the result of expanded programs preventing mother-to-child transmission (PMTCT). According to the World Health Organization (WHO), UNICEF, and UNAIDS report in 2010, antiretroviral therapy (ART) regimens for PMTCT are now reaching 45% of HIV-positive pregnant women globally, although only 25% in low- and middle-income countries.[21]

Children infected with HIV show a number of physical effects: They have higher mortality rates; are more likely to be malnourished, stunted, and wasted; and more likely to have a variety of infections.[22] Most studies show that children who are HIV positive have developmental delays; that is, they function more poorly on tests of cognitive and motor development compared to similar children who are not infected.[23]

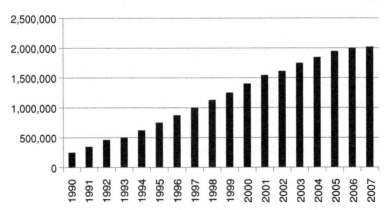

Figure 4.1 Number of children living with HIV globally, 1990–2007.[24]

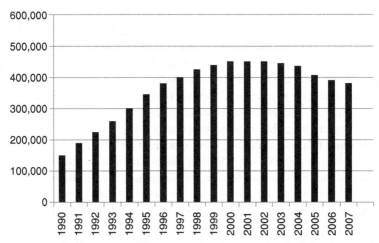

Figure 4.2 Number of new HIV infections among children under 15, 1990–2007.[25]

For example, in a study of HIV-positive children under 2.5 years in Soweto, South Africa, 72% had severe motor delay and 52% had severe cognitive delay. Motor development was affected more severely than cognitive development.[26]

The evidence of behavioral problems for these children is less clear. A study of HIV-positive 6- to 11-year-olds in India demonstrated behavioral problems,[27] but studies of preschool-aged children in Thailand did not report that children affected by AIDS displayed any more behavioral problems than nonaffected children.[28]

Young Children Affected by HIV and AIDS

Although a high percentage of children living with HIV tend to be very young, this is not the case for orphans. Among children aged 0–17 who were either single or double orphans, an estimated 16% (7 million children) are under 8 years old.[29] The percent of all young children who are orphans is low; for example, Hosegood et al. found that 3%–4% of children aged 0–4 in Malawi, Tanzania, and South Africa were paternal orphans, and 1%–2% were maternal orphans.[30]

However, these figures probably underestimate the percentage of young children made vulnerable by AIDS because children experience the effects of parent illness long before a parent dies.[31] When an adult in a household is ill, children receive far less attention than when all family members are well.[32] Heymann et al., using the Botswana Family Needs Survey, found that 86% of HIV-affected adults caring for children aged 0–5 reported experiencing difficulties, compared to 77% for school-aged children and 67% for adolescents.[33] Further, parents of young children caring for someone with AIDS spent only 76 hours per month caring for their children, compared to 96 hours per month for those who were not providing this care. Therefore, the estimate of 7 million young orphans neglects the number of young children who are vulnerable to the loss of caregiving associated with a family member suffering from AIDS.

The number of young children who are affected by HIV and AIDS should be of particular concern. First, as the previous section illustrated, younger children are particularly vulnerable to risks. In the earliest years, both the risks of poor growth and development, and the opportunities for good growth and development, are greatest. Second, younger children are less able to help than older children, and their care requires more time, effort, and skills than does care for older children. Third, rearing a young child requires skills and knowledge about nutrition, health, sanitation, stimulation, and psychosocial support that may not be known to older non-parental caregivers, who frequently take over care for AIDS-affected children. Fourth, these children are least able to protect themselves from poor treatment, stigma, or discrimination. It is not surprising, then, that children who are orphaned or made vulnerable because of HIV and AIDS have higher rates of mortality, malnutrition, and illnesses, and that they lack learning opportunities and psychosocial support.[34]

Vulnerability increases with poverty and low levels of parent education. The combination of being an orphan and being in poverty increases the likelihood of risk and negative outcomes.[35] Orphan and vulnerable child households are reported to be poorer, more stigmatized, and have less access to health care,[36] and OVCs are reported to be more likely to be in poorer health[37] and malnourished.[38] Several studies have found that HIV-affected families experience additional stresses[39] and become poorer as a result of adult illness and death.[40] Children are more likely to migrate or have to change residences, reducing the consistency of care.[41] Young children, in particular, may be subject to changes in residence and caregiving, and in some cases, as in Russia, more vulnerable to abandonment.[42]

UNICEF reported that, in communities with high levels of HIV and AIDS and extreme poverty, all children are vulnerable and should be helped, concluding that this approach is not only cost-effective but also helpful in reducing stigmatization.[43] Indeed, a review of national plans of action for children affected by HIV and AIDS in the 17 sub-Saharan African countries with the highest prevalence of HIV and AIDS found that most programs focus on vulnerable children rather than simply orphans.[44] The estimated numbers for orphaning and vulnerability are remarkably different in these national plans of action; for example, in Kenya, approximately 11% of children are orphaned by AIDS, but fully 40% are considered by the government to be vulnerable. In Zambia, 16% are orphans, but 67% live below the poverty line. In Tanzania, 2 million children are estimated to be orphans, but twice that number is estimated to be vulnerable. Therefore, national governments are targeting children other than those who are specifically single or double orphans,[45] and this focus should bring more attention to the specific issues of young children living in precarious circumstances.

INTERVENTIONS FOR ORPHANED AND VULNERABLE YOUNG CHILDREN

A Developmental Framework for Interventions

A developmental approach is needed because children respond very differently to their experiences at different ages, depending on their level of physical, cognitive, and psychosocial development. For example, the effects of the illness or death of a key caregiver will be different for infants, young children, children in the middle childhood years, and adolescents. The developmental level (including emotional maturity and level of understanding) of a child or adolescent will influence how he or she reacts to the death of a mother or father (or both) and to separation from siblings and other possible consequences of parental death. The first document to outline these age–appropriate responses clearly was the 2004 issue of *Children on the Brink*.[46]

The age-related needs of infancy and early childhood, middle childhood, and adolescence must inform interventional programming. However, most of the policies, programs, information, and literature concerning orphans and other children made vulnerable by HIV/AIDS have tended to regard them as an age-undifferentiated population. Data and programming recommendations have often failed to make key age-related distinctions, ignoring the physical, cognitive, emotional, and psychosocial differences that characterize children and adolescents in different stages of development. The primary issues, as they relate specifically to young AIDS-affected children, are described next.

HEALTH AND NUTRITION

Health and nutrition programs have long recognized the particular vulnerability of young children. A child's chances of survival are much lower if the mother becomes sick with AIDS and dies, or if the child himself is infected by HIV and AIDS. Boys and girls under age 5 in most circumstances are vulnerable to potentially fatal measles, diarrhea, and pneumonia. Malnutrition increases the chances of the child's dying from these diseases. Severe malnutrition during the first few years of life can cause irreversible stunting and impaired cognitive functioning.[47]

ATTACHMENT AND RELATIONSHIP WITH CAREGIVERS

In the first 1–2 years of life, young children need to feel attached to at least one consistent and concerned caregiver for their healthy development and, in fact, for their survival. In addition to the fulfillment of basic physical needs, the child needs touching, holding, emotional support, and love from this consistent caregiver. When a young child loses such a caregiver, he or she is at risk of losing the ability to make close emotional bonds—to love and be loved—and is as well at increased risk of illness and death. Even before the age of 2, children are sensitive to feelings of loss and stress in others and need reassurance.[48]

Between ages 3 and 6, young children remain vulnerable to disease and malnutrition, but their psychosocial needs are sometimes neglected because they appear to be more independent. They continue to need a sense of belonging and social and emotional support. They also need opportunities to learn, because this is the critical period for establishing curiosity, exploration, and fine motor skills.[49]

Young children may lose the opportunity for emotional attachment and closeness when a parent dies, when caregivers are distracted by other needs, or when they are placed in institutional care that does not provide a consistent caregiver. From a developmental perspective, institutionalization in a setting that does not provide the needed nurture and care can be particularly harmful.[50] There is thus a pressing need to ensure that family-based care is available for these children, either through support for relatives, foster care, local adoptive placement, or community organizations and faith-based organizations (FBOs) that are integrally linked to the community.[51]

BEREAVEMENT AND LOSS

The illness or death of a parent or other family member has different effects on children, depending in part on a child's age and stage of development. Children under age 5 may not understand the finality of death and may expect a person who has died to reappear. They may fear that they have caused a loved one's death.[52] Caregivers need to assure a child that this is not the case.

Children who are experiencing loss may feel anxiety and sadness, and may have outbursts of anger. Some regress or behave like younger children. These behavioral changes are almost always transitory, and caregivers should be able to recognize them as reflections of the loss and not respond negatively to them. Caregivers need to make the child feel safe and loved, be willing to talk about loss and the person who died, and provide clear information about death.

There is growing awareness of the importance of a developmental response in programs broadly designed for OVC. For example, the Family Health International Guide for Program Managers[53] includes a new awareness of the importance of meeting young children's needs. As Steinitz concludes, "It is important to reach very young children because early childhood programs help build a foundation for later life"[54].

A major goal across all programs is keeping children with families, and having orphanages serve as temporary refuges rather than as permanent options for many children. A body of research showing the negative effect of institutions, particularly for young children, has resulted in an increased effort to keep children in homes.[55] Orphanage care also is much more costly per capita than leaving the child in a home.[56] It usually results in the child's loss of contact with extended family, which is an essential part of long-term well-being. Therefore, the goal of many programs for young children is to provide enough support to the extended family so that the child can stay with them.

One must not, however, assume that being placed in an extended family necessarily means that the child is being well cared for. Stigma, bias, and family overload from caregivers and other children may result in challenges for the entering child. In a qualitative evaluation in KwaZulu-Natal, South Africa, the organization TREE and researchers Klavsvig and Taylor report a variety of challenges for poor families who take in additional orphans.[57] If the family is poor, children are an additional burden, and at a young age they provide little additional labor. In these circumstances, the children sometimes feel they are being exploited, and the adults feel resentful if the children are not compliant. In some cases, children attribute their parents' death to bewitchment by the family members who are now their official caregivers. In a number of cases, rivalries develop with the biological children, who may resent the appearance of additional needs. In extreme cases, children cannot be placed with relatives because of family rifts or because the children have severe health or behavioral problems. These children may be sent to rural areas, where the researchers reported that, in some cases, neglectful caregivers exploited them as domestic workers or cattle herders, thus occasionally beginning a slow process of alienation until the children left the home and took to the streets.[58] Thus, it is not surprising that children prefer to be with a grandparent, who may have a greater commitment to the child. In one study in Namibia that asked young children their preferences for who to live with, the most common placement request was with a grandmother or grandfather, even if that person was poorer than another relative.[59]

Interventions for Children Living with HIV

Medical responses to young children are slowly beginning to increase, but psychosocial responses have been slower. The likelihood that a child will receive antiretroviral drugs has increased as a result of improvements in a number of HIV treatment drugs for children, as well as because of reductions in their cost.[60] According to UNAIDS, the number of children initiated on ART has increased significantly over the past few years.[61] Whereas only 75,000 infected children under 15 years of age were receiving treatment in 2005, this number grew to 198,000 in 2007 and to 275,700 by the end of 2008, accounting for 38% of those children infected with HIV who are in need of treatment. UNAIDS recommends that children be screened and their HIV status identified as early as possible.[62] Many countries are therefore in the process of scaling up screening and intervention programs. In 2008, 83 of 123 reporting countries had the capacity to provide HIV testing to infants within 2 months of birth, up from 57 of 109 reporting countries in 2007.[63]

One of the major stumbling blocks to providing more support to infants who are HIV positive is the low rate of follow-up in PMTCT programs. One study in Cameroon found that the greatest loss to follow-up of infants in care (45%) occurred even before the mother received her child's positive test result.[64] In Rwanda, an experimental approach to increasing follow-up was to incorporate recommendations on early childhood development (ECD) into the PMTCT program.[65] In the pilot project, the ECD intervention was only tested in a few locations and results were not conclusive.[66] It remains an idea that requires testing.

There has been concern that caregivers will reduce their care of a child after learning that the child is HIV positive. A qualitative study on children aged 1–5 years in South Africa examined the effects of the caregivers' learning of their child's HIV status on their attitudes and aspirations for the child.[67] One year after learning the results of the HIV test, most caregivers exhibited positive attitudes toward knowing their child's status and maintained high aspirations for the child. The caregivers apparently learned to cope over the course of the year, mainly through counseling and spirituality. Knowledge of HIV status was perceived as valuable since it enhanced the caregiver's competency in providing care to the child.[68]

The perceived usefulness of knowing a child's HIV status is important, as it may promote acceptance and coping with the results and encourage caregivers' aspirations for the child's future, thereby improving the quality of care.[69] The finding of high aspirations for children in this study differs from views expressed in a Ugandan study, indicating that some mothers would not care for an HIV-positive child as they believed that child will die anyway.[70] Although the high aspirations could be real, they may also be unrealistic, as studies have documented higher levels of wishful thinking among caregivers of HIV-positive children than of HIV-negative children.[71]

Once a child's HIV status is known, improving his or her health status should improve his or her cognitive and motor development. Potterton et al. examined the association of ART and children's development in South African children under 2.5 years of age. Only 16% of the children were receiving highly active antiretroviral therapy (HAART).[72] Weight-for-age, age, and whether the child was on HAART were the most important factors in predicting cognitive and motor development. Delays in diagnosis and treatment and poor treatment coverage are obvious areas for attention to reduce the negative consequences of HIV infection on developmental outcomes.[73]

A major area of work to support children living with HIV is the provision of additional support to staff in pediatric wards, to help them best deal with children's pain and suffering while still feeling that they are able to do their job. Richter, Chandan, and Rochat developed strategies for helping pediatric staff cope with their own sense of loss, and designed strategies to help them reduce the children's experience of pain through techniques such as giving children a transitional object.[74] This is an area of work that deserves far more attention.

Finally, one study in South Africa looked at nonmedical interventions to improve developmental outcomes. In this study, HIV-infected babies randomly assigned to receive a psychosocial intervention program during clinic visits showed significantly greater improvement in cognitive and motor development after 6 and 12 months compared to those receiving standard care only. The program involved sharing simple activities with caregivers to promote motor, cognitive, and speech and language skills.[75]

Interventions for Young Children Affected by HIV and AIDS

Community organizations, including those supported by nongovernmental organizations (NGOs) and FBOs, provide a large amount of support for children vulnerable to HIV and AIDS. However, they are often overstretched.[76] Moreover, these community-based organizations tend to support a few needs while leaving others neglected. Foster found that many more programs supported school assistance (62%) than daycare or child care programs (10%).[77] These programs frequently overlooked young children,[78] even though, as Foster et al. observe, investments during this period of a child's life have long-term impacts.[79] In Uganda, one study of 612 beneficiaries showed that 18% of children of preschool age received support, compared to 44% of 6- to 14-year-olds and 38% of 15- to 18-year-olds.[80]

A review of case studies of programs run by NGOs and FBOs for young children affected by AIDS and of the experiences of five sub-Saharan countries on ECD and HIV/AIDS policy development showed that most programs for young children are small-scale, community-based interventions run by NGOs.[81] The quality and scale of these programs varies widely. Malawi is perhaps the most experienced country on ECD, with a national-level program of community-based child care centers; however, the bulk of orphan and psychosocial needs still falls upon community providers, not the government. At the moment, the number of community-based child care programs in most countries is far too small to meet children's needs.

Although a large number of small-scale programs are run by NGOs for young children, few have been evaluated. Schenk reports a similar difficulty in reviewing evaluations of community-based programs for OVC;[82] in a review of psychosocial support programs for OVC of all ages, King et al. found no evaluations that would indicate which of these programs contributed to children's well-being.[83] Therefore most of the results reported here are descriptions of program results. There is a great need for more systematic assessments of various approaches and for discovering how well they are reaching those most in need.

TYPES OF INTERVENTIONS
Interventions for young children include programs that provide services directly to children (e.g., daycare centers) or create indirect effects through changes in their caregiving environment, such as increasing caregiver capacity to provide care, external support, or access to services. These interventions may reduce biological and/or

psychosocial risk factors for poor development, such as providing feeding for mal-nourished children or a home visitor who reads books to children living in poverty. These interventions may also strengthen protective factors, such as by providing social support to a mother or additional funds to the family in the form of cash trans-fers. In general, interventions may promote good child development, prevent risks for poor child development, and reduce or ameliorate the negative effects of prob-lems such as low birth weight, developmental delay, or poverty. When the presence of HIV and AIDS in families is combined with poverty, the need for preventative interventions or amelioration is usually high.

Here, we describe interventions for children under 5 that are delivered through family strengthening, child care centers, and external support mechanisms. These interventions include focuses on food and nutrition, psychosocial support, early education, protection, and health.

FAMILY STRENGTHENING

Social support for families includes information, social, and economic support. Information and social support often come through home visiting programs. For example, both Speak for the Child in Kenya (see Box 4.1)[84] and the Grandmothers' Program in Uganda[85] provide regular home visiting, information, and help in access-ing resources. The Action for Children program in Uganda provides caregivers, usu-ally grandmothers, with a variety of services, including health and nutrition information, food supplements, and home visits. Nyenko finds that grandparents who received support from this program were more encouraged to take care of their grandchildren.[86]

Box 4.1

SPEAK FOR THE CHILD, KENYA[87]

Speak for the Child supports families and communities in western Kenya to improve the health, nutrition, and psychosocial care of young children orphaned and affected by HIV/AIDS using a combination of home visits by local women, "mentors" who have received training, and a village-level committee who can "speak for the child". Speak for the Child began serving 500 children in Kakamega and currently serves approximately 44,000 OVC in Western and Nyanza Provinces.

The program provides some resources (e.g., preschool fees) but also helps caregiv-ers to recognize and solve problems themselves. It combines interventions to improve caring and psychosocial development as well as health and nutrition, although the former are far less well understood.

Results in 2006 showed that, in comparison with a nonintervention area, the pro-gram was effective in increasing immunization rates, food intake, feeding frequency and quality, income generation for caregivers, attendance in preschool, and, to a degree, improved early stimulation activities; more recent pretest–posttest results have also shown positive effects. These results are suggestive but, as in the case of many of these reports, do not have the rigor of a randomized controlled trial.

Children in their preschool years have a concept of death such that, in the absence of an explanation, they have a developmental tendency to assume that they are to blame for the death of others, resulting in guilt in addition to loss. In their qualitative evaluation in South Africa, respondents from all communities described two different ways in which orphans aged 3–5 reacted to their bereavement and change of circumstances: depression and withdrawal on the one hand, and "acting out" on the other.[88] Too often, no information is given to the child. One study found that parents were unclear about how to disclose their own HIV status to their children, and many did not disclose until children were 11 or 12, at which point many children had already guessed it.[89] Programs are needed that provide help to families in dealing with disclosure of HIV status, particularly to young children.

Disclosure of the child's status is also difficult. Nam et al. found that most families did not disclose information about the child's HIV status to the child before adolescence, even when children were taking medications and probably wanted to know the reason.[90] Current best practice is to inform children of as much as they can understand when they appear ready to hear it, which is often shown by the questions they ask.

CHILD CARE CENTERS

Child care programs serve a number of purposes: They prepare children for school, provide respite for caregivers, support children's families, provide alternative care if none is available in families, and give psychosocial support to help families understand the challenges of having an ill family member. They can also provide access to a regular meals and health care, and can free older siblings to attend school.

A number of NGOs have developed a comprehensive approach to community development that incorporates a child care program or improved access to funding for preschool. Almost all have a health and nutrition component. However, they often vary widely in their implementation and quality: Programs may offer very basic child supervision by untrained volunteers, or may offer a highly structured early childhood curriculum delivered by skilled staff. In Swaziland, simple community-based child care centers were used as places where children could get food, play, and even obtain some basic learning, but the child development aspect was initially very limited. In Rwanda, a comprehensive approach provided child care for children 2–4 and 4–6, nutrition support, and access to health care, and also freed caregivers for income earning and older siblings for school.[91] Perhaps the best developed model is in Malawi, which has an extensive system of community-based child care centers that were developed before the AIDS pandemic. The centers are run by community volunteers, but the system for training and support for the volunteers has been improving over the past 15 years and now has a curriculum, a training system, and policy support. At this point, almost half of the children attending are orphans.[92] Research on child care programs has shown that these interventions, if of sufficient quality, can have a long-term impact on children's development and later productivity.[93]

INCREASED EXTERNAL SOCIAL SUPPORT

In an assessment of constraints to providing better care in South Africa, financial restrictions were a considered a major limitation. The financial and physical limitations these families face suggest that they need different kinds of income-generating strategies.[94] South Africa provides different types of child grants, which, although small, may make a huge difference for families. Although most respondents regarded the child grant as inadequate, most depended on it, especially since many of the mothers were also infected and their opportunities for formal employment were limited.

Cash transfers have demonstrated a strong potential to reduce poverty and strengthen children's education, health, and nutrition, especially when such transfers were received on behalf of younger children; therefore, cash transfers can form a central part of a social protection strategy for families affected by HIV and AIDS.[95] These programs have achieved impressive results with respect to increases in the quantity and quality of food consumption and improvements in nutritional status, although the latter varies more across countries and types of indicators. In all countries, the largest grant expenditures by far were on food.[96]

In Malawi, the National Action Plan for Orphans and Vulnerable Children (2004–2009) outlines programs and includes guidance for the establishment of meaningful social protection interventions, and the Malawi Growth and Development Strategy has social protection as a key theme.[97] The latter also includes the design, implementation, and evaluation of a social cash-transfer scheme linked to schools and child care centers that seek to reduce poverty and hunger in ultra-poor households. A pilot Social Cash Transfer Scheme is being administered in seven districts. As of April 2009, it had reached more than 23,000 households and 92,000 individual beneficiaries, of whom more than 48,000 were OVC.[98] The Social Cash Transfer Scheme also links with community-based organizations to provide access to early child development, psychosocial support, and home-based care services for cash transfer beneficiaries.[99] Miller et al. have reported improved health, improved food security, and greater school enrollment among beneficiaries of the Social Cash Transfer Scheme.[100] Despite these positive findings, only 12% of families with an OVC are receiving basic external support from governments or NGOs.[101] Most continue to receive support only from other family members or the local community.[102]

Government Programs and Policies in 17 Countries

In a comprehensive review of programs and policies for young children affected by HIV and AIDS in the 17 highest-prevalence countries in sub-Saharan Africa,[103] countries varied enormously in their recognition of the special needs of young children. Those that most effectively incorporated the needs and issues of young children were Rwanda, Malawi, Namibia, and Kenya. These countries were more likely to describe the situation of OVC in terms of child age, to incorporate age-appropriate recommendations in psychosocial and home visiting interventions, to have a community-based child care program, and to consider age appropriateness in health and nutrition programs.

Eleven countries proposed some form of organized early child care services, usually a community-based model. Some were more related to an educational concept. Nigeria proposed free pre-primary education in the schools for all, and specific counseling for OVC. Mozambique suggested developing a preschool strategy. Zambia proposed incorporating ECD into a school support system, but the description was not clear, and no funds were allocated in the first year, although it hopes to receive funds from the U.S. President's Emergency Plan for AIDS Relief. Fewer than half the countries perceived that community-based child care could serve a purpose in supporting families and providing access to services like food and health care, psychosocial support for children, and a respite for families. Although the idea is growing, it continues to need support. In fact, few countries included any capacity-building for this area, suggesting that they are not yet fully aware of what these community-based centers might require.[104]

Although all of the programs mentioned the importance of psychosocial support for all children, only Kenya recognized that young children have unique needs; it suggested one session per year to train caregivers in how to deal with young children. Zambia also recognized the importance of helping caregivers deal with young children, but the activities were still broad and not well defined. In Malawi, Rwanda, and Swaziland, Community Child Care Teachers (volunteers) are expected to provide this support.

Few suggested a holistic response for children infected by HIV; the medical model and provision of ART was the primary response. There is a great need for more information on children's course of development, the possible effects of the virus on their functioning, and their psychosocial as well as medical needs. These issues are only now beginning to be addressed.

There was a clear association between when the plan was prepared and the amount of concern for ECD. Plans emerging from 2006–2007, which included the four with the highest awareness, were much more focused on programming and policies for younger children than were those prepared in 2000–2005. It is likely that some of the earlier plans will change as they gain awareness of the needs of younger children.

GAPS IN EVIDENCE AND PROGRAMS

Many approaches for young children are available, but they are not at scale, and there are no major efforts to promote any one particular model. The most common interventions in this age range are the PMTCT programs, but these are limited to a short time period. Heymann, Clark, and Brewer argue that, unless we fundamentally reframe our approach to HIV prevention to fully address the health of families, the future for at-risk children is likely to remain bleak.[105] The approach to supporting young children affected by HIV and AIDS recommended here offers parallel recommendations: Only by addressing the needs of the family can we successfully meet the needs of the youngest children whose lives are, by definition, intertwined.

Other recognized gaps are the lack of systematic investigations of the effectiveness of any of these programs with respect to HIV and AIDS, in contrast to the increasing literature on the effects of ECD programs in developing countries.[106] This review, as well as others by King et al. and Schenk,[107] found few evaluation studies that could inform the development of policy. The Speak for the Child project remains one of the few that has done an adequate evaluation. There is a wealth of interesting descriptive data on programs, but the rigor of an effectiveness assessment is missing.

The analysis of policies suggests that many countries still do not see the specific needs of young children, or do not prioritize them, despite evidence of their long-term impact. We do not yet have a set of agreed-upon interventions to draw from, other than child care centers, although an increasing number of programs are working with young children. The ongoing choice of who to target—children who are orphaned by HIV and AIDS, children whose parents are ill, all orphans, or all vulnerable children—is slowly moving toward targeting all children. If this model were used, the visibility of young children's programming might increase. Poverty is an overwhelming risk factor, and all children are vulnerable when poverty and HIV/AIDS coexist.

Lack of coordination among programs hampers giving every child the best start in life. Incorporating ECD information into other programs offers many benefits. Linking ECD with PMTCT programs could not only improve young children's development, but also improve follow-up after childbirth, which has been a major problem in PMTCT programs.

External support appears to be an urgent need in many of these cases, but the scale of the problem has resulted in few children actually receiving this support. How can such support be expanded? And how is this support used by families? Families are recognized as the best caregivers, but the circumstances under which young children coming in to families are stigmatized and discriminated against should be examined to determine what external interventions might help to moderate the situation.

CONCLUSION

To meet young children's needs, two actions must be taken: first, clearly define the kinds of approaches that are most likely to be effective for young children who are vulnerable to the myriad risks of poverty and infection; and second, reflect these changes in national plans of action and programs at scale to provide the kinds of support these children and their families need to grow and prosper.

Despite a consistent effort to highlight differences created by a child's developmental level, attention and services for young children remain spotty and infrequent, far below the need. Young children who are experiencing the problems of poverty and lack of caregiving attention associated with adult sickness in a home, or who face orphan status, are still not on the development agenda. For example, the recommendations from the UNICEF Fourth Stocktaking Report in 2009 do not disaggregate children by age. A 2008 analysis of several national plans of action for OVC[108] revealed that many country plans did not incorporate developmental concerns into their thinking. Only with continued effort will all children during the critical 0–5 years of age receive the care and attention that is their right if they are to develop their fullest potential.

Specific recommendations for this age level include ensuring good infant and young child feeding, health care, and growth monitoring and promotion; preserving sibling relationships (particularly when a sibling has been a primary caregiver); supporting consistent and loving caregiving; and developing community child care and early learning programs. Parenting programs and family support programs should focus on the developmental changes children are undergoing. It is critical to recognize not only the physical needs of young children, but also their powerful psychological and emotional vulnerability in these first years of life.

NOTES
1. Grantham-McGregor, S. et al., and the International Child Development Steering Group. (2007). Developmental potential in the first 5 years for children in developing countries. *Lancet, 369*, 60–70.
2. Richter, L., Foster, G., & Sherr, L. (2006). *Where the heart is: Meeting the psychosocial needs of young children in the context of HIV/AIDS*. The Hague: Bernard van Leer Foundation.
3. Foster, G., Deshmukh, M., & Adams, A. (2008). *Strengthening community responses to children affected by HIV/AIDS* (pp. 1–27). Geneva: The Joint Learning Initiative on Children and HIV/AIDS (JLICA).
4. National Scientific Council on the Developing Child. (2007). *The science of early child development: Closing the gap between what we know and what we do.* Cambridge, MA: Centre on the Developing Child, Harvard University.
5. Belsky, J. et al. (2007). Are there long term effects of early child care? *Child Development, 78*, 681–701.
6. Heckman, J. J. (2006). Skill formation and the economics of investing in disadvantaged children. *Science, 312*, 1900–1902.
7. Eshel, N. et al. (2006). Responsive parenting: interventions and outcomes. *Bulletin of the World Health Organization, 84*(12), 991–998; Engle, P. L. et al., & the Lancet Child Development Series Steering Committee. (2007). Strategies to avoid the loss of developmental potential in more than 200 million children in the developing world. *The Lancet, 369*, 229–242.
8. Bradley, R. H., & Corwyn, R. F. (2005). Caring for children around the world: A view from HOME. *International Journal of Behavioural Development, 29*(6), 468–478.
9. Isabella, R. A. (1993). Origins of attachment: Maternal interactive behavior across the first year. *Child Development, 64*, 605–621; Bowlby, J. (1969). *Attachment and loss: Vol 1. Attachment.* New York: Basic Books.
10. Bornstein, M. H. et al. (2008). Mother-child emotional availability in ecological perspective: Three countries, two regions, two genders. *Developmental Psychology, 44*(3), 666–680.
11. Eluvanthingal, T. J. et al. (2006). Abnormal brain connectivity in children after early severe socio-emotional deprivation: A diffusion tensor imaging study. *Pediatrics, 117*, 2093–2100; Nelson, C. A., Zeanah, C., & Fox, N. A. (2007). The effects of early deprivation on brain-behavioral development: The Bucharest early intervention project. In D. Romer, & E. Walker (Eds.), *Adolescent psychopathology and the developing brain: Integrating brain and prevention society* (pp. 197–215). New York: Oxford University Press; Johnson, D. E., Gunnar, M. R., & Palacios, J. (2009, May). *Growth failure in institutionalized children.* Paper presented at the Leiden Orphanage Seminar, Leiden, Netherlands.
12. Rutter, M. (1998). Developmental catch-up, and deficit, following adoption after severe global early privation. English and Romanian Adoptees (ERA) Study Team. *Journal of Child Psychology and Psychiatry, 39*, 465–476.
13. Shonkoff, J. P., Boyce, W. T., & McEwen, B. S. (2009). Neuroscience, molecular biology, and the childhood roots of health disparities: Building a new framework for health promotion and disease prevention. *JAMA : The Journal of the American Medical Association, 301*(21), 2252–2259.
14. Walker, S. P. et al. (2007). Child development: risk factors for adverse outcomes in developing countries. *Lancet, 369*(9556), 145–157.

15. UNAIDS. (2008). *Report on the global AIDS epidemic.* Geneva: UNAIDS.
16. Ibid.
17. Ibid.
18. Mason, E. (2006). Positioning paediatric HIV in the child survival agenda. In *Proceedings of the UNICEF–WHO consultation.* New York: UNICEF; UNAIDS, *Report on the global AIDS epidemic*, 2008.
19. Bourne, D. E. et al. (2009). Emergence of a peak in early infant mortality due to HIV/AIDS in South Africa. *AIDS, 23*(1), 101–106.
20. UNAIDS. (2008). *Report on the global AIDS epidemic.*
21. WHO, UNAIDS, & UNICEF. (2010) Towards universal access: Scaling up priority HIV/AIDS interventions in the health sector 2010–Progress report 2010. Geneva: World Health Organization.
22. JLICA. (2009). *Home truths: Facing the facts on children, AIDS, and poverty.* Cambridge, MA: JLICA; Potterton, J. et al. (2009). Neurodevelopmental delay in children infected with human immunodeficiency virus in Soweto, South Africa. *Vulnerable Children and Youth Studies, 4*(1), 48–57.
23. McCombe, J. A. (2009). NeuroAIDS: A watershed for mental health and nervous system disorders. *Journal of Psychiatry and Neuroscience, 34*(2), 83–85; Van Rie, A. et al. (2007). Neurologic and neurodevelopmental manifestations of pediatric HIV/AIDS: A global perspective. *European Journal of Paediatric Neurology, 11*(1), 1–9; Drotar, D. et al. (1997). Neurodevelopmental outcomes of Ugandan infants with Human Immunodeficiency Virus Type 1 infection. *Pediatrics, 100*(1), e5; Boivin, M. J. et al. (1995). A preliminary evaluation of the cognitive an motor effects of pediatric HIV infection in Zairian children. *Health Psychology, 14*(1), 13–21; Bagenda, D. et al. (2006). Health, neurologic and cognitive status of HIV-infected, long-surviving, and antiretroviral naive Ugandan children. *Pediatrics, 117*(3), 729–740; Baillieu, N., & Potterton, J. (2008). The extent of delay of language, motor, and cognitive development in HIV-positive infants. *Journal of Neurologic Physical Therapy, 32*(3), 118–121; Gupta, S., Shah, D. M., & Shah, I. (2009). Neurological disorders in HIV-infected children in India. *Annals of Tropical Pediatrics, 29*, 177–181; Sadoh, W. E., Okunla, O. P., & Oviawe, O. (2007). Neurologic manifestations of childhood AIDS in Benin City, Nigeria. *Journal of Pediatric Neurology, 5*, 21–25; Tahan, T. T. et al. (2006). Neurological profile and neurodevelopment of 88 children infected with HIV and 84 seroreverter children followed from 1995 to 2002. *Brazilian Journal of Infectious Disease, 10*(5), 322–326; Sherr, L., Mueller, J., & Varrall, R. (2009). A systematic review of cognitive development and child human immunodeficiency virus infection. *Psychology, Health and Medicine, 14*(4), 387–404.
24. Data from UNAIDS. (2008). *Report on the global AIDS epidemic.*
25. Ibid.
26. Potterton et al. (2009). Neurodevelopmental delay in children.
27. Grover, G., Pensi, T., & Banerjee, T. (2007). Behavioural disorders in 6–11 year old, HIV-infected Indian children. *Annals of Tropical Pediatrics, 27*(3), 215–224.
28. Sanmaneechai, O. et al. (2005). Growth, development, and behavioural outcomes of HIV-affected preschool children in Thailand. *Journal of the Medical Association of Thailand, 88*(12), 1873–1879.
29. UNICEF and the Expert Working Group of the Global Partners Forum for Orphans and Vulnerable Children. (2004). *The framework for the protection,*

care, and support of orphans and vulnerable children living in a world with HIV and AIDS. New York: UNICEF.

30. Hosegood, V. et al. (2007). The effects of high HIV prevalence on orphanhood and living arrangements of children in Malawi, Tanzania, and South Africa. *Population Studies: A Journal of Demography, 61,* 327–336.

31. UNICEF, UNAIDS, WHO, & UNFPA. (2008). *Children and AIDS: Third stocktaking report.* New York: United Nations Children's Fund.

32. Gray, G. E. et al. (2006). The effects of adult morbidity and mortality on household welfare and the well-being of children in Soweto. *Vulnerable Children and Youth Studies, 1,* 15–28.

33. Heymann, S. J. et al. (2007). Extended family caring for children orphaned by AIDS: Balancing essential work and caregiving in a high HIV prevalence nations. *AIDS Care: Psychological and Socio-medical Aspects of AIDS/HIV, 19,* 337–345.

34. Fonseca, J. et al. (2008). New threats to early childhood development: Children affected by HIV/AIDS. In M. Garcia, A. Pence, & J. L. Evans (Eds.), *Africa's future, Africa's challenge: Early childhood care and development in sub-Saharan Africa* (pp. 93–114). Washington, DC: The World Bank.

35. UNICEF, UNAIDS, WHO, & UNFPA. (2009). *Children and AIDS: Fourth stocktaking report.* New York: United Nations Children's Fund.

36. Miller, C. M. et al. (2007). Emerging health disparities in Botswana: examining the situation of orphans during the AIDS epidemic. *Social Science & Medicine, 64,* 2476–2486.

37. Watts, H. et al. (2007). Poorer health and nutritional outcomes in orphans and vulnerable young children not explained by greater exposure to extreme poverty in Zimbabwe. *Tropical Medicine & International Health, 12,* 584–593.

38. Bridge, A. (2006). Nutritional status of young children in AIDS-affected households and controls in Uganda. *American Journal of Tropical Medicine and Hygiene, 74,* 926–931.

39. Heymann, et al. (2007). Extended family caring for children orphaned by AIDS.

40. Gillespie, S., Kadiyala, S., & Greener, R. (2007). Is poverty or wealth driving HIV transmission? *AIDS, 21,* S5-S16; Gray, et al. The effects of adult morbidity and mortality.

41. Floyd, S. et al. (2007). The social and economic impact of parental HIV on children in northern Malawi: Retrospective population-based cohort study. *AIDS Care: Psychological and Socio-medical Aspects of AIDS/HIV, 19,* 781–790; Ford, K., & Hosegood, V. (2005). AIDS mortality and the mobility of children in KwaZulu-Natal, South Africa. *Demography, 42,* 757–768; Hill, C., Hosegood, V., & Newell, M. L. (2008). Children's care and living arrangements in a high HIV prevalence area in rural South Africa. *Vulnerable Children and Youth Studies, 3,* 65–77.

42. Zabina, H. et al. (2009). Abandonment of infants by HIV-positive women in Russia and prevention measures. *Reproductive Health Matters, 17,* 162–170.

43. UNICEF, UNAIDS, WHO, & UNFPA. (2009). Children and AIDS: Fourth stocktaking report.

44. Engle, P. L. (2008). National plans of action for orphans and vulnerable children in sub-Saharan Africa: Where are the youngest children? (Working Paper no. 50). The Hague: The Bernard Van Leer Foundation.

45. Engle. (2008). National plans of action for orphans.

46. UNICEF & the Expert Working Group. (2004). The framework for the protection, care, and support of orphans.

47. Walker et al. (2007). Child development: Risk factors for adverse outcomes; Victora, C. G. et al. (2008). Maternal and child undernutrition: Consequences for adult health and human capital. *Lancet, 371*(9609), 340–357.

48. Bowlby. (1969). *Attachment and loss*; Bornstein et al. (2008). Mother-child emotional availability; Dyregrov, A. (2008). *Grief in young children: A handbook for adults*. London: Jessica Kingsley Publishers.

49. Engle, P. L., Dunkelberg, E., & Issa, S. (2007). ECD and HIV/AIDS: The newest programming and policy challenge. In J. Evans, A. Pence, & M. Garcia (Eds.), *Early child development in Africa*. Washington DC: World Bank; Richter, Foster & Sherr. (2006). *Where the heart is.*

50. Rutter, M. et al. (2010). Deprivation-specific psychological patterns: Effects of institutional deprivation. *Monographs of the Society for Research in Child Development, SRCD 295,*751, 1–252. Malden, MA: Wiley-Blackwell.

51. Firelight Foundation. (n. d.). *From faith to action: Strengthening family and community care for orphans and vulnerable children in sub-Saharan Africa* (2nd ed.). Santa Cruz, CA: Firelight Foundation. Retrieved October 24, 2010, http://www.firelightfoundation.org/pdf/fromfaithtoaction-ed2.pdf

52. Dyregrov. (2008). *Grief in young children.*

53. Steinitz, L. Y. (2009). The way we care: A guide for managers of programs serving vulnerable children and youth. Windhoek, Namibia: Family Health International.

54. Ibid., p. 70

55. The St. Petersburg-USA Orphanage Research Team. (2008). The effects of early social-emotional and relationship experience on the development of young orphanage children. *Monographs of the Society for Research in Child Development, 73*(3), pp vii–295; Nelson, Zeanah, & Fox. (2007). The effects of early deprivation on brain-behavioral development.

56. Desmond, C., & Gow, J. (2001). The cost-effectiveness of six models of care for orphan and vulnerable children in South Africa. South Africa: UNICEF; Dunn, A., & Parry-Williams, J. (2008). Assessment of alternative care in Sierra Leone. New York: UNICEF.

57. Kvalsvig, J. D., & Taylor, M. (2005). *Report to reach: Study on orphans and vulnerable children in Kwazulu-Natalphase I–Formative research.* KwaZulu-Natal, South Africa: Training & Resources In Early Education (TREE).

58. Ibid.

59. Haihambo, C. et al. (2004). HIV/AIDS and the young child: An assessment of services provided to children affected and infected by HIV/AIDS in Windhoek, Namibia. Windhoek, Namibia: University of Namibia Press.

60. UNICEF, UNAIDS, WHO, & UNFPA. (2009). Children and AIDS: Fourth Stocktaking report.

61. UNAIDS. (2008). Report on the global AIDS epidemic, 2008.

62. Ibid.

63. Ibid.

64. Clinton Foundation. (2009). *Initiative data provided to UNICEF, 2009.* Reported in UNICEF, UNAIDS, WHO, & UNFPA, 2009.

65. JLICA Learning Group 3. (2008). A learning collaborative on child health in Rwanda: Applying the breakthrough series model to PMTCT-plus and early childhood development. Technical report, JLICA Learning Group 3: Expanding

Access to Services and Protecting Human Rights. Retrieved from http://www.jlica.org

66. Personal communication.

67. Kimani-Murage, E. W. et al. (2010). 'You opened our eyes': Care-giving after learning a child's positive HIV status in rural South Africa. *Health and Social Care in the Community, 18*(3), 264–271.

68. Ibid.

69. Ibid.

70. Brouwer, C. N. et al. (2000). Psychosocial and economic aspects of HIV/AIDS and counseling of caretakers of HIV-infected children in Uganda. *AIDS Care, 12*, 535–540.

71. Klunklin, P., & Harrigan, R. C. (2002). Child-rearing practices of primary caregivers of HIV-infected children: An integrative review of the literature. *Journal of Pediatric Nursing, 17*, 289–296.

72. Potterton et al. (2009). Neurodevelopmental delay in children.

73. Potterton, J. et al. (2010). The effect of a basic home stimulation programme on the development of young children infected with HIV. *Developmental Medicine & Child Neurology, 52*, 547–551.

74. Richter, L., Chandan, U., & Rochat, T. (2009). Improving hospital care for young children in the context of HIV/AIDS and poverty. *Journal of Child Health Care, 13*(3), 198–211.

75. Potterton et al. (2010). The effect of a basic home stimulation programme.

76. Foster, Deshmukh, & Adams. (2008). Strengthening community responses to children.

77. Foster, G. (2004). *Study of the response by faith-based organizations to orphans and vulnerable children.* New York: World Conference of Religions for Peace and UNICEF. Retrieved from http://www.unicef.org/FBO_OVC_study_summary.pdf

78. Foster, Deshmukh, & Adams. (2008). Strengthening community responses to children.

79. Ibid.

80. Nsakira, H., & Taylor, N. (2008). Strengthening mechanisms for channeling resources to child protection and support initiatives: Learning from communities supporting vulnerable children in Uganda. JLICA Technical Report: Learning Group 2 on Community Action, FARST Africa, Kampala.

81. Engle, Dunkelberg, & Issa. (2007). ECD and HIV/AIDS.

82. Schenk, K. (2009). Community interventions providing care and support to orphans and vulnerable children: A review of evaluation evidence. *AIDS Care, 21*(7), 918–942.

83. King, E. et al. (2009). Interventions for improving the psychosocial well-being of children affected by HIV and AIDS. *Cochrane Database of Systematic Reviews, 15*(2), doi: 10.1002/14651858.CD006733.pub2.

84. *Speak for the Child.* Project of AED. Retrieved May 21, 2010, http://www.aed.org/Projects/Speak-for-the-Child.

85. Nyesigomwe, L. (2006). Strengthening the capacity of grandmothers in providing care to young children affected by HIV/AIDS. *Journal of Intergenerational Relationships, 4*(1), 55–63.

86. Nyenko, J., & Keishanyu, R. (2005). *A review report January–June 2005.* Kampala, Uganda: Grandparents Action Support Project, Action for Children.

87. Speak for the Child. (2010).

88. Kvalsvig & Taylor. (2005). Report to reach: Study on orphans and vulnerable children.

89. Nam, S. et al. (2009). Discussing matters of sexual health with children: What issues relating to disclosure of parental HIV status reveal. *AIDS Care, 21*(3), 389–395.

90. Ibid.

91. Kim, J. et al. (2008). *Expanding access to services and protecting human rights:* Integration and Expansion of Prevention of Mother-to-Child Transmission (PMTCT) of HIV and Early Childhood Intervention Services, Learning Group 3, The Joint Learning Initiative on Children and HIV/AIDS, 3, 1–37. Retrieved from http://www.jlica.org/userfiles/file/PMTCTECD_091508-FINAL-revised2.pdf

92. Engle, Dunkelberg, & Issa. (2007). ECD and HIV/AIDS.

93. Heckman. (2007). Skill formation and the economics.

94. Kompaore, M. (2004, July 11–16). Income-generating activities: Effective tools in the promotion of economic self-sufficiency to access ARV treatment among people living with HIV. International AIDS Conference, Abstract no. MoPeD3779, Bangkok, Thailand.

95. Adato, M., & Bassett, L. (2008). What is the potential of cash transfers to strengthen families affected by HIV and AIDS?: A review of the evidence on impacts and key policy debates. Cambridge, MA: JLICA.

96. Ibid.

97. UNICEF, UNAIDS, WHO, & UNFPA. (2009). Children and AIDS: Fourth stocktaking report.

98. Ibid.

99. Adato & Bassett. (2008). What is the potential of cash transfers.

100. Miller, C., Tsoka, M., & Reichert, K. (2008). *Impact evaluation report: External evaluation of the Mchinji social cash transfer pilot.* Boston: Center for International Health and Development (CIHD) at Boston University for the Government of Malawi, USAID and UNICEF Malawi.

101. UNICEF, UNAIDS, WHO, & UNFPA. (2009). *Children and AIDS: Fourth stocktaking report.*

102. Foster, Deshmukh, & Adams. (2008). Strengthening community responses to children.

103. Engle. (2008). National plans of action for orphans.

104. Ibid.

105. Heymann, S. J., Clark, S., & Brewer, T. (2008). Moving from preventing HIV/AIDS in its infancy to preventing family illness and death (PFID). *International Journal of Infectious Diseases, 12*(2), 117–119.

106. Walker et al. (2007). Child development: Risk factors for adverse outcomes; Engle et al. & The Lancet Child Development Series Steering Committee. (2007). Strategies to avoid the loss of developmental potential.

107. King et al. (2009). Interventions for improving the psychosocial well-being of children; Schenk. Community interventions providing care.

108. Engle. (2008). National plans of action for orphans.

5

Education in a Pandemic

The Needs of School-aged Children

XIAOMING LI AND YAN GUO ▪

Although in many countries the prevalence of HIV has decreased in the past decade, the number of children orphaned by HIV/AIDS continues to rise due to the time lag between HIV infection and HIV-related death.[1] In the worst affected countries, the number of children orphaned by HIV/AIDS increased almost three-fold between 2000 and 2006.[2] In sub-Saharan Africa, the hardest-hit region by HIV with 24 of the 25 countries with the highest HIV prevalence rates in the world, the number of children under 18 years of age orphaned by HIV/AIDS was estimated at 12 million in 2008, or roughly one in 20 children in sub-Saharan Africa.[3] The growing number of children orphaned or made vulnerable by HIV/AIDS (i.e., children affected by HIV/AIDS) and their psychosocial well-being remain a great concern in the region and to global society.

The majority of children affected by HIV/AIDS are school-aged children. An analysis of national surveys from 40 sub-Saharan African countries revealed that the age of orphans was fairly consistent across countries with about 85% being between 5 and 14 years old.[4] In 2004, UNICEF reported that, among the 143 million orphans in three regions (Africa, Asia, and Latin America), about 12% were younger than 6 years of age, 33% were 6 to 11 years old, and the remaining 55% were between 12 and 17 years old.[5]

The educational needs of school-aged children affected by HIV/AIDS therefore deserve greater attention worldwide. Education is widely recognized to be essential for child development and the prosperity of society. At the individual level, education is conceived as a key means for children to advance themselves.[6] School can play a crucial role for children affected by HIV/AIDS by improving their lives and economic prospects and securing their future. In addition to being a way out of poverty, a quality school education can also provide social and emotional support to children affected by HIV/AIDS and strengthen their resilience. In contrast, lack of education has severe and lifelong repercussions for children. Without an appropriate education, it is difficult, if not impossible, for children to maximize their potential to become capable and contributing citizens, or to enjoy as rich and meaningful lives as possible.[7]

The importance of education far outreaches the individual level. Education, as one of the fundamental structural elements of modern societies, also plays a critical role in securing sustainable social, economic, and political development.[8] Education has the potential to mitigate national and regional poverty and its negative impacts, and to contribute to nation- and community- building, which is especially important for developing countries. In a globalized economy, the ability of any country, particularly developing countries, to compete in global markets depends heavily on the success with education which develops human capital and social foundations.[9]

Recognizing the essential importance of education on a child's life, the United Nations (UN) Convention on the Rights of the Child (1989) advocated children's rights to education in article 28.[10] As of 2004, 194 countries had ratified this convention.[11] However, more than 7 years have passed, and the educational rights of millions of children are still at risk, especially those of children affected by the impact of the HIV pandemic.

The purpose of this chapter is to review global research on the impact of HIV/AIDS on children's education and interventions and/or practices by governments, nongovernmental organizations (NGOs), international and local humanitarian agencies, local communities, and community-based organizations in addressing the educational needs of school-aged children affected by HIV/AIDS. It is our hope that researchers, practitioners, and policy-makers will be informed by this global research on the educational needs of children affected by HIV/AIDS, and will be able to design and implement culturally appropriate and context-specific approaches to fulfill our collective promise to the educational rights of children affected by HIV/AIDS, and of all children.

This chapter first reviews existing evidence on the impact of the HIV/AIDS pandemic on education systems (teachers and school resources), the impact of HIV/AIDS on children, and the educational outcomes of school-aged children affected by HIV/AIDS, including their school enrollment, attendance, performance, behaviors, and completion. It is then followed by a review of global interventional practices that aim to address multiple threats to the educational needs of children affected by HIV/AIDS and other vulnerable children. Finally, it makes recommendations for future actions based on lessons learned from the existing research.

IMPACTS OF HIV/AIDS ON CHILDREN'S SCHOOLING

In order to understand why education is a primary strategy for protecting children and securing their future, as well as its role in advocating HIV prevention, it is necessary to be aware of the impacts of the HIV/AIDS pandemic on children's schooling at multiple levels of the education system and society.[12] Because HIV/AIDS has become the leading cause of death in sub-Saharan Africa,[13] its impact has reached beyond the health sector and has been felt particularly in the education sector, where HIV/AIDS is affecting both the providers and receivers of education.

Impact on Teachers and Other School Personnel

Throughout sub-Saharan Africa, HIV has infected a substantial number of teachers in the education system. HIV/AIDS prevalence among school teachers is even higher than in other adult populations in some regions of sub-Saharan Africa, ranging from

12% to 25% in southern African countries.[14] In Ghana, a western African country, the HIV/AIDS prevalence rate was 9.2% in the education sector in 2004, compared to the national seroprevalence rate of 3.0%.[15] An analysis by the Mobile Task Team at the University of KwaZulu-Natal estimated that teachers in South Africa were dying at a rate three to four times higher than would be the case without HIV, a significantly higher rate than that of many other adult populations.[16] Similarly, in Kenya, Uganda, and Zambia, AIDS-related deaths among teachers rose throughout the 1990s.[17]

AIDS is resulting in higher mortality and permanent loss of qualified teachers on a scale that has severely impaired the ability of school systems to provide quality education.[18] Furthermore, the HIV-related loss of professional life and productivity among infected teachers has compromised the quality of education. The World Bank estimated that, in Africa, a teacher living with HIV had an average net loss of 6 months of professional life before progressing to AIDS, and an additional year before dying from the disease, which resulted in significant instability and negative impacts on the education system.[19] Because of AIDS-related disability, the already stressed education system carries a large proportion of unproductive workforce and lacks enough qualified teachers to replace or substitute the infected teachers. In addition to reduced productivity and loss of experienced teachers, the loss of other personnel in education systems (e.g., education officers, planning and management personnel, and inspectors) to HIV/AIDS also compromises the efficiency and quality of the education system in many countries hard-hit by HIV, as these losses further impair the system's ability to plan, manage, and implement necessary educational policies and programs.[20]

Impact on Other School Resources

In response to high HIV prevalence, many nations may have to increase spending on their health sector; consequently, the education sector may receive a reduced proportion of the national or local budget. Limited resources in the system are further consumed by HIV-related expenditures at schools, such as treatment and care, insurance, and death benefits for teachers and other school personnel.[21] Likewise, at the household and community levels, more financial resources are drained by HIV-related treatment and care, and less money is allocated to pay for children's schooling.[22] Therefore, reduced national or local budgets for education and the diminished capacity of households and communities to finance schools may further compromise the quality of learning and teaching.

In countries hard-hit by HIV/AIDS, the overall population growth slows down due to HIV/AIDS; fewer children are being born because of the early death of a large number of young adults of reproductive age. Among children born to HIV-positive parents, some are born HIV positive and many may die before reaching school age if no proper treatment is provided. Some school-aged children have to stay at home and take care of sick parents or take care of younger siblings after the death of their parent; some have to work to supplement family income because of household economic deprivation caused by parental HIV-related illness and death. This leads to an overall lower school enrollment, or declined demand for education, which then leads to the closure of some schools and further reduces the accessibility of children affected by HIV/AIDS to formal schooling.[23]

Impacts on Children and Their Families

The HIV epidemic impacts children's schooling at both individual and family levels. At the individual level, children affected by HIV/AIDS are shouldering more burdens while pursuing their education. Many children affected by HIV/AIDS may not have the luxury of going to school, and those who manage to go to school bear additional economic, psychological, and social burdens. Economically, the illness and death of a parent or both parents mean a direct loss of family income, coupled with the draining of family savings on treatment and funeral services.[24] As mentioned in the previous section, children in these families may have to take time off from school to care for ill parents or younger siblings, help in the fields, or work outside the household to supplement family income and make up for the loss or reduced productivity of family labor.[25] Psychologically, these children show more negative symptoms and experience more difficulties concentrating on school work.[26] It is common for teachers to report that they find orphaned children daydreaming, missing school days, arriving at school late and unprepared, or being nonresponsive in the classroom. Socially, these children are likely to experience discrimination at schools or in the community due to HIV-related illness or death of a parent.

At the family level, after the death of one or both parents, orphaned children are usually adopted by their extended families, and many of the children are cared for by their grandparents.[27] Due to the drain of resources caused by HIV-related illness and death, and the increasing number of orphans, extended families may have limited resources to invest in these orphans and, consequently, children affected by HIV/AIDS may likely see a decline in the quantity and quality of food and a loss of educational opportunity, and may face stigmatization and labor exploitation from members of the extended family.[28]

For children who lose one of their parents to AIDS, existing research has shown differential effects of maternal death and paternal death on their educational attendance and outcomes. In general, the loss of a father was often associated with household economic deterioration and consequently resulted in children dropping out of school.[29] The loss of a mother, however, was a strong predictor of poorer schooling outcomes, including being less likely to be enrolled in school, being at a lower grade-for-age, and having poorer performance in school.[30] Children who had lost their mother were less likely to complete their primary school education than those who had lost their father.[31] The loss of a mother was shown to have a greater negative impact on children's educational achievement than the loss of a father, an effect that grew stronger over time.[32] Therefore, among AIDS orphans, maternal and double orphans were found to be the most disadvantaged in their educational outcomes, although the nature and size of differences in comparison with paternal orphans and other children vary from study to study.[33]

Educational Outcomes of Children Affected by HIV/AIDS

Because of the vulnerabilities associated with HIV-related parental illness and death, children affected by HIV/AIDS are likely to show poorer educational outcomes compared to other children. A number of recent studies, using large survey samples across countries and longitudinal data, have reported that children affected by HIV/

AIDS—compared to other children—experience educational disadvantages on a number of outcome measures, including school enrollment, attendance, retention, performance, and completion.

SCHOOL ENROLLMENT AND ATTENDANCE
HIV-related parental illness and death have long-term effects on children's school enrollment and attendance. Both before and after the death of one or both parents, children affected by HIV/AIDS were found to be less likely to go to school. Research showed that children living with HIV-positive parents (e.g., children who faced the potential loss of a parent) were less likely to attend school than were children of HIV-negative parents.[34] Existing research repeatedly reports that orphans were less likely to be enrolled in school.[35] In Eastern and Southern Africa, children who had lost their parents were only half as likely to go to school as those living with both parents.[36] Orphans in the extended family were less likely to be enrolled in school compared to nonorphans living in the same households; the enrollment gap between orphans and nonorphans increased with age.[37] Double orphans (i.e., children who have lost both parents to AIDS) were more likely to be disadvantaged in school attendance compared with single orphans (i.e., children who lost one parent to AIDS).[38] In Tanzania, for example, surveys show that the school attendance rate was 71% for non- and single orphans, but 52% for double orphans.[39] Research in Uganda found that, among orphans 15–19 years of age, only 29% continued their schooling undisrupted after the loss of their parents, 25% attended school irregularly, and 45% dropped out of school.[40]

Research has found that orphans are less likely to be at their proper educational level at school (grade-for-age) than nonorphans, especially for younger children and double orphans.[41] The households affected by HIV often delay school enrollment of younger children, while trying to maintain the enrollment of older children if possible.[42]

SCHOOL PERFORMANCE
Compared to research on school enrollment, there is less research regarding educational performance and school behaviors of children affected by HIV. A recent study among children affected by HIV/AIDS in China indicated that children affected by HIV/AIDS had poorer school performance in comparison to their peers from the same community who did not experience HIV-related illness and death in their families.[43] Particularly, AIDS orphans had the lowest academic marks among the three groups of children (orphans, vulnerable children, and comparison children), based on the reports from both children and teachers. From teachers' perspectives, educational expectation was significantly lower among children affected by HIV/AIDS (orphans and vulnerable children) than comparison children. In addition, AIDS orphans were found to be significantly more likely to demonstrate aggressive, impulsive, and anxious behaviors than were comparison children. They were also less confident in interacting with peers. Furthermore, children affected by HIV/AIDS had more learning difficulties, such as being less likely to be able to concentrate on their studies, which might also contribute to poorer school performance.[44]

SCHOOL COMPLETION
Children who had lost their parents were more likely to drop out of school due to a number of reasons, such as inability to pay the costs of schooling, stigma, or poor academic performance.[45] Orphans had lower levels of educational attainment than

other children in most sub-Saharan African countries.[46] A study in Zimbabwe suggested that AIDS orphans who had made it to school were less likely to complete school in comparison to nonorphans.[47] Longitudinal data from Africa showed a substantial decrease in primary school participation following a parental death from AIDS, especially for children who lost their mother or who had low baseline academic performance.[48] Research in Uganda comparing different living arrangements suggested that school-aged children who lived with a surviving parent were most likely to continue their education, whereas those fostered by grandparents had the least chance.[49]

Limitations of the Existing Research

There are several limitations in the existing research on educational outcomes of children affected by HIV/AIDS. First, the number and scope of the existing studies on the educational outcomes of HIV/AIDS-affected children are limited. Most studies were conducted in sub-Saharan Africa, and studies in other regions such as Asia and Latin America were lacking. Second, only a limited number of educational outcomes is examined, as most of the studies focused only on children's school enrollment and attendance. In the future, more studies are needed to examine children's school performance, school behavior, and school completion. Third, there are some methodological limitations related to research design, including lack of an appropriate control group in most studies for a valid comparison, lack of longitudinal design to assess changes in children's educational outcomes over time, and lack of culturally appropriate quantifiable indicators of educational outcomes. Finally, most of the existing studies relied on data collected from a single source rather than from multiple sources (e.g., students, teachers, caregivers). The incorporation of perspectives from school teachers and caregivers may triangulate the data from children affected by HIV/AIDS and improve the quality of the studies. Future research on the schooling needs of children affected by HIV/AIDS needs to be carefully designed and executed to address these limitations if it is to help us develop a better understanding of the scope, extent, and mechanism of the impacts of HIV/AIDS on the educational needs of these children.

Despite these limitations, the existing research clearly demonstrates the vulnerability and risks experienced by children affected by HIV/AIDS in terms of their schooling and related educational outcomes. Children affected by HIV/AIDS suffer economic, psychological, and social burdens that often have negative impacts on their various educational outcomes, including deprivation of opportunities for formal education, delayed school enrollment, lower grade-for-age status, irregular school attendance, poorer school performances, and increased dropout rates.[50] These educational disadvantages have been the foci of various intervention initiatives by governments, international agencies, NGOs, and local communities.

INTERVENTIONAL PRACTICES TARGETING EDUCATIONAL NEEDS OF CHILDREN AFFECTED BY HIV/AIDS

Based on the global research presented above, we propose a conceptual framework to guide the review of existing intervention initiatives implemented to address the educational needs of children affected by HIV/AIDS and other vulnerable children worldwide. The conceptual framework (Figure 5.1) delineates the relationships among the multiple threats that children affected by HIV/AIDS are facing (e.g., HIV/AIDS, poverty, droughts, armed conflicts, discrimination), children's diverse needs (e.g., education, economic, psychological, social), and support from various levels (e.g., family, community, governments, international agencies, local NGOs). In the framework, we identify those multiple threats to the educational and other needs of children affected by HIV/AIDS that require concerted efforts from all stakeholders. In addition to the HIV/AIDS epidemic, these threats include recurrent drought and food insecurity, longstanding and deepening poverty, wars, armed conflicts, political instability, and financial crises. The compounding effects of these threats not only increase the vulnerability of families and children, but also severely compromise the ability of the community and government to provide adequate education and other essential social services to vulnerable children.

Our conceptual framework also recognizes the necessity of addressing the educational needs of children affected by HIV/AIDS in the context of other needs, such as medical, economic, psychological, and social. The Convention on the Rights of the Child emphasized that "every child has the right to the enjoyment of the highest attainable standard of health and the right to a standard of living adequate for the child's physical, mental, spiritual, moral, and social development".[51] With this declaration, the Convention underscored that a wide range of needs are fundamental to

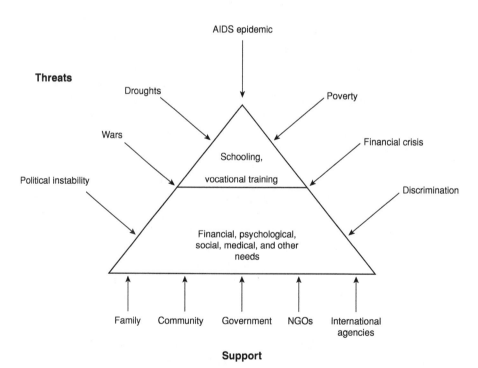

Figure 5.1 Conceptual framework of relationships among HIV/AIDS-affected children's educational and other needs, multiple threats, and levels of support.

children's development, and that only in concert with these needs can education enable them to reach their fullest potential. For example, food security is imperative for meeting the educational needs of children affected by HIV/AIDS; children who have to constantly worry about tomorrow's food naturally place only secondary importance on schooling.

Recognizing the extent of the HIV/AIDS epidemic, the multiple threats that accompany high HIV/AIDS prevalence, and the diverse needs of children affected by HIV/AIDS, many governments, NGOs, international agencies, and local communities have implemented initiatives to help children affected by HIV/AIDS attend, stay and succeed in school. However, few of these initiatives have been reported in global research and even fewer are well-documented and systematically evaluated. Based on the limited information available, we present a showcase of different types of intervention practices designed to address the educational needs of children affected by HIV/AIDS.

As shown in Table 5.1, the existing interventions vary both in scope (from universal policies to targeted projects) and in intervention strategies (from waiving school tuitions, to provision of alternative schooling, to mobilization of local community). Some of the interventions directly benefit children's schooling, whereas others support children's schooling indirectly by providing support and services to the caregivers or household of the children. Many of the interventions reviewed in this chapter take place in African countries, especially in eastern and southern African countries, where the HIV/AIDS epidemic has hit hardest. Interventions in other regions, such as China and Thailand, are also included.

Initiatives Directly Supporting Schooling

In the context of the HIV/AIDS epidemic, education for all is argued to "provide the policy framework and mandate for all learners to engage in the many benefits of schooling;" on the other hand, however, education is "neither universally accessible, equitable, nor free—for many Africans, and disproportionately so for girls."[52] Some programs address the schooling issue of children affected by HIV/AIDS within the larger scale of national education policy, such as free primary education (FPE) in Kenya. Since many families with children affected by HIV/AIDS would otherwise lack the means to send them to school because of their precarious economic status, children affected by HIV/AIDS thus benefit from the policy of free education for all and receive education otherwise denied to them. Instead of providing free formal education for all, some governments offer free education to specific groups of vulnerable children, such as AIDS orphans and rural children in China.

Free Primary Education (FPE) in Kenya
The Kenyan Minister of Education, Science, and Technology announced in January 2003 the initiation of FPE for all children nationwide. The introduction of FPE resulted in a substantial growth of Kenya's school enrollment by more than 1 million almost overnight. Many of those newly enrolled were children affected by HIV/AIDS and children living in poverty. This sudden enormous increase in school enrollment posed a challenge to the country's educational resources and capacity, which are key components that ensure the overall quality of free education.[53] It is critical for FPE

Table 5.1 Description of the 11 Intervention Programs to Improve Education of Children Affected by HIV/AIDS (CABA)

Country	Time	Program/Policy	Main Intervention Strategy	Coverage
Kenya	2003–	Free Primary Education (FPE) policy	Government abolished primary school fee and enabled children's access to education.	From 5.9 million to 7.2 million students; most are CABA*
China	2003–	Free compulsory education for vulnerable children	Government provided free schooling for children orphaned by AIDS, and economic assistance to households affected by HIV/AIDS. Since 2005, the Chinese government has started to provide free 9-year compulsory education to rural students.	School fee waiver 2006: more than 50 million rural students; 2007: 150 million rural students
Thailand	1962–	Rajaprajanugroh Foundation	The Thai monarchy created the foundation and built schools initially for children orphaned by disaster. Now, these schools provide educational opportunities for children made vulnerable by diverse causes, including HIV/AIDS.	N/A†
Zambia	2000–	Interactive Radio Instruction (IRI) program	Government -initiated distance-learning with broadcast lessons to primary and secondary school students, monitored by volunteer teachers.	2005: 900 centers and 60,000 students
	2003–	Better Education and Life Opportunities Through Networking and Organizational Growth (BELONG) program	International agencies collaborated to provide food to CABA at community schools and economic empowerment to female caregivers, and to promote advocacy on reduction in stigma and discrimination against CABA.	70,000 CABA; 7,800 child- and female-headed households

Country	Years	Program	Description	Results
United Republic of Tanzania	1997–	Complementary Basic Education (COBET) program	Government and UNICEF provided basic education and vocational training to out-of-school and older-for-grade children.	2000: 1,530 students, among whom 449 were orphans
	2000–	Most Vulnerable Child program	Government helped establish local committees to identify children made vulnerable by diverse causes including HIV/AIDS and to provide necessary assistance to these children.	2007: 100,000 most vulnerable children
Rwanda	2003–	Community Child Mentoring program	A local nongovernmental organization (NGO) initiated the program to match child-headed households with mentors in the community to provide psychological and practical support to children in the households.	2007: 11,123 children
	2003–	Children's Learning and Development (CHILD) program	An international humanitarian organization initiated the program to provide basic education and vocational training to out-of-school children and young adults aged 12–25 years, with a special emphasis on CABA.	2005: 2,000 students; 2006: 2,500 students
Swaziland	2003–2005	All Children Safe in School programs	A collaboration of international agencies and government helped pay school fees for CABA, provide school meals and school-based farming opportunities, and improve water and sanitation at school.	2003: more than 3,000 students brought back to school; 2004: 7,627 students
	2003–	Neighborhood Care Points (NCP) program	Government and UNICEF mobilized communities to provide meals, education activities, and psychological support to CABA and 4- to 12-year-old out-of-school children.	2007: 34,000 children

*CABA, children affected by AIDS (orphans and vulnerable children); †N/A, not available and other free education programs to build sufficient local human and financial capacity to ensure the quality of free education while providing an educational opportunity for children affected by HIV/AIDS and other needy children. Another challenge for the FPE program was to establish effective communication between the government and the public regarding the respective roles and responsibilities of government, schools, and parents.

FREE COMPULSORY EDUCATION FOR VULNERABLE CHILDREN IN CHINA

In response to the rapid increase of HIV infections in China, the Chinese government initiated the Four Frees and One Care national program in 2003 for the HIV-infected population, children affected by HIV/AIDS, and their families. "Four frees" refer to free antiretroviral treatment, free HIV counseling and testing, free prevention of mother-to-child transmission, and free schooling for children orphaned by AIDS. "One care" refers to the care and economic assistance provided to individuals living with HIV/AIDS and their families.[54] As part of this program, the Chinese government committed to providing free schooling for AIDS orphans and building village schools in areas heavily hit by AIDS.[55] In 2005, the Chinese government took a further step by implementing a nationwide policy to exempt rural students from paying school tuition for their 9-year compulsory education. In the first phase of the program, which started in 2006, more than 50 million rural students in China's western provinces benefited from the policy.[56] It was estimated that in the second phase of the program, starting in 2007, a total of 150 million rural students would be covered by the program.[57]

Although most of the children affected by HIV/AIDS resided in rural areas and benefited from this national policy, some barriers for successful schooling remained for them. For example, families were still responsible for expenditures such as books, uniforms, and school supplies, which could still be a significant financial burden for impoverished families, such as those affected by HIV/AIDS.

FREE SCHOOLING FOR VULNERABLE CHILDREN IN THAILAND

Thailand provides another example of a national initiative to provide free education to needy children, including children affected by HIV/AIDS. The Thai monarch, King Bhumibol Adulyadej, created the Rajaprajanugroh Foundation, which consisted of 36 boarding schools that initially cared for children orphaned by natural disasters (e.g., typhoons, tsunamis), in 1962.[58] Today, these schools are providing educational opportunities for children orphaned or made vulnerable by a variety of causes, including HIV/AIDS. These schools are tailored to meet the different needs of students. For example, the Phra Dabot schools provide professional or vocational training (e.g., radio repair, welding, construction, and electrical skills) to indigent students who are taught by knowledgeable forest monks. These schools provide necessary life skills and vocational training to vulnerable children. To ensure that quality education is being delivered to students in all regions of Thailand, the Distance Learning via Satellite Foundation, launched in 1995, links classrooms in His Majesty's private school, Wang Klai Kangwol in Hua Hin, with schools all over Thailand. One of the key features of the Thailand program was the utilization of existing resources and structures on a national scale to provide schooling to children affected by HIV/AIDS.

Initiatives Providing Complementary Education

As mentioned in the previous section, compared to other children, children affected by HIV/AIDS are more likely to drop out of school and be at lower grade-for-age. In addition, children affected by HIV/AIDS may also miss out on valuable life skills and vocational training that would have been passed on to them by their parents. Children may be more likely to face economic, psychological, social, and health problems later in life as they may lack the necessary skills and knowledge to cope with these problems. To meet these needs of children affected by HIV/AIDS, particularly out-of-school children, left-behind students, and those with extreme financial difficulties, some programs provide complementary or informal education to these children, including vocational and life skills training. The following are some examples of these programs.

COMPLEMENTARY BASIC EDUCATION PROGRAM IN TANZANIA

In 1997, in response to the country's poor primary school enrollment rates, Tanzania's Ministry of Education and Culture, with support from UNICEF, initiated the Complementary Basic Education (COBET) program, which offered a second chance at schooling for out-of-school and older-for-grade children for whom formal education at school was usually denied or unsuitable because of their age. The program was intended to help these children, most of whom were children affected by HIV/AIDS, return to the formal education system or pursue informal educational opportunities. Initially, children attending the program were brought by their parents or caregivers, or came on their own. With the expansion of the program, local community members were involved in identifying COBET learners.

A key component of the COBET program was its curriculum, which provided children with both basic education and vocational skills. Children attended classes for 3.5 hours per day, 5 days a week, in two 15-week terms, for 3 years. The program employed and trained current or retired teachers and paraprofessionals (e.g., community members who had at least some secondary school education) to teach these children in community-based learning centers. At the end of the 3-year pilot phase, COBET had enrolled 1,530 learners in 50 learning centers in five districts, including 449 orphans (173 girls and 276 boys) and 146 vulnerable children (78 girls and 68 boys) living in extreme poverty.[59] Furthermore, COBET learners in the 3-year curriculum achieved similar academic performance to that of children in regular 7-year primary schools, as evidenced by the results of national math and English tests.[60] In addition to basic academic curriculum, COBET students also learned vocational skills that helped them earn a living. The positive outcomes of COBET's 3-year pilot phase prompted the government to expand the program nationwide.[61]

Despite the initial success, the reactions toward the program from students, community members, and educational officials were mixed. On the one hand, they praised the program for the educational opportunity otherwise unavailable to these most vulnerable children. On the other hand, COBET was considered by some people to be an inferior but expensive system that paralleled regular primary schools, and a soft option for some parents to get free education for their children. Another challenge for the program was lack of community ownership, as the program was perceived as foreign and donor-driven. The issue of achieving and maintaining quality when rolling out the program nationwide was also a challenge.

INTERACTIVE RADIO INSTRUCTION PROGRAM IN ZAMBIA

In 2000, the Zambia Ministry of Education initiated a distance-learning innovation: the Interactive Radio Instruction (IRI) program, also called Learning at Taonga Market. It was designed to provide affordable and quality education to vulnerable children who had never been in school, had dropped out of formal education, or were too old for the appropriate grade. Although the program did not specifically target children affected by HIV/AIDS, these children were most likely to fall into the above categories, and therefore they were one of the main beneficiaries of the program.

The IRI program provided a set of radio lessons for primary school children in grades 1 to 7, which was broadcast Monday to Friday from 9 AM to 4 PM, with lessons for different grades being broadcast at different times during the day. One innovation of the IRI program was the incorporation of life skills education, including education on HIV/AIDS prevention. In 2005, the IRI program was delivered to approximately 900 learning centers throughout the country and reached about 60,000 students.[62] The interactive radio instruction was further complemented through face-to-face mentoring with volunteers trained by the program. Local communities, faith-based organizations, and NGOs were mobilized together with the government to support the program. Although the government paid for the costs of the development and broadcasting of the curriculum, communities provided the venues and selected and supported the volunteer mentors.[63] The major challenge of the IRI program was the lack of adequate financial and material support for volunteer mentors in some resource-poor communities, which undermined the sustainability of these IRI centers. Other challenges included the high cost of airtime, technical difficulties such as poor radio reception in some areas, and lack of program supervision and monitoring, especially in hard-to-reach remote areas.[64]

COMMUNITY HARNESSED INITIATIVES FOR CHILDREN'S LEARNING AND DEVELOPMENT PROGRAM IN RWANDA

The Community Harnessed Initiatives for Children's Learning and Development (CHILD) program began in 2003 and was run by CARE International in Rwanda. The CHILD program provided basic education (e.g., lessons on literacy and numeracy) and vocational training (e.g., vocational skills and simple business development skills) in low-cost and informal education centers in the community (e.g., churches, community centers). The program was designed for out-of-school children and young adults 12–25 years of age, with a particular emphasis on children affected by HIV/AIDS. At the time of students' graduation, the program helped students establish income-generating activities by providing them with initial toolkits. It was estimated that the number of graduates from the program was around 2,000 in 2005 and 2,500 in 2006.[65]

Challenges to implementing the program included the high costs of vocational training; the impact of poverty, which prevented children from fully participating in the program (e.g., poor attendance, dropping out of the program); and the lower priority of literacy and numeracy education (e.g., an impossible luxury, a waste of time) for HIV/AIDS-affected children. Lessons learned from the program included the importance of strengthening trainees' entrepreneurial skills and business acumen to meet the demands of the job market, and the importance of involving local governments in the sustainability of the program (e.g., stable funding and other support).

Programs Addressing Educational Needs in a Larger Context of Multiple Threats

As a recurrent theme in the research, multiple aspects of the lives of children have been negatively affected by HIV/AIDS. Consequently, these vulnerable children are facing multiple threats, such as poverty and stigma. Children living in impoverished and/or marginalized households due to HIV-related parental illness and death are much less likely to go to school, as the treatment and care for parental HIV infection increasingly absorb already limited household resources and leave little or no savings for children's educational and other needs.[66] Without addressing other threats, such as psychological disruption, food insecurity, poverty, and social stigmatization, approaches to improving the educational outcomes of children affected by HIV/AIDS may not be effective or sustainable. Some programs encourage children affected by HIV/AIDS to attend and remain in school by providing school meals and food to their families. Others rely heavily on community mobilization to meet the diverse needs of children affected by HIV/AIDS. Intervention strategies in these initiatives include effectively identifying and assisting the most vulnerable children, providing mentors for child-headed households, and providing daily feeding and informal schooling to children affected by HIV/AIDS. The following are some examples of these programs.

BETTER EDUCATION AND LIFE OPPORTUNITIES THROUGH NETWORKING AND ORGANIZATIONAL GROWTH PROGRAM IN ZAMBIA

To lessen the impact of the food and drought crisis that hit Southern Africa in 2002, Project Concern International (PCI), with support from the World Food Program (WFP), the United States Agency for International Development (USAID), and UNICEF, initiated the Better Education and Life Opportunities Through Networking and Organizational Growth (BELONG) program in January 2003. The centerpiece of the BELONG program was the delivery of food commodities to children affected by HIV/AIDS in community schools (an alternative to regular primary schools) and households with children affected by HIV/AIDS. In return, parents and caregivers were encouraged to help children affected by HIV/AIDS attend school and maintain regular attendance. The BELONG program provided school feeding and other services to 70,000 children affected by HIV/AIDS in mostly urban community schools every day. In addition, 7,800 child- and female-headed households received a take-home ration every month.

In addition to food and nutritional support, the BELONG program, in collaboration with Pact Zambia (an international NGO), also implemented the WORTH economic empowerment model (a global women's empowerment program) for female caregivers of children affected by HIV/AIDS. It focused on literacy and small-business training to improve household financial security. Another key feature of the BELONG program is its advocacy—using participating children as role models (e.g., street children who now study at school or have good employment) as a way of advocating the program and reducing stigma and discrimination against children affected by HIV/AIDS. A 2004 evaluation suggested an 18% increase in overall school attendance among the assisted communities from 2003 to 2004.[67] Since 2005, with funding from USAID and the U.S. President's Emergency Plan for AIDS Relief (PEPFAR), the program expanded its services for children affected by HIV/AIDS to include psychosocial support, improvement in water and sanitation, provision of sports equipment, better access to basic health care, assistance with school-based agriculture, and life skills training.[68]

Challenges faced by the BELONG program included logistic problems in delivering food in a timely fashion, abuse of food commodities (e.g., food theft and attempts to sell food to needy children affected by HIV/AIDS or families rather than provide it without charge), and difficulty in maintaining regular monitoring visits, especially in remote areas. There were several lessons learned from the BELONG program. First, it was important to increase the range of services to accommodate the various needs of children affected by HIV/AIDS, including HIV prevention activities, household food security, access to medical services, and legislation that protects the rights of children affected by HIV/AIDS. Second, it was necessary to create effective partnerships among a wide range of stakeholders, including international agencies and programs (e.g., USAID, PEPFAR) and local NGOs and communities. Third, it was feasible to use participating children as role models to address the issues of stigma and discrimination against children affected by HIV/AIDS.[69]

ALL CHILDREN SAFE IN SCHOOL PROGRAM IN SWAZILAND
Between 2003 and 2005, the All Children Safe in School program was developed by UNICEF in partnership with the Ministry of Education in Swaziland, the WFP, the Food and Agriculture Organization, and Save the Children Fund. The program was designed to address the specific needs of children affected by HIV/AIDS, increase their access to quality education, and mitigate the impact of poverty and AIDS on their school attendance by providing grants to schools, meals for all school children, and farming opportunities and improvements in water and sanitation in schools.

By paying school fees for children affected by HIV/AIDS, the program brought 3,000 children back to school in 44 communities, with many in grades 1 and 2, as indicated in a 2004 midterm review.[70] A community Education for All (EFA) grant was also used to recruit additional teachers from local communities to accommodate increased enrollment and to provide basic psychosocial support to children affected by HIV/AIDS. A main meal and a mid-morning snack were offered in 80 schools for 29,245 children in 2003. An additional 95 schools were covered in 2004. The provision of meals greatly reduced hunger-related learning problems such as restlessness and fainting in class, improved children's timely arrival in the morning, and largely eliminated dropouts in the program schools.

Besides paying school fees and providing school meals, the program also supported schools in establishing school farms and gardens to engage students in learning agricultural skills, and to provide training to those residents of drought areas who lacked sufficient expertise. The establishment of school farms served as a base for future expansion of community expertise and ability in food production. In addition, the program improved water and sanitation conditions in 20 schools by building new facilities or renovating existing facilities, which was enthusiastically embraced by the local communities.

The program encountered the challenges of ensuring continued disbursements to guarantee HIV/AIDS-affected children's access to and retention in school, and the potential stigma toward children affected by HIV/AIDS from members of the community whose children did not receive a waiver of school fees. Lessons learned from the program included the importance of meeting the nonmaterial needs of children affected by HIV/AIDS (e.g., psychosocial and emotional), improving financial accountability in the disbursement of school grants to help children affected by HIV/ AIDS, and establishing transparent and efficient systems of monitoring and evaluation to address problems in a timely manner.[71]

Programs Focusing on Community Mobilization and Empowerment

The importance of mobilizing local communities as a cost-effective and sustainable approach to address the educational needs of children affected by HIV/AIDS and other vulnerable children has been increasingly recognized. Several programs focused on building local capacity by mobilizing and empowering various sectors of the local communities including local schools, community centers, churches, and neighborhoods, so that they could effectively collaborate with government and/or international agencies to address the educational and other needs of children affected by HIV/AIDS. The following are some examples of these initiatives.

NEIGHBORHOOD CARE POINTS (NCP) PROGRAM IN SWAZILAND
The Neighborhood Care Points (NCP) program was initiated by the government of Swaziland in 2003 and supported by UNICEF. A key feature of the program was community mobilization. The government and UNICEF mobilized communities to establish care centers, train caregivers, provide education activities to young children, and offer daily hot meals and psychosocial support to children affected by HIV/AIDS. By 2007, 34,000 children were served by 5,000 trained caregivers in 625 neighborhood care points spread throughout the four regions of Swaziland that received material support from UNICEF.[72] The neighborhood care points could be located at any place in the community (e.g., homes, churches, schools, community sheds, or sites under trees) where residents could come together to provide care and support to children from the neighborhood. The targets of the program were preschool-aged children affected by HIV/AIDS and 4- to 12-year-old out-of-school children. A 2006 evaluation of the program found that the most important activity at care points was the provision of food: at least one hot meal each weekday. The evaluation also revealed that the general quality of care provided at some communities was often low.[73] One challenge to the program was the difficulty in implementing the program in a sustainable way because of insufficient community participation and its dependence on outside donors for funding.

MOST VULNERABLE CHILD PROGRAM IN TANZANIA
The Most Vulnerable Child program was also initiated by the government—the Ministry of Health and Social Welfare in Tanzania—in 2000. A key component of the program was the establishment of a local 'most vulnerable child committee' that consisted of local people who understood the community, including members of local governments, communities, and schools, as well as two children identified as being most vulnerable and two caregivers. Besides AIDS orphans and vulnerable children, the program also targeted children made vulnerable by a wide range of causes, including children living with families that had taken in orphans, children with a disability, children engaging in child labor, and children of neglectful or abusive parents.

The committee identified the most vulnerable children in the community using national criteria that were adapted to the local context. The committee developed a plan of action that included raising money or in-kind assistance from members of the local community for the most vulnerable children. Money raised by a community was matched to varying degrees by the district council and UNICEF. The committee addressed issues such as education, hunger, lack of shelter, lack of health service access, and causes of child neglect (e.g., parental alcohol intoxication).[74]

By the end of 2007, more than 390,000 children had been identified as being "most vulnerable," with around 100,000 of them receiving support. Program evaluations in 2004 and 2007 cited education as "one of the major successes" of the program.[75] The program helped children by purchasing uniforms and books, paying fees for secondary school education, and building or renovating classrooms. The committees were also responsible for following up on these children's school enrollment and attendance. Challenges faced by this program included a lack of efficient process monitoring and a lack of sufficient financial support from either the communities or UNICEF. Lessons learned from the program included the importance of expanding the program from the narrow focus on "orphans" to "most vulnerable children," enhancing intersectoral coordination and collaboration at all levels, especially between the local government and the most vulnerable children committee, and accommodating children's multiple needs in the areas of education, health, shelter, and others.

COMMUNITY CHILD MENTORING PROGRAM IN RWANDA

Due to the 1994 genocide and the AIDS epidemic, there were a large number of orphans in Rwanda, and many of them lived in child-headed households. Bamporeze Association, an NGO in Rwanda, launched the Community Child Mentoring program in 2003. The program matched child-headed households with mentors in the community who gave the children advice and support and served as advocates for the children to ensure their access to education, health, shelter, property, etc. By 2007, the program had supported 11,123 children in five districts of Kigali Rural province: Buliza, Bicumbi, Nyamata, Gashora, and Ngenda.

In each district, the program employed a social worker to work with community leaders, teachers, and other members of the community to identify child-headed households. Children living in child-headed households and community members could suggest potential mentors who had a strong interest in child welfare and wished to undertake the role of mentoring these children. Bamporeze staff then interviewed those nominees, introduced potential mentors to children in child-headed households for approval, helped to establish the mentor–household relationship, and provided training for mentors. Mentors were expected to meet with the children once or twice a week, or as often as necessary, and to provide attention, encouragement, and other psychological support, as well as practical advice and assistance to the children.

The mentoring program helped children with their education in a number of ways. Mentors motivated children to grasp educational opportunities and supported their ongoing participation in education. They helped children to navigate administrative systems (e.g., applying for school fee exemptions) and to mediate between school and children if any conflicts arose. Mentors also helped children understand their right to utilize community resources, including education and health care services.

In addition, mentors helped connect children with the community to reduce the stigma and discrimination against them. Whenever necessary, mentors could also request professional help from Bamporeze social workers.

Challenges faced by the program included limited financial resources to pay for the mentors, concerns about the sustainability of the NGO operation, and a lack of process monitoring. Lessons learned from the program included the importance of improving the awareness in the local community of the needs of children living in child-headed households and of designing a holistic approach, including poverty reduction and psychosocial support, for the children in need.

CONCLUSION

Global research indicates that children affected by HIV/AIDS suffer from various educational disadvantages compared to other children in terms of their school enrollment, attendance, behaviors, performance, and completion. Specifically, children affected by HIV/AIDS were found to be less likely to be enrolled in school, to be older in age for their appropriate grade, to show poorer school performance and more behavioral problems at school (e.g., learning difficulties, aggressive, impulsive, and anxious behaviors, less confidence interacting with peers), to be more likely to drop out of school, and to have a lower level of educational attainment.

Recognizing the importance of education for HIV/AIDS-affected children's current and future well-being and for the future of their communities and nations, stakeholders at all levels, including governments, international agencies, local communities, and NGOs, have started taking action to address the educational needs of children affected by HIV/AIDS. The existing interventional practices take a variety of approaches, including direct assistance (e.g., paying school tuitions), provision of complementary education (e.g., vocational skills training), provision of foods and other services to children affected by HIV/AIDS or their households, and mobilization and empowerment of local communities. However, the number and scope of the existing interventional practices are limited and far from meeting the educational and other needs of children affected by HIV/AIDS. We would like to point out again that the intervention initiatives reviewed in this chapter were selected mainly based on the limited data and information available in existing global research. They are not necessarily reflective of the current state-of-the art or best practices in the field. The lack of rigorous program evaluation and appropriate outcome data in most of these programs further limited our ability to critically evaluate current practices. Nevertheless, based on the limited empirical evidence, we would like to make the following recommendations for future interventional practices to address the educational needs of children affected by HIV/AIDS.

Address the Educational Needs Within the Larger Context of Poverty Eradication

To make the best use of the limited resources that are committed to children's education, especially in developing countries, it is important to identify the focus of assistance appropriately. The experience of a number of existing practices suggests that it is more appropriate to place the educational needs of children affected by HIV/AIDS within the larger context of poverty eradication and economic and organizational capacity-building in the local community. Poverty, although measured differently in various studies, was believed to be a major constraint on children's schooling.[76]

Since poverty is usually a primary threat for communities with a large number of children affected by HIV/AIDS, it prevents children from receiving education and preparing for their future. As the World Bank argues, for most economic assistance programs, poverty is a better target than orphanhood.[77] On the one hand, assistance is urgently needed to meet the basic needs of children affected by HIV/AIDS, such as food, shelter, clothing, medical care, and schooling. On the other hand, the focus of the assistance should be on building the capacity and infrastructure of local communities to cope with the negative effects of HIV/AIDS and overall poverty, instead of only short-term resource-intensive assistance to children affected by HIV/AIDS.[78] In addition, targeting overall poverty and assisting children impoverished from diverse causes reduces the possibility of unintended stigma and resentment from members of the community toward those who have received varied assistance (e.g., school fees exemption and food commodities) from the intervention initiatives.

Take a Holistic Approach

In response to the multiple threats to the educational attainment of children affected by HIV/AIDS, a holistic, dynamic, and contextualized strategy is needed. In addition to direct assistance for these children's formal education (e.g. school fees exemption), various types of supports that meet the diverse needs of children affected by HIV/AIDS are also required. Existing interventional practices provide valuable experiences in addressing these children's educational needs in conjunction with other needs.

Because of the intensity and scope of the HIV/AIDS pandemic and the resulting consequence of large numbers of children affected by HIV/AIDS, treating the situation as only an emergency that demands rapid and short-term actions to mitigate its immediate consequences is short-sighted; addressing the multiple needs of children affected by HIV/AIDS, particularly their educational advancement, has been increasingly recognized as a long-term effort that requires holistic and strategic efforts from multiple sectors and organizations. Since the improvement of these children's educational outcomes (e.g., enrollment, retention, performance, and completion) hinges on the satisfaction of other needs, such as food security and nutrition, poverty reduction, and psychological health, different sectors, agencies, and practitioners can all play a unique role in improving the well-being of children affected by HIV/AIDS and collectively work toward achieving the UN's Millennium Development Goals (MDGs) of improved children's health and education. As an essential condition to provide a systematic, integrated, and holistic solution for these children's educational needs, our conceptual framework calls for intersectoral coordination and partnership.

Engage Multiple Shareholders

The importance of a sector-wide approach has been increasingly recognized in many existing intervention initiatives. An intersectoral approach is the development of cooperation among all related sectors to support a single-sector policy under government leadership.[79] Likewise, effective intervention also requires coordination among governments, local communities, and international agencies in dealing with policies, actions, and resources. By drawing on the comparative advantages of different stakeholders, the overall capacity to achieve the MDG of improved children's health and education can be strengthened. For example, governments' collaboration with the WFP and/or the Food and Agriculture Organization may likely strengthen school feeding programs and school-based agriculture programs. In collaboration with international or local NGOs with specialized ability and expertise (e.g., food assistance and distribution, agriculture knowledge, distance education, poverty reduction), the intervention programs' capabilities to implement corresponding interventional practices are likely to be strengthened. Previous experience indicates the importance of effective and efficient communication and coordination among a wide range of stakeholders throughout the process to avoid potential conflicts and strengthen the united action.[80]

Involve and Empower Communities and Families

Existing research and interventional practices have repeatedly underscored the role of family and community in caring for and providing support to children affected by HIV/AIDS. Families (including extended families or foster families) provide direct protection and support to children affected by HIV/AIDS before and after parental illness and death. Strengthening families' ability to provide adequate care for children affected by HIV/AIDS and increasing the quality of family-based care are crucial for the well-being of these children. Intervention programs with strong community involvement and commitment are more likely to succeed in meeting these children's educational needs in a cost-effective and sustainable way. Therefore, the importance of improving communities' awareness of the needs of children affected by HIV/AIDS and commitment to taking care of them cannot be overstated for the long-term sustainability of any successful intervention program. Local community-based organizations may also play an important role in helping these children's education. They may have a better understanding of the problems and potential solutions in the cultural setting and are strongly motivated to provide much needed help for children affected by HIV/AIDS and their families within the communities.

Ensure Long-term Sustainability

The long-term sustainability of an effective program relies on the availability of at least two types of resources: financial and human capital resources. In addition to continuous external financial and expertise support, a critical element for the sustainability of any successful program is local capacity building. Broad-based community mobilization and empowerment that give communities a strong sense of program ownership often prove to be a key to a program's success and long-term sustainability. Only when the local communities are willing and able to consider the educational needs of children affected by HIV/AIDS as their own responsibility can the situation of these children be expected to improve and advance over the long term.

Effective and Rigorous Program and Outcome Evaluation

One of the limitations identified among almost all of the existing intervention programs is the lack of rigorous evaluation efforts. King and colleagues have recently conducted a Cochrane Review of the global literature to assess the effectiveness of interventions that aim to improve the psychosocial well-being of children affected by HIV. They employed broad inclusion criteria to include all possible study designs (e.g., randomized controlled trial, crossover trials, cluster-randomized trials, factorial trials, nonrandomized trials, pre–post design, cohort design, case–control studies), a range of outcome measures (psychological measures including mental health status, suicide, mental illness, and criminal behaviors, and social measures including schooling, quality of life, and socioeconomic status), and different intervention strategies (psychological therapy, psychosocial support and/or care, medical intervention, and social intervention). They searched electronic databases, internet/websites of relevant organizations involved in HIV/AIDS work, and contacted the experts in the field; they started with a total of 1,038 non-duplicated citations. They found that although many programs tried to improve the psychosocial well-being of these children, no studies rigorously assessed the effectiveness of such programs. The authors concluded that most of the existing practices were based on anecdotal knowledge, descriptive studies, and situational analyses without providing strong empirical evidence for the effectiveness of the interventions.[81]

Likewise, regular and effective process monitoring for quality assurance of program implementation is lacking in many programs, especially those dealing with food and grant distribution.[82] Factors that impede the process monitoring of many programs include difficulty in reaching geographically remote areas and a lack of baseline data for evaluation. Without rigorous monitoring and evaluation of the feasibility, fidelity, and effectiveness of existing programs, evidence-based practices and policies are seriously weakened and limited, which may hamper future efforts to scale up the programs. In the future, the effective monitoring of intervention processes and the rigorous evaluation of intervention outcomes are urgently needed; this requires increased partnerships between program implementers and researchers. Only by doing so may we implement evidence-based interventional practices and policies that can meet the educational and other needs of children affected by HIV/AIDS while preventing unintended harm to these children and the unintentional waste of our limited and valuable financial and human resources.

We would like to complete this chapter by pointing out one simple argument, defended by economics Nobel Laureate and Columbia University professor Joseph Stiglitz: A willing world can afford universal education for all children.[83] Stiglitz estimated that the average annual cost of education for developing countries was about US$40 per student.[84] To achieve the second MDG of universal primary education by 2015, the additional cost was estimated to be US$9.1 billion annually. To put this number in perspective, he pointed out that it only amounted to 1% of global military spending (US$956 billion) in 2003. Therefore, one thing is made clear: The educational rights of all children, including children affected by HIV/AIDS, are not a matter of affordability, but a matter of willingness and commitment.

NOTES

1. Salaam, T. (2005). *AIDS orphans and vulnerable children (OVC): Problems, responses, and issues for Congress* (CRS report for Congress no. RL32252). Washington DC: The Library of Congress.

2. UNICEF. (2009). *Promoting quality education for orphans and vulnerable children: A sourcebook of programme experiences in eastern and southern Africa.,* New York: UNICEF.

3. UNICEF. (2004). *Children on the brink 2004: A joint report of new orphan estimates and a framework for action.* New York: UNICEF.

4. Monasch, R., & Boerma, J. T. (2004). Orphanhood and childcare patterns in sub-Saharan Africa: An analysis of national surveys from 40 countries. *AIDS, 18*(Suppl. 2), S55–65.

5. UNICEF. (2004). *Children on the brink 2004.*

6. UNICEF. (2009). *Promoting quality education for orphans and vulnerable children.*

7. Stiglitz, J. E. (2005). A willing world can end child poverty. In C. Bellamy (Ed.), *The state of the world's children: Childhood under threat.* New York: UNICEF.

8. Bredie, J. W. B., & Beeharry, G. K. (1998). *School enrollment decline in sub-Saharan Africa: Beyond the supply constraint* (Discussion paper no. 395). Washington DC: World Bank.

9. Stiglitz J. E. (2005). A willing world can end child poverty.

10. UNICEF. (2009). *Promoting quality education for orphans and vulnerable children.*

11. Bell, D., & Murenha, A. (2009.) *Re-thinking schooling in Africa: Education in an era of HIV and AIDS* (AIDS2031 working paper No. 23). New York: AIDS2031 Social Drivers Working Group.

12. UNICEF. (2004). *Children on the brink 2004.*

13. Ibid.

14. Bell & Murenha. (2009). *Re-thinking schooling in Africa.*

15. Tamukong, J. (2004). *The impact of HIV/AIDS on teachers and other education personnel in West and Central Africa: A Synthesis of the Literature from 2000 to 2004.* Yaoundé, Cameroon: ERNWACA.

16. Badcock-Walters, P., et al. (2003). *Educator mortality in-service in Kwazulu Natal: A consolidated study of HIV/AIDS impact and trends.* Paper presented at Demographic and Socio-Economic Conference, Durban, South Africa, 28 March.

17. Amenyah, A. M. (2005). *The importance of learning for changing sexual practices in response to HIV/AIDS crisis in Ghana.* PhD dissertation, University of Georgia; Kelly, M. (2000). *The impact of HIV/AIDS on the education sector in Africa sub-regional outlook and best practices.* Synthesis paper for African Development Forum, Addis Ababa, Ethiopia.

18. Badcock-Walters et al. (2003). *Educator mortality in-service in Kwazulu Natal.*

19. World Bank. (2000). *Exploring the implications of the HIV/AIDS epidemic for educational planning in selected African countries: The demographic question.* Washington DC: World Bank.

20. Gachuhi, D. (1999). *The impact of HIV/AIDS on education systems in the Eastern and Southern Africa region and the response of education systems to HIV/AIDS: Life skills programmes.* New York: UNICEF.

21. Ibid.
22. Ibid.
23. Ibid.; Carr-Hill, R., et al. (2002.) *The impact of HIV/AIDS on education and institutionalizing prevention education.* Paris, France: International Institute for Educational Planning/UNESCO.
24. Andrews, G., Skinner, D., & Zuma, K. (2006). Epidemiology of health and vulnerability among children orphaned and made vulnerable by HIV/AIDS in sub-Saharan Africa. *AIDS Care, 18,* 269–276; Nyambedha, E. O., Wandibba, S., & Aagaard-Hansen, J. (2001). Policy implications of the inadequate support systems for orphans in Western Kenya. *Health Policy, 58,* 83–96.
25. Heymann, J., et al. (2007). Extended family caring for children orphaned by AIDS: Balancing essential work and caregiving in a high HIV prevalence nations. *AIDS Care, 19,* 337–345.
26. Tu, X., et al. (2009). School performance and school behavior of children affected by acquired immune deficiency syndrome (AIDS) in China. *Vulnerable Children and Youth Studies, 4,* 199–209; Zhao, G., et al. (2009). Psychosocial consequences for children experiencing parental loss due to HIV/AIDS in Central China. *AIDS Care, 21,* 769–774.
27. Salaam. (2005). *AIDS orphans and vulnerable children (OVC).*
28. Ibid.
29. Case, A., Paxson, C., & Ableidinger, J. (2004). Orphans in Africa: Parental death, poverty, and school enrollment. *Demography, 41,* 483-508; Yamano, T., & Jayne, T. S. (2004). Measuring the impact of working-age adult mortality on small-scale farm households in Kenya. *World Development, 32,* 91–119.
30. Case, A. & Ardington, C. (2006). The impact of paternal death on school outcomes: Longitudinal evidence from South Africa. *Demography, 43,* 401–420.
31. Nyamukapa C., & Gregson, S. (2005). Extended family's and women's roles in safeguarding orphans' education in AIDS-afflicted rural Zimbabwe. *Social Science and Medicine, 60,* 2155–2167.
32. Ibid.
33. Birdthistle, I., et al. (2009). Is education the link between orphanhood and HIV/HSV-2 risk among female adolescents in urban Zimbabwe? *Social Science and Medicine, 68,* 1810–1818.
34. Mishra, V., et al. (2005). *Education and nutritional status of orphans and children of HIV-infected parents in Kenya* (DHS working paper no. 24). Calverton, MD: USAID.
35. Case & Ardington. (2006). The impact of paternal death on school outcomes; Case, Paxson, & Ableidinger. (2004). Orphans in Africa; UNICEF. (2009). *Promoting quality education for orphans and vulnerable children;* Yang, H., et al. (2006). Living environment and schooling of children with HIV-infected parents in Southwest China. *AIDS Care, 18,* 647–655.
36. UNICEF. (2009). *Promoting quality education for orphans and vulnerable children.*
37. Case, Paxson, & Ableidinger. (2004). Orphans in Africa.
38. Ibid.; Monasch & Boerma. (2004). Orphanhood and childcare patterns in sub-Saharan Africa; UNICEF. (2004). *Children on the brink 2004.*
39. UNICEF. (2004). *Children on the brink 2004.*
40. Sengendo, J., & Nambi, J. (1997). The psychological effect of orphanhood: A study of orphans in Rakai District. *Health Transition Review, 7*(Suppl.), S105–124.

41. Bicego, G., Rutstein, S., & Johnson, K. (2003). Dimensions of emerging orphans crisis in sub-Saharan Africa. *Social Science and Medicine, 56*, 1235–1247.

42. Ainsworth, M., Beegle, K., & Koda, G. (2005). The impact of adult mortality and parental deaths on primary schooling in North-Western Tanzania. *Journal of Development Studies, 41*, 412–439; Bicego, Rutstein, & Johnson. (2003). Dimensions of emerging orphans crisis in sub-Saharan Africa.

43. Tu, X., et al. (2009). School performance and school behavior.

44. Ibid.

45. Ainsworth, Beegle, & Koda. (2005). The impact of adult mortality and parental deaths; Case & Ardington. (2006). The impact of paternal death on school outcomes.

46. Monasch & Boerma. (2004). Orphanhood and childcare patterns in sub-Saharan Africa.

47. Nyamukapa & Gregson. (2005). Extended family's and women's roles in safeguarding orphans' education.

48. Evans, D. K., & Miguel, E. (2007). Orphans and schooling in Africa: A longitudinal analysis. *Demography, 44*, 35–57.

49. Sengendo & Nambi. (1997). The psychological effect of orphanhood.

50. UNICEF. (2009). *Promoting quality education for orphans and vulnerable children*; Evans & Miguel. (2007). Orphans and schooling in Africa; Tu et al. (2009). School performance and school behavior of children.

51. UNICEF. (2009). *Promoting quality education for orphans and vulnerable children*.

52. Bell & Murenha. (2009). *Re-thinking schooling in Africa*.

53. UNICEF. (2009). *Promoting quality education for orphans and vulnerable children*.

54. China Ministry of Health, UNAIDS, & WHO. (2005). *2005 Update on the HIV/AIDS Epidemic and Response in China*. Beijing: China Ministry of Health.

55. Ibid.

56. China Daily. (2006, December 13). Fees waived for 150 million rural kids. Retrieved March 23, 2010, http://www.jongo.com/articles/06/1213/525/NTI1fe9c03m5.html

57. Ibid.

58. Ministry of Foreign Affairs, Government of Thailand. (2010). Father of the Land – Education. Retrieved March 30, 2010, http://www.mfa.go.th/royalweb/5-e.html

59. UNICEF. (2009). *Promoting quality education for orphans and vulnerable children*.

60. Ibid.

61. Ibid.

62. Ibid.

63. Ibid.

64. Ibid.

65. Ibid.

66. Salaam. (2005). *AIDS orphans and vulnerable children (OVC)*.

67. UNICEF. (2009). *Promoting quality education for orphans and vulnerable children*.

68. Ibid.

69. Ibid.

70. Ibid.

71. Ibid.

72. Ibid.

73. Ibid.

74. Ibid.

75. Ibid.

76. Oleke, C., et al. (2007). Constraints to educational opportunities of orphans: A community-based study from Northern Uganda. *AIDS Care, 19,* 361–368.

77. Ainsworth, M., & Filmer, D. (2002). *Poverty, AIDS and children schooling: A targeting dilemma.* Policy research working paper 2885. Washington, DC: World Bank.

78. Schenk, K. (2009). Community interventions providing care and support to orphans and vulnerable children: A review of evaluation evidence. *AIDS Care, 21,* 918–942.

79. UNICEF. (2009). *Promoting quality education for orphans and vulnerable children.*

80. Ibid.

81. King, E., et al. (2009). Interventions for improving psychosocial well-being of children affected by HIV and AIDS. *Cochrane Database of Systematic Reviews* (2) CD006733. DOI: 10.1002/14651858.CD006733.pub2.

82. UNICEF. (2009). *Promoting quality education for orphans and vulnerable children.*

83. Stiglitz, J. E. (2005). A willing world can end child poverty.

84. Ibid.

6

Healthy Minds

Psychosocial Interventions for School-aged Children Affected by HIV/AIDS

LUCIE D. CLUVER, MALEGA C. KGANAKGA,
MARK E. BOYES, AND MIHYUNG PARK ■

For any child, the school years are essential in the transition into young adulthood. During these years, children establish friendships, form relationships, and build resilience to cope with life's challenges. For young children, the family and primary caregiver are often the strongest influences; however, during the school years, this situation rapidly and irreversibly expands to include the influence of teachers, peers, and the wider community. Importantly, for children in families affected by HIV/ AIDS these formative years often take place alongside familial experiences of severe illness and death. The psychosocial difficulties associated with growing up in an AIDS-affected family are only just beginning to be understood and are the focus of this chapter. Specifically, the chapter has three major aims: first, the psychosocial needs of children affected by AIDS will be discussed; second, potential mechanisms through which familial HIV/AIDS may influence children's psychosocial development will be described; and third, the evidence base for psychosocial interventions targeting AIDS-affected children will be reviewed. Throughout the chapter, we will discuss real-world examples, with a particular focus on sub-Saharan Africa, as well as identify gaps in the research literature.

We use the ecological model of Bronfenbrenner[1] as a broad conceptual framework. This model was specifically developed to further the understanding of risk and protective factors associated with children's psychosocial health. Recently, Richter, Foster, and Sherr[2] have adapted this model for use with AIDS-affected children. The model sees children at the center of multiple, interacting layers of influence. Most proximal to the child are relationships with caregivers and their everyday caregiving environment. More distal to the child are school and community influences, followed by the wider political, policy, and cultural factors that contribute to the contexts in which children live. The model suggests that the impact of severe adversity (such as belonging to an AIDS-affected family) in a particular "sphere" of a child's life can be mitigated by positive factors in another "sphere." This theory has been supported by research examining children's resilience, or their capacity to maintain psychosocial well-being despite the major life events to which they are exposed.[3] The chapter will specifically focus on children who have lost a parent or caregiver to

AIDS, children who are caring for an AIDS-sick caregiver ("young caregivers"), children who are HIV positive themselves, and children who live on the streets due to bereavement or HIV/AIDS-related family problems. It is important to note that many children may fall into two or more categories, or may move between categories over time.

PSYCHOSOCIAL NEEDS OF SCHOOL-AGED CHILDREN AFFECTED BY AIDS

Until the early 2000s, there was almost no research into the psychosocial needs of AIDS-affected children, and the literature on child mental health in the context of parental illness or death did not yet address AIDS-affected families. As the number of AIDS-affected children has risen into the millions,[4] a new body of research has developed. The majority of this research is clustered in sub-Saharan Africa and the United States, although new research in China and India is currently under way.[5] Almost all of this research is still focused on understanding the problems experienced by children affected by AIDS, an area in which our knowledge is far from complete.

Children Orphaned by AIDS

Remarkably consistent evidence comes from both America and sub-Saharan Africa that losing a parent to AIDS is negatively associated with children's psychological and social well-being. Emerging evidence from China suggests a similar pattern. Although there were early fears that orphans might be "potential rebels" or a "delinquent generation,"[6] recent findings suggest that children orphaned by AIDS are much more likely to suffer symptoms of depression or anxiety than to have behavior problems. In sub-Saharan Africa, multiple studies have reported that being orphaned by AIDS is associated with high levels of emotional distress, particularly symptoms of depression, anxiety, and post-traumatic stress. Children orphaned by AIDS also report difficulties in socializing with their peers.[7] Similar findings have been obtained in the United States, although children there are more likely to also report behavior problems, such as aggression.[8] Recently, a controlled study in China also reported heightened psychological distress in children orphaned by AIDS.[9] However, few of the studies cited are able to compare the impact of being orphaned by AIDS with the impact of being orphaned by other causes. A recent South African study compared children orphaned by AIDS, children orphaned by other causes, and nonorphans on mental health outcomes. Results revealed that being orphaned by AIDS was consistently associated with more depression, posttraumatic stress disorder (PTSD), and peer problems (see Figure 6.1) than parental death by other causes.[10]

New evidence also suggests that orphaned children may be at greater risk of becoming infected with HIV in later life. A recent review[11] found four studies worldwide reporting higher levels of HIV infection among adolescent orphaned children in Zimbabwe,[12] South Africa,[13] and Russia.[14] Three more studies reported higher levels of risky sexual behavior in orphaned children.[15] Although we do not yet know the mechanisms through which orphanhood may be influencing sexual behavior

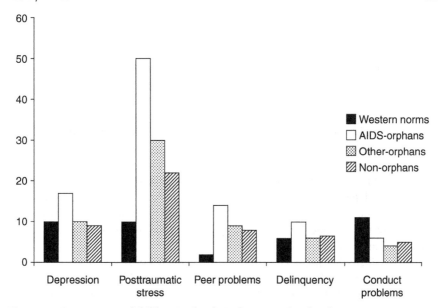

Figure 6.1 Proportions of children in the clinical range in South Africa.

and HIV infection, one study does suggest that psychological distress may be contributing to risky sexual behavior among orphaned children.[16]

Children Living with HIV-positive or AIDS-sick Adults

Orphanhood by HIV/AIDS is not a single acute event; rather, it is a process preceded by a parent's chronic and debilitating illness.[17] In sub-Saharan Africa, health systems are often overburdened by HIV-related illnesses. This has resulted in most terminal AIDS patients remaining in the home. Therefore, children in AIDS-affected families are likely to witness a caregiver's debilitating illnesses and death.

It has been established that HIV is often a "family secret" and that this can reduce a child's opportunities to seek support from school or peers.[18] Research also shows that HIV-positive mothers find disclosure of their status to their children stressful and worrying. A particular worry is whether or not school-aged children will be able to keep their parents' status confidential, and this prevents many mothers from disclosing.[19] The evidence on the effects of disclosure to children is mixed, and most of it comes from the United States, which may limit its generalization to the developing world. The few studies conducted in sub-Saharan Africa have focused on parents' views of the effects of disclosure, and there is a clear need for research exploring children's perspectives.[20] The little research that has been conducted suggests that disclosure to children is often left toward the terminal stage of the disease, as parents are often not ready to disclose in the initial stages of the illness. In most cases, non-disclosure is linked to avoidance of stigma and protection of the children.[21] We do know that children who are not told of their parent's status often suspect that something is wrong and may become confused and anxious.[22] Similarly, some studies report more behavior problems and depression in children after mothers disclose HIV-positive status.[23] On the other hand, disclosure to children may be helpful and essential for long-term family coping. When disclosure does happen, some parents report that it increases family closeness.[24] It is imperative that we better understand how to make parental disclosure as positive as possible for children and parents.

We know very little about the psychosocial needs of children living with HIV-positive or AIDS-sick caregivers in the developing world. In the United States, studies have found both emotional and behavioral difficulties for children whose parents are HIV positive.[25] In China, children with AIDS-affected parents showed higher distress than children in healthy families.[26] In the developing world, qualitative evidence certainly suggests that these children suffer from distress, and this is supported by some initial quantitative studies.[27] In South Africa, the extent of caregiver sickness was found to be a mediator of children's mental health problems,[28] and a small study found more psychological distress among children whose parents had full-blown AIDS than among children whose parents did not.[29]

It is also likely that many children who live with AIDS-sick adults are acting as "young caregivers;" taking on medical care (including tasks such as washing and bathing the sick adult), household tasks, and care of younger siblings.[30] Evidence from the West suggests that young caregivers of parents with other illnesses and disability are at risk of psychosocial problems.[31] However, almost no research to date examines psychological outcomes for young caregivers in the contexts of AIDS or in the developing world. Bauman and colleagues[32] compared 50 young caregivers of AIDS-sick parents in Zimbabwe to 50 young caregivers in the United States. Results showed high levels of depression in both groups. In qualitative studies, children report both emotional distress and positive experiences and competencies associated with responsibility and contribution to the household.[33] Understanding the

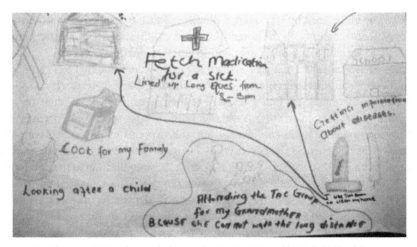

Figure 6.2 Things which I do: cook for my family, looking after a child, fetching medication for a sick person—lined up in long queues from 8 AM to 3 PM, getting information about diseases, attending the HIV support group for my grandmother because she cannot walk the long distance.[34]

extent to which the psychosocial problems experienced by children orphaned by AIDS are established during the period of parental sickness is of the utmost importance for future research.

HIV-positive Children

For school-aged children, being HIV positive brings specific psychosocial needs and risks; however, again, these are not yet well understood. This section will only focus on children who have been infected perinatally (i.e., by an HIV-positive parent at birth) as psychosocial outcomes may be different for children who are infected via abuse, injection drug use, infected blood, and consensual or forced sexual contact. This is a newly recognized group of children. Before the introduction of pediatric antiretroviral treatment (ART), few perinatally infected children survived infancy.[35] Recent estimates for Africa suggest that mortality among HIV-positive perinatally infected children is 36% by age 1, 62% by age 5, and 83% by age 15.[36] A 2010 review finds that this low rate of survival is due to variable access to pediatric ART, delayed diagnosis, and poorly resourced health systems.[37] However, as more children are surviving beyond early childhood, it is important to consider their specific psychosocial needs during the school-aged years.

The very limited evidence suggests that being infected by HIV may cause developmental, motor, and emotional delays for children.[38] However, a recent review found almost no studies that looked at HIV-positive children over the age of 2, or at the psychosocial effects of children's HIV infection.[39] Studies of young children found that HIV-positive children scored lower on the personality-social domain of the Denver scale[40] and had less secure attachment to their mothers.[41] A recent qualitative study in South Africa of HIV-positive children found psychosocial challenges, including dealing with the loss of biological parents, coming to terms with their HIV status, external stigma and discrimination, and disclosure difficulties.[42] For all studies of HIV-positive children, it is difficult to distinguish effects of HIV infection from the social, economic, and family impacts of the illness.

In the United States, pediatric ART provision since the mid-1990s has resulted in a cohort of HIV-positive children who are now progressing through adolescence.[43] Research with this group suggests that they experience emotional challenges in adjusting to a chronic, highly stigmatized, and parentally acquired disease.[44] These children are also at greater risk of psychiatric hospital admissions for depression and behavior problems (with an incidence rate of 6.17 cases per 1,000 person-years, as opposed to 1.70 cases per 1,000 person-years in the general population).[45] In particular, disclosure to children of their HIV status remains a major issue. Most children who have been infected at birth are not told of their own status until they are thought to be old enough to understand (and often to keep the family secret). Disclosure to the child also often means disclosure of the parent's HIV status, and the causes of infection. Studies in the United States suggest that this can be a stage of great disruption for families, although children feel strongly that disclosure is important, and many have already guessed by the time they are told.[46] The school-aged years are also those in which adolescents develop relationships and often have their first sexual experiences. HIV-positive children report concerns about relationships and safe sex,[47] and fear that disclosure to sexual partners could lead to social stigmatization or rejection.[48] Research also suggests that this can be a time of rejection or inconsistent use of ART medication, due to unpleasant side effects (such as development of embarrassing fat deposits), and adolescent "acting out."[49] Lack of medication adherence can have severe individual and public health outcomes in regards to opportunistic infections and viral resistance.

Rollout of ART to children in the developing world has been far slower than in developed countries. But the next 5 years will see increasing numbers of perinatally infected children on long-term ART surviving through adolescence. The experiences of these children will certainly be in a different context to that of the United States, but it is essential that the developing world (particularly sub-Saharan Africa) does not ignore the possibility of similar challenges in the future.

Children Living on the Streets

The stress of familial HIV/AIDS can contribute to children living or working on the streets. The word "street-child" is often used for two groups of children: those who live with their families, but spend time on the street (often to earn money), and those who sleep on the streets (but may have occasional or regular contact with families). Although evidence is scattered and on a small scale, research does suggest that a disproportionate number of children orphaned by AIDS are living as street-children.[50] There is very little empirical research on the effects of living on the streets in the developing world, but qualitative work and a small number of quantitative studies suggest major daily risks of violence, drugs, transactional sex, and abuse.[51]

POTENTIAL MECHANISMS THROUGH WHICH FAMILIAL HIV/AIDS MAY INFLUENCE PSYCHOSOCIAL DEVELOPMENT

What is it about living in an AIDS-affected family that makes the lives of these children even more difficult than those of other orphans? Research is beginning to elucidate potential mechanisms through which familial HIV/AIDS may influence psychosocial outcomes. These are briefly summarized below. Understanding the mechanisms through which familial HIV/AIDS impacts child well-being will have important implications for the development of effective interventions.

- *Caregiver sickness.* HIV diagnosis and illness in parents are often associated with depression and reduced social support.[52] Although we could find no studies exploring the direct effects of HIV on parenting, there is strong evidence from other groups that children are negatively affected by parental depression and reduced social support.[53] In one South African study, the extent of caregiver illness positively predicted the level of psychological problems for children,[54] and in Uganda, having a chronically ill adult in the household was strongly associated with child psychosocial distress.[55]
- *Extreme poverty.* Many studies in the developing world have shown that suffering from AIDS has major financial impacts on households. These include

loss of income from the sick person and the caregiver, medical costs, and funeral expenses.[56] In South Africa and Ethiopia, mental health problems for children orphaned by AIDS were shown to be mediated by poor nutrition, school exclusion for financial reasons, and lack of access to social grants,[57] although in Uganda hunger was not found to be a key mechanism.[58] We know less about the effects of poverty on children whose parents are alive but unwell, or the effects of poverty on HIV-positive children. Some qualitative evidence suggests that extreme poverty may result in children engaging in transactional sex to support their families or pay school fees.[59]

- *AIDS-related stigma.* Stigma is one of the strongest mechanisms accounting for mental health problems such as depression and post-traumatic stress in children orphaned by AIDS.[60] Qualitative evidence suggests that AIDS-related stigma is also a cause of great distress for children whose parents are visibly sick with AIDS, with people gossiping about them or labeling their parents as promiscuous or prostitutes.[61] Families of HIV-positive people may also be stigmatized due to inaccurate fears of infection through touching or sharing food with a person from an AIDS-affected household.[62] Bullying is also an important mechanism accounting for psychological distress, and seems to be directed both at children with parents sick with AIDS, and children orphaned by AIDS.[63]

- *Social support and family support.* Research suggests that social support from family, friends, and school staff can mitigate the effects of trauma among children orphaned by AIDS.[64] Attitudes of fostering families toward orphaned children and ill-treatment in their homes were also predictive of child psychosocial adjustment.[65] Importantly, a recent review and study of caregivers of children orphaned by AIDS (mostly grandmothers) found high levels of mental and physical health problems, suggesting that foster families may need increased support themselves.[66]

- *Cumulative factors.* The Bronfenbrenner model and other theories of child well-being, use a cumulative risk approach.[67] This means that a child may be able to cope with one stressor, but multiple stressors can interact to increase risk of psychosocial problems. This is supported by evidence from a large ($n = 1,025$) South African study, in which poverty and AIDS-related stigma interacted to increase the likelihood of child psychological disorder (defined as scoring above Western clinical cutoffs on widely used measures of depression, anxiety, or PTSD) from 19% to 83%, and bullying increased the likelihood of disorder for children orphaned by AIDS more than for others.[68]

INTERVENTION FOR AIDS-AFFECTED CHILDREN

Over the past 20 years, there has been a particular focus on developing and funding intervention programs for AIDS-affected children. Many of these programs focus on children's psychosocial well-being; however, there is an almost total lack of rigorous evaluation of these intervention programs. A 2009 Cochrane systematic review of interventions for improving the psychosocial well-being of children affected by HIV and AIDS found no studies for inclusion. The authors concluded that current practice is based on anecdotal knowledge, descriptive studies, and situational analyses, and that such studies do not provide a strong evidence base for the effectiveness of these interventions.[69] Additionally, there is a lack of longitudinal data that would allow stronger inferences regarding *causal* relationships between potential risk and protective factors and child outcomes. Understanding the mechanisms through which familial HIV/AIDS impacts upon children's well-being is vital for both intervention programs and social policy design.

Debates in Intervention Design

An important and hotly debated issue regarding interventions for AIDS-affected children is that of "targeting." Many nongovernmental organizations (NGOs) and government-led programs are targeted specifically at orphaned children (or children orphaned by AIDS). With regard to psychosocial health, this presents two important questions. First, is there sufficient evidence to show that AIDS-affected children have psychosocial needs that differ from those of other children living in poverty? The evidence presented earlier in this chapter suggests that children orphaned by AIDS and HIV-positive children are suffering from greater psychosocial problems than other children. We do not yet have enough research to know whether this is also true for children with parents sick with AIDS, but qualitative studies suggest that this may be the case. Second, are targeted interventions feasible in the context of stigma? There have been strong objections to this approach. These objections have highlighted the differing definitions of "orphan" in different communities[70] and children's reports of stigma associated with receiving HIV-targeted or orphan-targeted relief.[71] This has led to a drive for programs that instead focus on improving outcomes for all "vulnerable" children. With very limited resources in the developing world, it is difficult to know how we can reconcile the need to help this specific group of children with the need to avoid the stigma that may come with targeted interventions.

Another important debate in programming for AIDS-affected children is whether or not psychosocial problems in the developing world should be addressed using traditional models of psychosocial interventions. The Western therapeutic model of approaching child mental health is resource intensive and often requires skilled professionals to conduct intervention programs. Policy-makers, and increasingly the research community, are accepting that interventions are not sustainable in developing countries unless they are scaleable and feasible in resource-poor communities, are able to be based within existing structures (such as NGOs), and make use of existing capacity.[72] There are no simple answers to these issues, and they are currently being debated by researchers and policy-makers. The following section discusses some widely used interventions in terms of their evidence-base and feasibility in resource-poor communities.

Interventions Where Evidence Suggests Effectiveness

- *School-based peer group support.* King and colleagues' review[73] found no studies that tested the effectiveness of interventions for children orphaned by

AIDS or AIDS-affected children under the age of 18. Since this was published, our literature searches have identified one published study; a cluster randomized controlled trial (n = 326) of a school-based peer group support program in Uganda.[74] This program was for children orphaned by AIDS, and it included 16 group sessions of psychosocial exercises, as well as monthly physical health assessments and treatment (e.g., antimicrobial medication) or referral to a pediatrician. The group sessions were facilitated by trained teachers who were supervised by a psychologist and the researcher. At 10-week follow-up, children involved in the program showed reduced levels of depression, anger, and anxiety. This program certainly shows promise, although its scaleability may be limited by the human resources required (i.e., an experienced counselor as supervisor) and the cost of medical care and treatment.

• *Mentoring.* Another potentially valuable new study involved a mentoring program for heads of youth-headed households in Rwanda.[75] The quasi-experimental study included 593 heads of households, of which 441 received regular visits from trained mentors. After 18 months of mentoring, youth reported greater perception of adult support and less feeling of marginalization. Although feelings of grief in the comparison group rose, grief in the mentored group stayed stable. There was also a slight decrease in depressive symptoms in the mentored group. Although most of the youth in this study were over school-age, these generally positive findings suggest that this intervention could also be helpful for younger groups.[76]

• *Solution-focused stories.* Many interventions focus on therapeutic storytelling. Importantly, storytelling has a high level of cultural acceptability in sub-Saharan Africa, and this kind of intervention can be done by lay people. In particular, hero books (which use storytelling and drawing to encourage children to develop problem-solving skills) and memory work (in which parents/caregivers develop a "life history" and discuss post-bereavement plans with their families) have gained increasing popularity.[77] There are no published studies of the effectiveness of hero books in relation to AIDS-affected children; however, the Regional Psychosocial Support Initiative (REPSSI) has recently conducted a controlled trial of hero books in schools with 285 children in South Africa.[78] This found that the intervention group showed improved educational outcomes and reported less worries, although there were no differences on children's reports of resolution of self-identified major problems in their lives. It would be very valuable to use standardized tools to test these interventions.

Popular Interventions That Lack Sufficient Evidence

• *Residential camps.* A study (not yet published but with a report available online)[79] in Zimbabwe compared 1,258 orphaned and vulnerable youth aged 14–20 years who received either community psychosocial support (formal and informal services that address psychosocial well-being either directly, e.g. counseling, or indirectly, e.g. school and nutritional support programs), attended the Salvation Army Masiye Camp (a residential, faith-based program for vulnerable children), or no intervention. Unfortunately, no preintervention scores were collected, the groups were not randomized, and no standardized measures of mental health were used, so these findings are difficult to interpret.[80]

• *Broad-based psychosocial support programs.* Many programs use a combination of material support and "psychosocial support." This is often loosely defined, and can include organized therapeutic or nontherapeutic groups, HIV-prevention education, individual counseling, and mentoring or home visits.[81] Unfortunately, there is almost no evidence to allow us to know whether these programs are making an impact on children's mental health or social networks. A study in Zimbabwe used UNICEF guidelines to develop a teacher-led psychosocial support program (including counseling, a buddy system, provision of school uniforms and supplies, and scripture lessons). Teachers reported better classroom behavior. Unfortunately, the study was small, without a control group, and did not use child-report or mental health measures, so we do not know whether this intervention has positive impacts on children's psychological well-being.[82]

• *School-based activity groups and school strengthening.* In South Africa, a cluster randomized controlled trial is currently evaluating the impact of two linked interventions by Soul City. Soul Buddyz clubs are groups, facilitated by teachers, which meet weekly and follow curricula based on developing skills such as safety, increasing children's self-esteem, and encouraging preventative behaviors for HIV and future violence. The Schools as Nodes of Care and Support program aims to enable schools to identify and support vulnerable children. Findings will be available in 2011–2012 (from the University of Witwaterstrand and the University of Oxford).

Similarly, the Caring Schools Project aims to support South African schools by offering sustainable physical, social, and emotional care to orphans and vulnerable children. Youth facilitators are placed in the school to identify orphans and vulnerable children and provide support for these children. In a recent evaluation of the programs, school principals and youth facilitators in 25 schools were interviewed. Overall, they reported improved school attendance and lower rates of drop out.[83] However, rigorous evaluation of the project, using pre- and post intervention measures, as well as control schools, is required before firm conclusions regarding its effectiveness can be made.

Community-based psychosocial support programs. The National Association of Child Care Workers (NACCW) *Isibindi* program is a community-based child and youth care service in South Africa. Community members are recruited to be trained as Community Child and Youth Care Workers (CYCW) to work holistically and developmentally in the "life space" of children and ensure children's rights are met. Through home visits, CYCWs provide a caring and reliable adult presence for children. Caregivers are assisted with accessing social security grants, basic child care, advice, and counseling. An external evaluation showed some positive impact on the targeted children and families.[84] Unfortunately, as the evaluation was not designed to provide evidence of children's well-being outcomes, it is not possible to make a firm conclusion about the *Isibindi* model's effectiveness. However, as the evaluation suggested some positive potential for delivering effective support services to affected children and families, it will be worthwhile to undertake a more rigorous evaluation to determine the model's effect on children's psychosocial well-being.

Additionally, USAID is currently conducting a series of evaluations of their community-based programs, which differ by location but include elements such as community volunteer home-visits, community-based social workers, health centers, and schools.[85] However, as yet, no results regarding mental health outcomes have been published.

Interventions Which Address Proven Mechanisms of Psychosocial Problems

We are clearly far behind where we need to be in terms of evidence-based interventions for AIDS-affected children. However, we do have useful knowledge of some of the potential mechanisms that are leading to psychosocial problems for AIDS-affected children, and some of the preventable risk factors associated with psychosocial distress. If we can find evidence-based interventions targeting these mechanisms and risk factors, even if they have not yet been tested with AIDS-affected children, it could help to guide the development of effective interventions. Targeting these mechanisms may also force us to think "outside the box" of our established psychosocial interventions and theories.

- *Providing antiretrovirals to parents.* We know that both parental death from AIDS and parental AIDS-sickness are directly linked to children's psychosocial well-being. The provision of antiretroviral (ARV) medication to parents or caregivers can prevent HIV-infection from progressing to AIDS and death. Therefore, providing ARVs to HIV-infected parents can be viewed as a primary preventative psychosocial intervention for children. The use of ARVs can also reduce visible signs of AIDS in parents, and evidence suggests that this could reduce community-level stigma for their families.[86] No known studies have tested the psychological impact of parental ART on children, but an ongoing study in South Africa will have findings on this by 2011.[87] Importantly, in the developing world, only 42% of people eligible for ARVs currently receive medication.[88] Interventions focusing on increasing this proportion are likely to result in benefits to the children of these adults.
- *Prevention of parent-to-child transmission and provision of pediatric ART.* Research suggests that HIV infection can lead to cognitive and neurological problems for children. In addition, the emotional impacts of diagnosis and the social impacts of being HIV positive put children at risk of psychosocial distress. A major preventative measure of these outcomes would be to stop transmission of HIV to children in the perinatal period. A short course of highly active antiretroviral therapy (HAART) to both mother and child can reduce transmission rates from 35% in sub-Saharan Africa to below 2%.[89] In 2008, prevention of mother-to-child transmission (PMTCT) in low- and middle-income countries was 32%.[90] It is important that this be combined with either sole breastfeeding or sole formula-feeding to reduce likelihood of infection in infancy.[91] For those children who are HIV positive, early and sustained ART

may have positive impacts on motor development, although findings on cognitive development are less clear.[92]

• *Reducing AIDS-related stigma and bullying.* To the best of our knowledge, no research has specifically tested interventions to reduce stigma for the families of HIV-positive people. However, there have been reviews of programs to reduce stigma associated with HIV more generally. Findings suggest that there may be positive results such as legal protection for HIV-positive individuals, availability and accessibility of ARV medication,[93] and sensitization to and contact with HIV positive people.[94] Stigma seems to be closely connected to lack of accurate HIV knowledge,[95] which suggests that public health measures to increase understanding of how HIV is, and just as importantly is not, transmitted may be helpful. However, recent longitudinal evidence from South Africa has found stigma to be higher among those who know someone who has died of AIDS. It also found that increased personal contact with an HIV-positive person did not reduce levels of stigma.[96] An ongoing study in South Africa has found positive effects of a U.S.-designed program called CHAMP, which aims to strengthen family relationships and enhance problem-solving and youth peer negotiation skills. This led to reductions in HIV-stigmatizing attitudes among both adolescents and caregivers.[97] It is clear that much more research is needed to understand how we can best combat AIDS-related stigma.

• *Anti-bullying.* The effectiveness of a number of interventions to reduce bullying has also been evaluated. Most of these have been in schools, and almost all have been in the developed world. A recent systematic review[98] examined curriculum-based interventions, "whole-school" interventions, social skills groups, mentoring, and social worker support. Only four of the ten curriculum-based studies were associated with decreases in bullying. With the "whole-school" approach, seven out of ten studies decreased bullying. Three of the four social skills interventions showed no reductions in bullying. Both mentoring and increased numbers of school social workers showed decreases in bullying. A year later, a meta-analysis of developed-world school-based anti-bullying programs concluded that most did not have meaningful effects on bullying reduction.[99] In sub-Saharan Africa, one small evaluation study of a school-based anti-bullying intervention suggests it had no impact, but the number of participants was too small ($n = 54$ in three comparison groups) for meaningful conclusions.[100]

The evidence from the developed world does suggest that whole-school approaches, mentoring, and increased numbers of social workers have the potential to reduce bullying. Whole-school approaches involve some combination of school-wide rules, teacher training, classroom curriculum, conflict resolution training, and individual counseling. Transferring these concepts to the developing world requires adaptation to different school structures and cultures, developing low-cost approaches, and allowing for human resource shortages (especially in sub-Saharan Africa). It is also important to incorporate the issues of HIV and AIDS into anti-bullying programs.

• *Increasing social support and caregiver–child connectedness.* Evidence suggests that improving social support and caregiver–child connectedness has the potential to buffer the impact of belonging to an AIDS-affected family. It is important to remember that both of these factors work in a two-way dynamic: Children who are more resilient and personable are more able to gain support and affection than children who are depressed, anxious, traumatized, or have behavior problems.[101] There is evidence from both the developed and developing world that parenting programs encourage positive parenting and improve parent–child relationships.[102] In Zimbabwe, qualitative research with teenagers suggested that disclosure and discussion of parental HIV status was seen as helpful for family closeness.[103]

It may be especially important to encourage connectedness in foster families for AIDS-affected children. Although the vast majority of children remain in the kin network, there is evidence of a reduced sense of responsibility for children when biological links are not direct.[104] For children who are HIV positive, it is especially important that caregivers have the skills and motivation to ensure treatment adherence. We were only able to find one evaluation of such an intervention. In South Africa, grandmothers were trained in HIV/AIDS knowledge, intergenerational communication, basic nursing skills, accessing social services and grants, and relaxation. Participants reported greater knowledge and competence, but actual care was not tested and no control group was included, so this only remains indicative of a potentially useful intervention.[105]

We could find no quantitative evidence to date of higher levels of child abuse of AIDS-affected children. However, some researchers do report heightened risks of abuse in families with extreme stressors, poverty, or fostered children.[106] Anecdotal and qualitative evidence also suggests that abuse may be more prevalent for AIDS-affected children. The field of child abuse prevention is extensive, but a recent systematic "review of reviews" found that home visiting, parent training, and child sexual abuse prevention appear to be effective in reducing child maltreatment.[107] However, the authors noted that only 0.6% of the evidence came from the developing world, and that more research was needed there. It is also important to ensure that adequate capacity exists for child protection services to investigate and address cases of abuse. This is often made especially challenging in the developing world by staff shortages, lack of resources such as vehicles for social workers, and long distances in rural areas.[108]

• *Reducing poverty.* A number of interventions aim to improve economic well-being in AIDS-affected homes. These include microfinance schemes, provision of food parcels, "sponsoring" of children, and education support. One study of economic empowerment and a savings scheme in Uganda found some positive impacts on child mental health.[109] A widely debated method of poverty reduction is the social welfare grant system. In South Africa, sustained state efforts to increase grant uptake for families with children has resulted in increased numbers of orphaned children receiving grants.[110]

• *Home- and community-based care.* We do not yet understand fully the mechanisms by which having an AIDS-sick adult in the home can lead to children's psychosocial distress. But qualitative evidence suggests that children's caregiving responsibilities can mean that they are not able to attend school, do homework, or see friends.[111] New data from South Africa reports that children are preoccupied with worry about their sick parents: "There are times I can't hear clearly because I think about her, how she is doing, whether she is eating her tablets" (boy, 12 years).[112] One potential intervention (to date not yet studied in children) is the provision of home and community-based care. Home-based care involves trained lay workers who visit homes to provide nursing assistance and psychosocial support for AIDS-affected families. This could reduce the burden on children of both caregiving responsibilities and of worrying for the safety of a sick person left alone. The case study in Box 6.1 provides a description of home-based care in the South African context.

  • *Street-children.* To the best of our knowledge, no interventions specifically targeting street-children have been empirically evaluated. However, a number of theoretical and descriptive studies do provide guidelines for working with street-children. These include the need to recognize the independence and capabilities of street-children.[115] Anthropological studies highlight the strong social networks that street-children develop among themselves.[116] Many studies stress the heterogeneity within the group of street-children, and how it is important for interventions to distinguish between children "on the street" and "of the street" (i.e., living at home but working on the street versus living and sleeping on the streets).[117] Some studies suggest that street-children are at no greater mental health risk than other poor children, but they certainly have higher

---

Box 6.1

CASE STUDIES: INTERVENTIONS IN SOUTH AFRICA

Within South Africa, three innovative programs have been widely promoted—all are potential targets for future evaluation studies.

Home and Community-based Care
The Home and Community-Based Care (HCBC) program aims to support and empower families in caring for AIDS-affected children. Lay community caregivers facilitate the early identification of orphans and vulnerable children; make referrals to social workers for specialized services including alternative placements; provide supervision and ongoing support to vulnerable households; assist families to discuss and actively get involved in succession planning activities; provide psychosocial support; assist children and their families to access basic services, including social grants and other material assistance; assist children and families to access legal documents; and help children attend school and restore normal schooling.

Drop-in Centers/Community Care Centers
Community Care centers are local sites that provide psychosocial support such as before- and after-school feeding schemes, homework clubs, laundry services, recreational facilities, training on skills for domestic work, life skills programs, and holiday programs including camps. The center identifies children and families in need of care and links such families to appropriate services, such as access to grants, referrals to legal services and vital registration documents, writing of wills, health care

services, and referrals to social workers for alternative care placement in places of safety, foster care, and adoption.

Child Care Forums

Child Care Forums (CCFs) are locally based organized groups who are committed to advocating for the needs of children within their community. Community mobilization can include facilitating activities to reduce stigma, community income-generating projects, community-based day care facilities, after-school care, and holiday programs to provide relief for caregivers. These forums are established in the HIV and AIDS and STI Strategic Plan for South Africa, 2007–2011.[113] A recent review of CCFs found a total of 400 CCFs in South Africa, but the total number of child beneficiaries reached less than 200,000.[114]

---

levels of exposure to violence and sexual risk.[118] Suggested interventions for street-children include preventative measures within families to reduce children leaving for the streets and outreach work to engage street-children, help with re-entering school, and provide vocational training. They specifically do *not* include reunification of children with families without addressing the circumstances that made them leave.[119]

RECOMMENDED ACTIONS AND INTERVENTIONS

To date, there is an almost total lack of rigorously tested interventions for AIDS-affected children. This means that recommendations for action must be cautious. It also clearly highlights the need for a rapid expansion in high-quality research specifically focusing on interventions for this group of children. Qualitative work suggests that it is important to be aware of the potential for stigmatizing AIDS-affected children through targeted programs. However, universal access to support programs may be impossible to achieve in resource-poor settings.

One preventative approach to psychosocial distress among AIDS-affected children is by provision of ARVs, thereby preventing the progression from HIV infection to AIDS in caregivers, preventing the early death of caregivers, protecting children from mother-to-child-transmission, and maintaining physical health for HIV-positive children. Studies do suggest that peer group support, mentoring, and solution-focused stories may be helpful in reducing psychosocial distress, and ongoing studies are currently examining school-based peer groups, family-centered training, and community-based strategies. In addition, there is good epidemiological evidence to suggest the value of interventions targeting specific mechanisms of psychosocial problems in AIDS-affected children. These could include programs that aim to reduce AIDS-related stigma at a community level, to reduce bullying at a school level, and to improve nutrition and reduce extreme poverty in AIDS-affected households. Increasing child–caregiver connectedness, and HCBC for families are also potentially protective interventions.

All of these potential interventions unquestionably need further research. We need to understand whether they do impact upon children's psychosocial well-being, whether these impacts last over time, and whether or not these interventions are feasible and sustainable in the developing world. However, it is also important to remember that research (especially high-quality research such as randomized controlled trials) is time-consuming, expensive, and requires specific skills. It is likely to be years before we have a strong enough body of research to guide truly evidence-based practice. In the meantime, the number of AIDS-affected children is rising by millions, raising a dilemma. Do we wait until we know "what works" for AIDS-affected children before we act and ignore children who are clearly experiencing great psychosocial distress? Or, do we continue to scale up programs and interventions for which we do not have enough evidence to determine whether they help or harm children? There are no clear or easy answers to these questions, but we propose the following recommendations.

First, a concerted and immediate effort is needed to develop a body of evidence testing the effectiveness of psychosocial interventions for AIDS-affected children. This will require the collaboration of governments, NGOs, researchers, and funding bodies. It will need coordination to ensure that the interventions tested are acceptable and sustainable, and that they are feasible to reproduce if they are proved effective. It will also need a willingness to be open about interventions that do not work. These are not easy demands. To date, NGOs are under great pressure to prove the "success" of programs, and reporting lack of effectiveness is seen as a failure by funding bodies rather than as an important step in developing our understanding of what will work. Researchers are unlikely to write up negative or ineffective results, and journals are unlikely to publish them. Such a program of research would need coordination; and a good model for this may be the Joint Learning Initiative on Children and HIV/AIDS.[120]

Second, the need to continue providing interventions while this evidence base is being developed should be recognized. However, it is essential that these interventions use the most up-to-date evidence to maximize their potential effectiveness. Many groups and individuals working with AIDS-affected children are motivated by love, protectiveness, and a sense of duty. These are important and should not be undervalued. But it is also important to channel these essential motivating factors into promoting interventions with a strong evidence base. It is also essential that funding bodies, which hold much of the power in determining programs of intervention in the developing world, commit to supporting programs that are shown to be beneficial.

The outlook is good. We are, for the first time, in a strong position to develop the essential body of evidence needed to evaluate psychosocial interventions for AIDS-affected children. We have research outlining the needs of children orphaned by AIDS, and we have ongoing research identifying the needs of children whose caregivers are sick with AIDS. Although research addressing the psychosocial needs of HIV-positive children in the developing world is still required, we have evidence from the developed world to guide us in this endeavor. We also have an expanding body of research identifying potential mechanisms through which belonging to an AIDS-affected family may impact on children's psychosocial well-being. By using the evidence we have already, and making a concerted and combined effort to develop new evidence, we can promote resilience and positive outcomes for AIDS-affected children.

NOTES

1. Bronfenbrenner, U. (1979). *The ecology of human development: Experiments by nature and design.* Cambridge, MA: Harvard University Press.
2. Richter, L., G. Foster, G., & L. Sherr, L. (2006). *Where the heart is: Meeting the psychosocial needs of young children in the context of HIV/AIDS.* Toronto: Bernard Van Leer Foundation.
3. Rutter, M. (2006). Implications of resilience concepts for scientific understanding. *Annals of the New York Academy of Sciences, 1094,* 1–12; Luthar, S., & Cicchetti, D. (2000). The construct of resilience: Implications for intervention and social policy. *Development and Psychopathology, 12,* 857–885.
4. UNAIDS. (2008). *Report on the global AIDS epidemic.* Geneva, Switzerland: UNAIDS.
5. Fang, X., et al. (2009). Parental HIV/AIDS and psychosocial adjustment among rural Chinese children. *Journal of Pediatric Psychology, 34*(10), 1053–1062.
6. T. Barnett, T., & Whiteside, A. (2002). *AIDS in the twenty-first century: Disease and globalization.* Basingstoke: Palgrave Macmillian; Hunter, S. (1990). Orphans as a window on the AIDS epidemic in Sub-Saharan Africa: Initial results and implications of a study in Uganda. *Social Science and Medicine, 31*(6), 681–690.
7. Atwine, B., Cantor-Graae, E., & Bajunirwe, F. (2005). Psychological distress among AIDS orphans in rural Uganda. *Social Science and Medicine, 61*(3), 555–564; Bhargava, A. (2005). AIDS epidemic and the psychological well-being and school participation of Ethiopian orphans. *Psychology, Health and Medicine, 10*(3), 263–275; Cluver, L., Gardner, F., & Operario, D. (2007). Psychological distress amongst AIDS-orphaned children in urban South Africa. *Journal of Child Psychology and Psychiatry, 48*(8), 755–763; Kaggwa, E. B., & Hindin, M. J. (2010). The psychological effect of orphanhood in a matured HIV epidemic: An analysis of young people in Mukono, Uganda. *Social Science & Medicine, 70*(7), 1002–1010; Makame, V., Ani, C., & McGregor, S. (2002). Psychological well-being of orphans in Dar El-Salaam, Tanzania. *Acta Paediatrica, 91,* 459–465; Makaya, J., et al. (2002). *Assessment of psychological repercussions of AIDS next to 354 AIDS orphans in Brazzaville, 2001.* Paper presented at the XIV International AIDS conference, Barcelona; Manuel, P. (2002). *Assessment of orphans and their caregivers' psychological well-being in a rural community in central Mozambique.* London: MSc, Institute of Child Health; Nyamukapa, C., et al. (2008). HIV-associated orphanhood and children's psychosocial distress: Theoretical framework tested with data from Zimbabwe. *American Journal of Public Health, 98*(1), 133–141; Pelton, P., & Forehand, R. (2005). Orphans of the AIDS epidemic: An examination of clinical level problems of children. *Journal of the American Academy of Child and Adolescent Psychiatry, 44*(6), 585–591; Poulter, C. (1996). Vulnerable children: A psychological perspective. Uppsala, Sweden: The Nordic Africa Institute; J. Sengendo, J., & Nambi, J. (1997). The psychological effect of orphanhood: A study of orphans in Rakai District. *Health Transitions Review, 7*(Suppl.) 105–124; Volle, S., et al. (2002). *Psychosocial baseline survey of orphans and vulnerable children in Zambia.* Paper presented at the XIV International AIDS Conference, Barcelona.

8. Forehand, R., et al. (2002). Noninfected children of HIV-infected mothers: A 4-year longitudinal study of child psychosocial adjustment and parenting. *Behavior Therapy, 33,* 579–600; Rotheram-Borus, M.-J., et al. (2004). Six-year intervention outcomes for adolescent children of parents with the human immunodeficiency virus/ *Archives of Pediatric and Adolescent Medicine, 158,* 742–748; Rotheram-Borus, M.-J., Stein, J. A., & Lin, Y.-Y. (2001). Impact of parent death and an intervention on the adjustment of adolescents whose parents have HIV/AIDS. *Journal of Consulting and Clinical Psychology, 69*(5), 763–773.

9. Fang et al. (2009). Parental HIV/AIDS and psychosocial adjustment.

10. Cluver, L., Fincham, D., & Seedat, S. (2009). Predictors of post-traumatic stress symptomology amongst AIDS-orphaned children. *Journal of Traumatic Stress, 22,* 102–112; Cluver, Gardner, & Operario. (2007). Psychological distress amongst AIDS-orphaned children.

11. Cluver, L., & Operario, D. (2008). Review: Intergenerational linkages of AIDS: Vulnerability of orphaned children for HIV infection. *Institute of Development Studies Bulletin, 39*(5), 28–35.

12. Birdthistle, I., et al. (2008). From affected to infected? Orphanhood and HIV risk among female adolescents in urban Zimbabwe. *AIDS, 22,* 759–766; Gregson, S., et al. (2005). HIV infection and reproductive health in teenage women made vulnerable by AIDS in Zimbabwe. *AIDS Care, 17*(7), 785–794.

13. Operario, D., et al. (2007). Prevalence of parental death among young people in South Africa and risk for HIV infection. *Journal of Acquired Immune Deficiency Syndromes, 44,* 93–98.

14. Kissin, D., et al. (2007). HIV seroprevalence in street youth, St. Petersburg, Russia. *AIDS, 21,* 2333–2340.

15. Campbell, P., et al. (2008). A situation analysis of orphans in 11 Eastern and Southern African Countries. Nairobi: UNICEF ESARO. Juma, M., Askew, I., & Ferguson, A. (2007). Situation analysis of the sexual and reproductive health and HIV risks and prevention needs of older orphaned and vulnerable children in Nyanza Province, Kenya. Nairobi: Department of Children's Services, Government of Kenya; Nyamukapa et al. (2008). HIV-associated orphanhood and children's psychosocial distress; Operario et al. (2007). Prevalence of parental death among young people in South Africa; Palermo, T., & Peterman, A. (2009). Are female orphans at risk for early marriage, early sexual debut, and teen pregnancy? Evidence from Sub-Saharan Africa. *Studies in Family Planning,* 40, 101–112; Thurman, T., et al. (2006). Sexual risk behavior among South African adolescents: Is orphan status a factor? *AIDS and Behavior, 10*(6), 627–635.

16. Nyamukapa et al. (2008). HIV-associated orphanhood and children's psychosocial distress.

17. Richter, Foster, & Sherr. (2006). *Where the heart is.*

18. Strode, A., & Barrett Grant, K. (2001). The role of stigma and discrimination in increasing the vulnerability of children and youth infected with and affected by HIV/AIDS. London: Save The Children.

19. Pilowsky, D., Wissow, L., & Hutton, N. (2000). Children affected by HIV: Clinical experience and research findings. *Child and Adolescent Psychiatric Clinics of North America. Special Children and Adolescents Affected by HIV/AIDS: A Mental Health Challenge, 9,* 451–464.

20. Nam, S., et al. (2009). Discussing matters of sexual health with children: What issues relating to disclosure of parental HIV status reveal. *AIDS Care, 21*(3), 389–395.

21. Kganaka, M. (2003). Construction of a model for home-based palliative care for people living with HIV/AIDS. Pretoria, South Africa: Medical University of Southern Africa.

22. Forsyth, B., & Damour, L. (1996). The psychological effects of parental human immunodeficiency virus infection. *Archives of Pediatric and Adolescent Medicine, 150*, 1015–1020.

23. Murphy, D., Marelich, W., & Hoffman, D. (2002). A longitudinal study of the impact on young children of maternal HIV serostatus disclosure. *Clinical Child Psychology and Psychiatry, 7*(1), 55–70; Murphy, D. A. (2008). HIV-positive mothers' disclosure of their serostatus to their young children: A review. *Clinical Child Psychology and Psychiatry, 13*(1), 105–122; Shaffer, A., et al. (2001). Telling the children: Disclosure of maternal HIV infection and its effects on child psychosocial adjustment, *Journal of Child and Family Studies, 10*(3), 301–313.

24. Delaney, R., Serovich, J., & Lim, J. (2008). Reasons for and against maternal HIV disclosure to children and perceived child reaction. *AIDS Care, 20*(7), 876–880.

25. Armistead, L., & Forehand, R. (1995). For whom the bell tolls: Parenting decisions and challenges faced by mothers who are HIV infected. *Clinical Psychology: Science and Practice, 2*, 239–250; Forehand, R., et al. (1998). The Family Health Project: An investigation of children whose mothers Are HIV infected. *Journal of Consulting and Clinical Psychology, 66*(3), 513–520; Forehand et al. (2002). Noninfected children of HIV-infected mothers, pp. 579–600; Hudis, J. (1995). Adolescents living in families with AIDS. In S. Geballe, J. Gruendal, & W. Andiman (Eds.), *Forgotten children of the AIDS epidemic* (pp. 83–94). New Haven, CT: Yale University Press; Rotheram-Borus, M.-J., Lightfoot, M., & Shen, H. (1999). Levels of emotional distress among parents living with AIDS and their adolescent children. *AIDS and Behaviour, 3*(4), 367–372.

26. Fang et al. (2009). Parental HIV/AIDS and psychosocial adjustment.

27. Gwandure, C. (2007). Home-based care for parents with AIDS: Impact on children's psychological functioning. *Journal of Child and Adolescent Mental Health, 19*(1), 29–44; Poulter. (1996). Vulnerable children.

28. Cluver, L., Gardner, F., & Operario, D. (2009). Caregiving and psychological distress of AIDS-orphaned children. *Vulnerable Children and Youth Studies, 4*(3), 185–199.

29. Gwandure. (2007). Home-based care for parents with AIDS.

30. Bauman, L., et al. (2006). Children caring for their ill parents with HIV/AIDS, *Vulnerable Children and Youth Studies, 1*(1), 56.

31. Becker, S. (2007). Global perspectives on children's unpaid caregiving in the family: Research and policy on 'young carers' in the UK, Australia, the USA and Sub-Saharan Africa. *Global Social Policy, 7*(1), 23–50; Becker, S., Dearden, C., & Aldridge, J. (2000). Young carers in the UK: Research, policy and practice. *Research, Policy and Planning, 8*(2), 13–22; Levine, C., et al. (2005). Young adult caregivers: A first look at an unstudied population. *American Journal of Public Health, 95*(11), 2071–2075.

32. Bauman et al. (2006). Children caring for their ill parents with HIV/AIDS.

33. Evans, J., & Becker, S. (In press). *Children caring for parents with HIV and AIDS: Global issues and policy responses*. Bristol: Policy Press; Robson, E. (2000).

Invisible carers: Young people in Zimbabwe's home-based healthcare. *Area,*
32(1), 59–69; Skovdal, M., et al. (In press). Young carers as social actors: Coping
strategies of children caring for ailing or ageing guardians in western Kenya.
Social Science and Medicine.

34. Young Caregivers Study Teen Advisory Group, 2010 www.youngcaregivers.
org.za.

35. Newell, M.-L., et al. (2004). Mortality of infected and uninfected infants
born to HIV-infected mothers in Africa: A pooled analysis. *The Lancet, 364,*
1236–1243.

36. Stover, J., et al. (2006). Projecting the demographic impact of AIDS and the
number of people in need of treatment: Updates to the Spectrum Projection
Package, *Sexually Transmitted Infections, 82,* 45–50.

37. Gray, G. E. (2010). Adolescent HIV - Cause for concern in Southern Africa,
PLoS Med, 7(2), doi:10.1371/journal.pmed.1000178.

38. Richter, L., Stein, A., & Cluver, L. (2009). Infants and young children affected by
AIDS. In P. Rohleder, et al. (Eds.), *HIV/AIDS in South Africa 25 years on:*
Psychosocial perspectives (pp. 69–88). Cape Town, South Africa: L Springer
Press.

39. Jaros, E., Myer, L., & Joska, J. (2009). *HIV/AIDS and mental health in*
Sub-Saharan Africa: A systematic review. Unpublished thesis.

40. Boivin, M., et al. (1995). A preliminary evaluation of the cognitive and motor
effects on pediatric HIV infection in Zairian children. *Health Psychology, 14*(1),
13–21.

41. Peterson, N., et al. (2001). The relationship of maternal and child HIV infection
to security of attachment among Ugandan infants. *Child Psychiatry and Human*
Development, 32(1), 3–17.

42. Ibid.

43. Bush-Parker, T. (2000). Perinatal HIV: Children with HIV grow up. *Focus, 15,*
1–4.

44. Mellins, C., et al. (2006). Rates of psychiatric disorder in perinatally HIV-
infected youth. *Pediatric Infectious Disease Journal, 25,* 432–437.

45. Gaughan, D., et al. (2004). Pediatric AIDS clinical trials group 219c team.
Psychiatric hospitalizations among children and youths with human immunodeficiency virus infection. *Pediatrics, 113,* 544–551.

46. Armistead, L., et al. (1999). Understanding of HIV/AIDS among children of
HIV-infected mothers: Implications for prevention, disclosure and bereave-
ment. *Children's Health Care, 28*(4), 277–295; Green, G., & Smith, R. (2004).
The psychosocial and health care needs of HIV-positive people in the
United Kingdom: A review. *HIV Medicine, 5*(Suppl 1), 5–46; Letteney S., & Heft
LaPorte, H. (2004). Deconstructing stigma: Perceptions of HIV-seropositive
mothers and their disclosure to children. *Social Work in Health Care, 38*(3),
105–123.

47. McKay, M., et al. (In press). Adapting a family-based HIV prevention program
for HIV-infected preadolescents and their families: Youth, families and health
care providers coming together to address complex needs. *Social Work &*
Mental Health.

48. Paiva, V., Ayres, J., & Frana, I. (2007). *The impact of AIDS related stigma and*
discrimination on AIDS orphans and their caretakers in Sao Paulo, Brazil.
Presented at the AIDS Impact Conference, Marseilles, France.

49. Mellins, C., et al. (2004). The role of psychosocial and family factors in adherence to antiretroviral treatment in human immunodeficiency virus-infected children. *The Pediatric Infectious Disease Journal, 23*, 1035–1041.
50. Stein, J. (2004). Streets as school and home to orphans in the Transkei. *AIDS Bulletin, 13*(2), 44–46.
51. Ennew, J. (1996). Difficult circumstances: Some reflections on street children in Africa. *Africa Insight, 26*(3), 203–212; Ennew, J., & Swart-Kruger, J. (2003). Introduction: Homes, places and spaces in the construction of street children and street youth. *Children, Youth and Environments, 13*(1) Spring 2003. Retrieved August 30, 2011, from http://colorado.edu/journals/cye.; Kissin et al. (2007). HIV Seroprevalence in street youth, St. Petersburg, Russia; Swart-Kruger, L., & Richter, L. (1997). AIDS-related knowledge, attitudes and behaviour among South African street youth: Reflections on power, sexuality and the autonomous self. *Social Sciences and Medicine, 45*(6), 957–966.
52. Stein, A., et al. (2005). Babies of a pandemic: Infant development and HIV. *Archives of the Diseases of Childhood, 90*, 116–118.
53. Stein, A., Ramchanani, P., & Murray, L. (2008). Impact of parental mental illness or mental disorder. In M. Rutter (Ed.), *Child and Adolescent Psychiatry* (pp. 407–420). Malden, MA: Wiley-Blackwell.
54. Cluver, Gardner, & Operario. (2007). Caregiving and psychological distress of AIDS-orphaned children.
55. Kaggwa & Hindin. (2010). The psychological effect of orphanhood in a matured HIV epidemic.
56. Booysen, F. (2004). Income and poverty dynamics in HIV/AIDS-affected households in the Free State Province of South Africa. *South African Journal of Economics, 72*(3), 522–545.
57. Bhargava. (2005). AIDS epidemic and the psychological well-being; Cluver, L., Gardner, F., & Operario, D. (2009). Effects of poverty on the psychological health of AIDS-orphaned children. *AIDS Care, 21*(6), 732–741; Cluver, L., & Orkin, M. (2009). Stigma, bullying, poverty and AIDS-orphanhood: Interactions mediating psychological problems for children in South Africa. *Social Science and Medicine, 69*(8), 1186–1193.
58. Atwine, Cantor-Graae, & Bajunirwe. (2005). Psychological distress among AIDS orphans in rural Uganda.
59. Robson. (2000). Invisible carers: Young people in Zimbabwe's home-based healthcare.
60. Cluver, L., Gardner, F., & Operario, D. (2008). Effects of stigma and other community factors on the mental health of AIDS-orphaned children. *Journal of Adolescent Health, 42*, 410–417.
61. Strode & Barrett Grant. (2001). The role of stigma and discrimination.
62. Deacon, H. (2006). Towards a sustainable theory of health-related stigma: Lessons from the HIV/AIDS literature. *Journal of Community & Applied Social Psychology, 16*(6), 418–425; Nyblade, N. (2006). Measuring HIV stigma: Existing knowledge and gaps. *Psychology, Health and Medicine, 11*(3), 335–345; Kganaka. (2003). Construction of a model for home-based palliative care for people living with HIV/AIDS.
63. Cluver, L., Bowes, L., & Gardner, F. (In press). Risk and protective factors for bullying victimisation amongst AIDS-affected and vulnerable children in South Africa, *Child Abuse and Neglect*

64. Cluver, Fincham, & Seedat. (2009). Predictors of post-traumatic stress symptomology.
65. Atwine, Cantor-Graae, & Bajunirwe. (2005). Psychological distress among AIDS orphans; Kaggwa & Hindin. (2010). The psychological effect of orphanhood.
66. Kuo, C., & Operario, D. (2009). Caring for AIDS-orphaned children: A systematic review of studies on caregivers. *Vulnerable Children and Youth Studies, 4*(1), 1–12.
67. Appleyard, K., et al. (2004). When more is not better: The role of cumulative risk in child behaviour outcomes. *Journal of Child Psychology and Psychiatry, 46*(3), 235–245; Rutter, M. (2000). Psychosocial influences: Critiques, findings, and research needs. *Development and Psychopathology, 12*, 375–405.
68. Cluver & Orkin. (2009). Stigma, bullying, poverty and AIDS-orphanhood.
69. King, E., et al. (2009). Interventions for improving the psychosocial well-being of children affected by HIV and AIDS. *Cochrane Collaboration Systematic Review, 2*, Art. No.: CD006733. DOI: 10.1002/14651858.CD006733.pub2.
70. Meintjies, H., & Giese, S. (2006). Spinning the epidemic: The making of mythologies of orphanhood in the context of AIDS. *Childhood, 13*(3), 407–430.
71. Giese, S., et al. (2003). Health and social services to address the needs of orphans and other vulnerable children in the context of HIV/AIDS in South Africa: Research Report and Recommendations., Cape Town, South Africa: Children's Institute, University of Cape Town.
72. Baker-Henningham, H., et al. (2009). A pilot study of the Incredible Years Teacher Training Programme and a curriculum unit on social and emotional skills in community preschools in Jamaica. *Child Care Health and Development, 33*, 624–631.
73. King, et al. (2009). Interventions for improving the psychosocial well-being of children.
74. Kumakech, E., Cantor-Graae, E., & Maling, S. (2009). Peer-group support intervention improves the psychosocial well-being of AIDS orphans: Cluster randomized trial. *Social Science and Medicine, 68*(6), 1038–1043.
75. Brown, L., et al. (2009). Impact of a mentoring program on psychosocial well-being of youth in Rwanda: Results of a quasi-experimental study. *Vulnerable Children and Youth Studies, 4*(4), 288–299.
76. Ibid.
77. Morgan, J. (2004). Memory work. Preparation for death? Legacies for orphans? Fighting for life? One size fits all, or time for product differentiation. *AIDS Bulletin, 13*(2), 36–41.
78. Rabinowitz, L., & Goldberg, R. (2009). An evaluation of an intervention using hero books to mainstream psychosocial care and support into South African schools via the curricula. Johannesburg, South Africa: REPSSI.
79. Gilborn, L., et al. Orphans and vulnerable youth in Bulawayo, Zimbabwe: An exploratory study of psychosocial wellbeing and psychosocial support programs. Retrieved from http://www.popcouncil.org/pdfs/horizons/zimorphans.pdf
80. Gilborn, L., et al. (2006). Orphans and vulnerable youth in Bulawayo, Zimbabwe: An exploratory study of psychosocial well-being and psychosocial support programs. Bulawayo, Zimbabwe: Horizons/Population Council Report.

81. Strebel, A. (2004). The development, implementation and evaluation of interventions for the care of orphans and vulnerable children in Botswana, South Africa and Zimbabwe: A literature review of evidence-based interventions for home-based child-centred development. Cape Town, South Africa: Human Sciences Research Council.

82. Chitiyoa, M., Changarab, D., & Chitiyo, G. (2008). Providing psychosocial support to special needs children: A case of orphans and vulnerable children in Zimbabwe. *International Journal of Educational Development, 28*, 384–392.

83. Strauss, J. P. (2007). An evaluation of the Caring Schools Project in the Free State Schools. Bloemfontein, South Africa: University of the Free State.

84. National Association of Child Care Workers (NACCW). (2009). *Isibindi model of care for children affected by HIV and AIDS.* Prepared for the Department of Social Development, UNICEF and NACCW for discussion at the Isibindi Partners Network Meeting.

85. MEASURE Evaluation, et al. (2007). Kilifi Orphans and Vulnerable Children Project: A case study. Chapel Hill, NC: USAID with support from Catholic Relief Services Kenya.

86. Kalichman, S., & Simbayi, L. (2004). Traditional beliefs about the cause of AIDS and AIDS-related stigma in South Africa. *AIDS Care, 16*(5), 572–580.

87. The Young Carers Project. Retrieved from www.youngcarers.org.za

88. WHO. (2009). Towards universal access: Scaling up priority HIV/AIDS interventions in the Health Sector Progress Report. Geneva, Switzerland: WHO.

89. Siegfried, N., van der Merwe, L., Brocklehurst, P., & Sint, TT. (2011). Antiretrovirals for reducing the risk of mother-to-child transmission of HIV infection. *Cochrane Database of Systematic Reviews, 7,* Art. No.: CD003510. DOI: 10.1002/14651858.CD003510.pub3.

90. WHO. (2009). Towards universal access.

91. Horvath, T., Madi, B., Iuppa, I., Kennedy, G.E., Rutherford, G.W., & Read, J.S. (2009). Interventions for preventing late postnatal mother-to-child transmission of HIV. *Cochrane Database of Systematic Reviews, 1,* Art. No.: CD006734. DOI: 10.1002/14651858.CD006734.pub2.

92. Potterton, J. (2006). A longitudinal study of neurodevelopmental delay in HIV infected children. Johannesburg, South Africa: University of Witwatersrand.

93. Abadıa-Barrero, C., & Castro, A. (2006). Experiences of stigma and access to HAART in children and adolescents living with HIV/AIDS in Brazil. *Social Science and Medicine, 62*, 1219–1288.

94. Brown, L., Macintyre, K., & Trujillo, L. (2003). Interventions to reduce HIV/AIDS stigma: What have we learned? *AIDS Education and Prevention, 15*(1), 49–69; Klein, S., Karchner, W., & O'Connell, D. (2002). Interventions to prevent HIV-related stigma and discrimination: Findings and recommendations for public health practice. *Journal of Public Health Management and Practice, 8*(6), 44–53.

95. Kalichman & Simbayi. (2004). Traditional beliefs about the cause of AIDS; Van Empelen, P. (2005). What is the impact of HIV on families? Copenhagen, Denmark: WHO.

96. Maughan-Brown, B. (2009). *Changes in HIV-related stigma among young adults in Cape Town, South Africa.* CSSR Working Paper, University of Cape Town.

97. Bell, C., et al. (2008). Building protective factors to offset sexually risky behaviors among black youths: A randomized control trial. *Journal of the National Medical Association, 100*, 936–944.

98. Vreeman, R. C., & Carroll, A. E. (2007). A systematic review of school-based interventions to prevent bullying. *Archives of Pediatric and Adolescent Medicine, 161*(1), 78–88.

99. Merrell, K., et al. (2008). How effective are school bullying intervention programs? A meta-analysis of intervention research. *School Psychology Quarterly, 23*(1), 26–42.

100. Meyer, N., & Lesch, E. (2000). An analysis of the limitations of a behavioural programme for bullying boys from a subeconomic environment. *South African Journal of Child and Adolescent Mental Health, 12*, 56–69.

101. Rutter. (2000). Psychosocial influences.

102. Bhana, A., et al. (2004). Children and youth at risk: Adaptation and pilot study of the Champ (Amaqhawe) Programme in South Africa. *African Journal of AIDS Research, 3*, 33–41.

103. Wood, K., Chase, E., & Aggleton, P. (2006). 'Telling the truth is the best thing': Teenage orphans' experiences of parental AIDS-related illness and bereavement in Zimbabwe. *Social Science & Medicine, 63*(7), 1923–1933.

104. A. Case, I. Lin, & S. McLanahan. (2000). How hungry is the selfish gene? *Economic Journal, 110*, 781–804.

105. Boon, H., et al. (2009). The impact of a community-based pilot health education intervention for older people as caregivers of orphaned and sick children as a result of HIV and AIDS in South Africa. *Journal of Cross-Cultural Gerontology, 24*(4), 373–389, online issue.

106. Dawes, A., Borel-Saladin, J., & Parker, Z. (2004). Measurement and monitoring. In L Richter, A. Dawes, & C. Higson-Smith (Eds.), *Sexual abuse of young children in South Africa* (pp. 176–205). Cape Town, South Africa: HSRC Press.

107. Mikton, C., & Butchart, A. (2009). Child maltreatment prevention: A systematic review of reviews. *Bulletin of the World Health Organization, 87*, 353–361.

108. Giese et al. (2003). Health and social services to address the needs of orphans.

109. Ssewamala, F., Han, C.-K., & Neilands, T. (2009). Asset ownership and health and mental health functioning among AIDS-orphaned adolescents. *Social Science & Medicine, 69*(2), 191–198.

110. Kganaka. (2003). Construction of a model for home-based palliative care.

111. Robson. (2000). Invisible carers.

112. The Young Carers Project. Retrieved from www.youngcarers.org.za.

113. Government of South Africa, 2007. Retrieved from http://www.unicef.org/southafrica/SAF_resources_ecdrapid.pdf.

114. Mathambo, ongoing; retrieved from http://www.hsrc.ac.za/Research_Project-915.phtml.

115. Panter-Brick, C. (2002). Street children, human rights, and public health: A critique and future directions. *Annual Review of Anthropology, 31*, 147–171.

116. Davies, M. (2008). A childish culture?: Shared understandings, agency and intervention: An anthropological study of street children in northwest Kenya. *Childhood, 15*(3), 309–330.

117. Ward, C. (2005). Monitoring the well-being of street children from a rights perspective. In A. Dawes, R, Bray, & A. Van der Merwe (Eds.), *Monitoring child well-being: A South African rights-based approach* (pp. 233–246). Cape Town, South Africa: HSRC Press.

118. Panter-Brick. (2002). Street children, human rights, and public health.

119. Ward. (2005). Monitoring the well-being of street children.

120. Joint Learning Initiative on Children and HIV/AIDS. Retrieved from www. jlica.org.

7

Transition Into Adulthood

The Changing Needs of Youth

SIMONA BIGNAMI-VAN ASSCHE AND VINOD MISHRA ■

Young people are especially vulnerable to HIV, but they are also our greatest hope for changing the course of the AIDS epidemic.[1]

Tackling HIV/AIDS among youth lies at the core of the international response to the epidemic, as it has been explicitly recognized in the Declaration of Commitment on HIV/AIDS adopted by the United Nations General Assembly Special Session (UNGASS) in 2001,[2] and reiterated in its 2006 Political Declaration on HIV/AIDS[3] as well as in the 2009–2011 Outcome Framework of the Joint United Nations Program on HIV/AIDS (UNAIDS).[4] This is because young people represent a population subgroup that is particularly vulnerable to HIV/AIDS. At the end of 2008, the latest available estimates indicate that almost 5 million young people aged 15–24 years were living with HIV/AIDS, which represented about 15% of all people living globally with the virus.[5] In addition, HIV incidence is highest in this age group. In 2008, new HIV infections among young adults aged 15–24 represented 54% of the 2.7 million of all new infections worldwide.[6]

In sub-Saharan Africa, where they represent the largest segment of the population, young people are especially vulnerable to HIV. In 2008, this region contained almost 60% of all 2.9 million young adults living with HIV/AIDS, 70% of whom were female.[7] Furthermore, data from the most recent Demographic and Health Surveys (DHSs)[8] indicate that HIV prevalence among sub-Saharan African youth is above the global average, being 3.7% overall, and 1.8% and 5.5%, respectively, for boys and girls.

Since about half of the world's population is under 25[9] and youth account for almost half of new HIV infections worldwide,[10] reducing the incidence and prevalence of HIV among young people has long been recognized as crucial to curbing the spread of the HIV/AIDS pandemic. In addition, experience shows that HIV prevention interventions for and in partnership with young people are among the most effective measures to achieve these goals.[11] Following the UNGASS Declaration of Commitment, HIV/AIDS interventions targeted at young adults have multiplied, and progress toward the specific goals set by the UNGASS has been monitored through a new system of key indicators. Recent trends in these indicators reveal that progress has been made, although comprehensive and correct HIV knowledge among youth remains low. There is also evidence of positive behavior modification and diminishing HIV prevalence among youth in at least a few countries in sub-Saharan Africa.[12] To what extent do these trends represent a real change? And, if they do, how can they be linked to existing interventions? What has worked, and what still needs to be done to expand successful interventions to other settings, and to properly monitor progress toward stated goals?

In this chapter, we attempt to answer these questions. Our starting point is the specific needs and vulnerabilities of young adults in the context of the HIV/AIDS epidemic, which we summarize in the next section. We then review available actions and interventions to tackle youth's needs and vulnerabilities, with a focus on two broad types: interventions targeted at behavior modification to improve health and access to health care (for example, HIV/AIDS information and education; interventions to improve sexual and reproductive health; interventions to encourage HIV testing; and interventions to improve access to treatment, care, and support for HIV-infected youth); and social interventions to help young adults establish sustainable livelihoods in a safe and supportive environment (for example, tuition support and vocational training). We illustrate the effectiveness of available interventions using real examples from global and regional contexts. On the basis of this review, we identify remaining gaps in the existing evidence, and we conclude with recommendations for future actions and interventions.

OVERVIEW OF THE NEEDS AND VULNERABILITIES OF YOUTH IN THE CONTEXT OF THE HIV/AIDS EPIDEMIC

Unique Needs, Unique Vulnerabilities

Youth have unique needs as they mature and adopt new social roles while being exposed to HIV/AIDS. The foundation of available HIV prevention efforts for youth is that meeting these needs is essential to reducing youth's vulnerability to risky sexual behaviors and, ultimately, HIV infection, as well as to mitigating the impact of HIV among infected youth. This framework for action has been formally endorsed through a global consultation held in May 2004 by the UNAIDS Inter-Agency Task Team on HIV and Young People (IATT/YP), which has identified four main needs of youth in the context of HIV/AIDS: to receive information about HIV/AIDS and the available protective measures; to have access to youth-friendly sexual and reproductive health care services, including voluntary counseling, testing and treatment; to have the life skills to make empowered choices and decisions about their health and their future; and to be provided with a safe and supportive environment in which they can access and use information, services, and life skills.[13]

We adopt this classification, and, in this section, we briefly review the evidence that links these needs to young people's vulnerabilities in the context of HIV/AIDS. We also appraise the specific needs and vulnerabilities of two subgroups of young adults: those who are HIV-infected, and those who were orphaned by HIV/AIDS. This allows us, in later sections, to properly evaluate available interventions that have targeted youth affected by HIV/AIDS, to better assess the gap in the existing evidence, and to make recommendations for future actions to stem the tide of HIV among youth.

NEED TO RECEIVE HIV/AIDS INFORMATION AND TO HAVE
ACCESS TO HEALTH SERVICES FOR HIV PREVENTION

Physical and sexual maturity is one of the key development phases that all young adults face. To understand intimacy and relationships is an important need that arises with this maturation.[14] In the context of the HIV/AIDS epidemic, young adults on the brink of their sexual maturity thus need, first and foremost, comprehensive and correct information about the modes of transmission and prevention of HIV, as well as additional information about sexual and reproductive health and where to obtain sexual and reproductive health services.[15] Lack of HIV/AIDS information and education makes youth vulnerable to risky behaviors such as early sexual debut, multiple sexual partners, and unprotected sexual intercourse, and thus ultimately to HIV infection and other sexually transmitted infections (STIs).[16] Limited access to basic information about sexual and reproductive health because of gender inequality highlights in particular young women's vulnerability to HIV infection, beyond their heightened biological susceptibility to the virus.[17]

When young adults are sexually active, the knowledge of prevention methods alone (particularly, condoms) is, however, not enough to reduce their exposure to risky sexual behaviors if they do not have access to these preventatives. In addition to appropriate HIV/AIDS information and education, it is also essential that youth have access to adequate sexual and reproductive health care services for HIV prevention, including HIV voluntary counseling and testing (VCT).[18]

It is important to stress that, although HIV/AIDS knowledge and access to health services are necessary conditions to reduce youth's vulnerability to HIV/AIDS, they are seldom sufficient, as documented by a large body of literature in psychological theory. Sexual behavior is widely diverse and deeply embedded in individual desires, social and cultural relationships, and environmental and economic processes. For instance, gender norms may undermine women's authority in sexual decision-making even if they have access to appropriate HIV/AIDS-related information and services, and thus limit their ability to negotiate abstinence or condom use with their partners or even put them at risk of sexual and physical violence.[19]

NEED TO ESTABLISH SUSTAINABLE LIVELIHOODS

Youth is a phase in an individual's life during which it is critical to acquire the skills necessary to become productive members of society. To establish sustainable livelihoods and develop their economic independence, youth need access to education and employment opportunities. In the context of HIV/AIDS, young adults may become vulnerable to poverty and social exclusion if they lack these skills and opportunities, and their sexual and reproductive health may be significantly compromised.[20]

Concerning education, it is well established that youth who are or have been in school are more likely to delay sexual initiation and have higher levels of contraceptive use.[21] A systematic review of recent studies has also found a link between higher educational levels and lower HIV risk as well as a greater decline in HIV prevalence among the most educated young adults in less developed countries.[22] Schooling offers an excellent means of reducing HIV risk and vulnerability, especially for young women. Girls who complete primary education are more than twice as likely to use condoms with their partners, while girls who finish secondary education are between four and seven times more likely to use condoms than girls with no education, and are less likely to be infected with HIV.[23] These studies suggest four possible pathways that link education and reduced HIV risk. First, education may prompt changes in a youth's sexual network structure, particularly in terms of number of sexual partners and age difference between partners. Second, attending school might promote confidence, self-efficacy, and the adoption of safer sexual behaviors by affecting communication within sexual networks. Third, young people attending school interact with each other in a structured environment, which may favor group negotiation of positive attitudes toward protective behaviors. Finally, education contributes to human capital formation that can encourage more positive future expectations, which in turn could support the adoption of protective behaviors. Conversely, the same studies indicate that school dropout leads young people to enter adult sexual networks in which the "rules" of sexual engagement are dictated by older partners with more experience.

Other circumstances that contribute to HIV vulnerability are high levels of youth unemployment, because these may force young people into marginal, dangerous, or illegal jobs, including sex work.[24] On the contrary, "access to career planning and job opportunities may lead to less favorable attitudes towards risky sexual behavior, and lower likelihood to engage in such behaviors."[25]

NEED TO BE PROVIDED WITH A SAFE AND SUPPORTIVE ENVIRONMENT

Young people need to be provided with a safe and supportive environment to effectively receive HIV/AIDS-related information, access services, and develop life skills. The two key elements of this environment are lack of discrimination and support through caring and close relations with families.[26]

"Family connectedness" has indeed been shown to be an important protective factor for initiation of sexual intercourse among Caribbean youth.[27] Guiella and Bignami-Van Assche have also found that family networks play a crucial role in influencing youth's HIV risk perception, and that the lack of familial support may negatively impact HIV risk perception and, in turn, protective behavior.[28] Indeed, not having parents is one of the missing protective factors that has been suggested to account for orphans' heightened vulnerability to HIV/AIDS[29] (we return to this point in the section "Specific Vulnerabilities of Orphaned Youth").

In general, communities and social environments beset by HIV-related stigma and discrimination can create obstacles to HIV prevention efforts by making people reluctant to access information and health care services, including voluntary counseling and testing, or even to use condoms with their partners for fear of being associated with the disease.[30]

These issues may be exacerbated by one's own HIV infection, as we discuss in detail in the following section.

Specific Needs and Vulnerabilities of HIV-infected Youth

The needs and vulnerabilities of youth that we reviewed in the previous section have different connotations for young adults who have already been infected with HIV. For instance, the content of HIV/AIDS information to be delivered to HIV-infected youth should focus on "positive living (good nutrition and healthy lifestyles), the likely progression of disease, treatment and care options, and how to prevent transmission to others, including mother-to-child transmission of HIV."[31]

Furthermore, the importance of accessing health care services is paramount for young adults who are living with HIV. Early diagnosis of HIV infection through timely access to HIV testing facilitates medical interventions and enables infected persons to reduce high-risk behavior and the likelihood of further HIV transmission. Access to treatment, care, and support are also needed to improve their quality of life and that of their families. In addition to leading to undue suffering, untreated symptoms reduce youth's ability to carry on with their lives and may result in frequent visits to health facilities, ultimately placing an excessive burden on health resources.[32]

Finally, a safe and supportive environment for young adults who are already HIV-infected is one in which they do not face stigma, discrimination, and social marginalization. Yet, this ideal is often far from reality. A qualitative study in Ethiopia, Tanzania, and Zambia indicated that youth are often blamed for bringing HIV into their community through their promiscuous, immoral and "improper" behavior that stems from their lack of control over their sexual desires.[33] A study in South Africa also revealed that families themselves may have strong stigmatizing attitudes toward their "evil" young children who contracted the disease. Young people are thus not comfortable sharing their HIV status with their parents, because they are ashamed and because they fear punishment and lack of care.[34] In general, studies have found that fear of rejection by family, friends, and community reduces the likelihood that people living with HIV will seek care and treatment, adhere to treatment, use condoms, or disclose their HIV status to their sexual partners.[35] Girls who are suspected to be HIV-positive bear the brunt of AIDS-related discrimination as they are more likely than boys to be denied access to education and health care.[36]

Specific Vulnerabilities of Orphaned Youth

Youth's vulnerabilities while still exposed to HIV or already HIV-infected may be compounded by the death or sickness of a family member, especially a parent. In countries heavily affected by HIV/AIDS, the number of young adults who experience these adverse circumstances has been growing, and youth orphaned by HIV/AIDS have come to represent a large share of orphans worldwide. According to the most recent global estimate, about 55% of all orphans are aged 12 to 17.[37] Estimates for seven sub-Saharan African countries with available data collected during the period 2003–2006 (Cameroon, Cote d'Ivoire, Lesotho, Malawi, Tanzania, Uganda, and Zimbabwe) place the number of orphans aged 15–17 at around 8 million, which represents 26% of the total for all orphans age 0–17.[38]

Despite these demographics, only a small number of cross-sectional studies have investigated the consequences of orphanhood (although they do not distinguish orphanhood caused by AIDS from orphanhood from other causes) for the health and well-being of young adults in the context of the HIV/AIDS epidemic. This research indicates that, for youth, the death of one or both parents is a risk factor for early and higher rates of sexual activity,[39] multiple sexual partners,[40] unprotected sexual activity,[41] unintended pregnancy,[42] and STIs, including HIV.[43]

Even though the data used in these studies are generally cross-sectional, so causal links are difficult to establish, they indicate that a number of factors contribute to negative outcomes for orphaned youth. The absence of parental control is their first source of vulnerability because, as noted earlier, it generally implies the lack of a safe and supportive environment. The economic and psychosocial distress following the death of one or both parents is the second source of vulnerability for orphaned youth. Young adults who have lost one or both parents often need to become household caretakers or income earners, so they have more demands placed on them than their peers. Financing secondary and higher education may thus become challenging for youth who have to pay fees themselves while helping support their family.[44] Indeed, existing studies indicate that orphaned adolescents are less likely to be in school than nonorphaned adolescents, and that lower schooling opportunities represent their main source of vulnerability compared to younger orphans and nonorphaned children.[45] Common reactions to these adverse circumstances are feelings of depression and hopelessness, as well as risky behaviors, which need special attention and strong protective measures.[46] Most notably, depressive symptoms have been shown to reduce adherence to treatment among HIV-infected youth.[47] Since a critical relation exists between adverse psychological outcomes among AIDS-orphaned adolescents and AIDS-related stigma, reducing the latter could be important to addressing the former.[48]

AVAILABILITY, FEASIBILITY, AND EFFECTIVENESS OF INTERVENTIONS FOR YOUTH AFFECTED BY HIV/AIDS

Youth: At the Center of the International Commitment on HIV/AIDS

The international community formally acknowledged for the first time the specific needs and vulnerabilities of youth affected by HIV/AIDS in the 2001 UNGASS Declaration of Commitment on HIV/AIDS.[49] The Declaration dedicated governments to meeting specific goals to fight HIV/AIDS among youth, in particular to "ensure that at least 95 per cent of young men and women aged 15 to 24 have access to the information, education, including peer education and youth-specific HIV education, and services necessary to develop the life skills required to reduce their vulnerability to HIV infection by 2010".[50] Five years later, the new Political Declaration on HIV/AIDS, adopted by the UNGASS in 2006, renewed the commitment of the Member States "to ensure an HIV-free future generation through the implementation of comprehensive, evidence-based prevention strategies, responsible sexual behavior, including the use of condoms, evidence and skills-based youth specific HIV education, mass media interventions, and the provision of youth friendly health services."[51] Empowering young people to protect themselves from HIV/AIDS has also more recently been set as one of the eight priority focus areas in UNAIDS' 2009–2011 Outcome Framework.[52]

"The Declaration of Commitment has galvanized global action, strengthened advocacy by civil society, and helped guide national decision-making about youth by placing their needs and vulnerabilities at the core of the international response to the epidemic."[53] One of the crucial efforts underlying these developments has been to build a consensus about the most effective programs and interventions to implement in order to meet the Declaration's targets for young people. This effort has been led by the UNAIDS IATT/YP, a working group created in December 2001 purposively "to support an accelerated, harmonized and expanded global, regional, and country-level response to the HIV/AIDS epidemic among young people."[54]

The UNAIDS IATT/YP began reviewing the evidence about the efficacy of interventions to prevent the spread of HIV among young people in developing countries through a global consultation held in May 2004. This meeting led to identifying the series of youth's needs and vulnerabilities that we have presented in the previous section, as well as the actions and interventions available and effective to address them. The results of this study are contained in a report[55] and have been updated by a series of briefs aimed to provide guidance to policy-makers.[56] The consensus that has emerged from this body of work is that "we know what works in preventing HIV among young people."[57] The remainder of this section summarizes the evidence and key arguments that support this conclusion, as well as the obstacles that still need to be overcome to halt the spread of the epidemic among youth.

Available and Effective Interventions to Tackle HIV/AIDS Among Youth

The IATT/YP identifies four core areas of action to prevent the spread of HIV and to attenuate its consequences among youth.[58] These are represented in Figure 7.1, alongside the needs and vulnerabilities that they address and that we presented in the previous section. We use this framework to review available and effective interventions to tackle HIV/AIDS among youth in developing countries.

The first core area of action is to provide young people with correct and appropriate information on how to protect themselves and their partners from HIV transmission. These strategies address youth's need for HIV/AIDS information and education

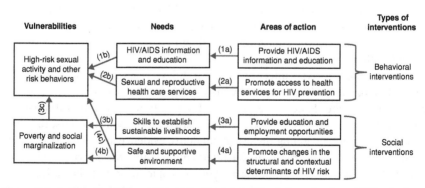

Figure 7.1 Actions and interventions to address youth's needs and vulnerabilities in the context of HIV/AIDS

(*pathway 1a*) with the goal of reducing their vulnerability to high-risk sexual activity and other risk behaviors (*pathway 1b*) and thus, ultimately, to HIV infection. Available interventions in this area may include some combination of the following: providing comprehensive and correct information about HIV prevention, modes of transmission, and common misconceptions about HIV and AIDS; providing information about sexual and reproductive health (sexuality and intimacy, contraceptive use for dual protection, safer sex, sexually transmitted infections) and where to obtain sexual and reproductive health services; and informing HIV-infected youth about treatment and care options, and about how to reduce the risk of transmission to others.[59] Although schools are the key setting for providing information and teaching youth the life skills necessary to prevent HIV, a number of other channels are available, including parents, peers, workplaces and job centers, health service providers, and the media.[60]

The second core area of action is to promote access to health services for HIV prevention among youth. These services include providing access to information, condoms, and harm reduction (where injecting drug use is prevalent) and access to diagnosis (testing) and treatment for STIs and HIV.[61] Strategies in this area address youth's need for health services (*pathway 2a*) with the goal of reducing their vulnerability to high-risk sexual activity and other risk behaviors (*pathway 2b*) and thus, ultimately, to HIV infection. Available interventions may include some combination of the following:[62] improving the knowledge and skills of health care providers; making facilities more responsive to the specific needs of young people, for example by changing the physical environment or opening hours; reaching out from the facility into the community to provide information, generate demand, and create community support; and involving other sectors, such as schools and the media, to provide information about the services, their location, and their availability, as well as to mobilize community support.

The third core area of action is to provide education and employment opportunities to young people. Strategies in this area address youth's need to develop life skills to establish sustainable livelihoods and develop their economic independence (*pathway 3a*), in order to limit their vulnerability to poverty and social marginalization (*pathway 3b*) and, by doing so, also limit their vulnerability to high-risk sexual activity and other risk behaviors that lead to contracting STIs, including HIV (*pathway 3c*). Interventions to promote access to education and employment opportunities may combine tuition support, peer education, and vocational training through schools and communities.[63]

The fourth area of action is to promote changes in the structural and contextual determinants of HIV risk at the family, community, and national levels. These include a range of factors that undermine young people's individual development and human rights, such as inequity, stigma, and discrimination; exploitation and abuse, in particular for women; and social unrest and migration.[64] Strategies in this area address young people's need for safe and supportive environments in which they can access and use information, services, and life skills (*pathway 4a*), in order to reduce their vulnerability to HIV risk behavior and infection, to poverty and social exclusion, or to both (*pathways 4b–4c*). Changes to the structural and contextual determinants of HIV risk are thus fundamental to making HIV prevention sustainable[65] and can be implemented through interventions at different levels: close to the young adult (parents, peers and teachers); at the community level (religious leaders, civil society organizations, youth centers, schools, workplaces and other institutions); or at the wider levels of the media and policy-making.

Interventions and programs that correspond to the first and second areas of action are ultimately aimed at changing individual behavior and the risks associated with sexual activity in the context of HIV/AIDS. Social interventions, on the other hand, aim to create social conditions that facilitate health promotion and risk reduction in the other two areas of action identified. In the following section, we review which interventions in these areas have been effective among those available and identified here.

"What We Know Works"

The evidence about "what we know works" for HIV prevention among youth is vast and increasing. As Dick et al. summarized, "during the past 20 years, and despite the continued lack of an effective vaccine, the armamentarium for preventing the transmission and decreasing the impact of HIV and AIDS has slowly grown."[66] Although most of the evidence about the effectiveness of this "armamentarium" of HIV interventions and programs comes from developed countries, an increasing body of research has become available for developing countries as well, especially for youth. Behavioral interventions have been by far the greatest focus of this research. Social interventions, on the contrary, are more rarely studied because few rigorously tested approaches are available and because they are seldom carried out in isolation from behavioral interventions, which makes it difficult to disentangle their specific effects.

It should be recognized that assessing the effectiveness of behavioral and social HIV interventions among youth poses delicate problems of definitions and faces important limitations of available evaluation methods, which we address later in the section "The Gaps in the Available Evidence." Here, we rather summarize general conclusions about the effectiveness of these interventions that can be drawn from the existing evidence in spite of their inherent problems and limitations.

EFFECTIVENESS OF INTERVENTIONS AIMED TO INCREASE HIV/AIDS AWARENESS AND KNOWLEDGE

HIV prevention programs and interventions among youth in developing countries have benefited from the experience gathered in developed countries since the early 1980s. There, youth HIV prevention programs have gone through two main phases. At the beginning of the 1980s, the first generation of HIV prevention programs promoted HIV/AIDS awareness and knowledge alone (*pathway 1a* in Figure 7.1), with the hope that it would produce the necessary behavioral changes. These programs successfully increased accurate knowledge about HIV transmission and prevention strategies, but unfortunately they did not lead directly to behavior change.[67] To address this issue, the second generation of HIV prevention programs in developed countries tried to go beyond simply increasing knowledge, and rather addressed "perceptions of risk, safer-sex intentions, assertive communication, and condom use skills, in addition to HIV/STI knowledge"[68] (*pathways 1a* and *1b* in Figure 7.1). This latter group of programs has represented the blueprint for youth HIV prevention programs in developing countries, which have thus generally been built to fulfill three main objectives: (1) raise HIV/AIDS awareness and knowledge, (2) promote attitudes and intentions toward low-risk sexual behaviors as a proximal determinant of behavioral change, and (3) promote a change in the behavior of youth in a direction that would decrease their risk of HIV infection.

Existing research shows that these programs have been successful in improving HIV/AIDS awareness and knowledge among youth in developing countries through two main channels: schools and the media. According to a recent review, the most effective interventions through schools have employed a range of activities such as lectures, plays, songs, and poems that are included in the school curriculum to deliver HIV/AIDS-related information and sensitize youth to HIV risk through peer educators and teachers, and have used a "cascade" approach to train teachers as widely as possible.[69] The most effective interventions through the media have taken the form of sustained multichannel mass media campaigns through radio and television programs that were adapted to the social context.[70] Globally, progress has indeed been made: in 17 out of 45 countries with available data, comprehensive HIV knowledge among females aged 15–24 has increased by 10 percentage points during the period 1999–2008; HIV knowledge has shown an increasing trend among men as well in 7 out of 12 countries with similar trend data. However, less than 50% of young people in developing countries had achieved comprehensive and correct knowledge about HIV/AIDS.[71]

Nonetheless, the evidence about the effectiveness of these interventions in changing attitudes toward HIV and, ultimately, sexual behavior is mixed. The two studies cited above suggest that the interventions they reviewed have been overall effective in changing sexual behavior and social norms surrounding HIV/AIDS, but other studies do not.[72] As we explain later, the main difficulty in drawing general conclusions from existing studies seems to be one of evaluation methods and definitions used. In spite of these limitations, it is well established that reductions in risky behaviors among youth, including condom use, have been occurring in a number of developing countries. HIV prevalence among young women attending antenatal clinics in urban or rural areas (or both) has also declined between 2000 and 2008 in 14 of the 17 countries with available data.[73]

EFFECTIVENESS OF INTERVENTIONS THAT PROMOTE ACCESS
TO HEALTH SERVICES FOR HIV PREVENTION

A separate literature has shown the effectiveness of interventions that promote access to health services for HIV prevention, including VCT. A consensus exists that the key characteristics of successful programs have been: (1) to adequately train service providers to offer a comprehensive package of services that may extend to adolescents' sexual and reproductive health; (2) to make improvements to clinic facilities in order to offer youth-friendly health services; (3) to involve multiple service providers such as nongovernmental organizations (NGOs), private practitioners, pharmacists, and traditional providers; and (4) to offer services in a range of different settings, including schools, the workplace, and community-based distribution points. To maximize effectiveness, improvements in health services have been generally accompanied by activities in the community to increase awareness of available HIV services, to generate youth demand for such services, and to increase access to and use of services through referral systems and support.[74]

Yet, "to date there are no studies that have rigorously followed youth in the developing world to determine whether they reduce their HIV risk behaviors as a result of undergoing VCT."[75] In addition, existing research about adults has reached mixed conclusions about this topic. Earlier studies have generally shown that adults accessing VCT in developed and developing countries reduced their HIV risk behavior by delaying intercourse, having a more limited number of sexual partners, and using condoms consistently.[76] Later studies, however, have rather observed an increase in risky sexual behaviors following HIV testing for HIV-negative adults, which was in part explained by increased access to and availability of HIV treatment.[77]

In addition, existing studies of behavioral change preventive interventions have almost entirely targeted people who are not infected with HIV. Little evidence thus exists about the effectiveness of behavioral prevention interventions focusing on people who are HIV positive, especially in developing countries.[78]

SOCIAL INTERVENTIONS AND COMPREHENSIVE APPROACHES TO HIV PREVENTION

There is a growing consensus that HIV prevention interventions that focus only on changing individual behavior are unlikely to produce long-term behavioral changes. Efforts to achieve more robust and durable effects have thus led to broader conceptualizations of adolescent sexual risk behavior in the context of their family, community, and the larger social environment.[79] The most recent recommendations for HIV intervention programs in developing countries are thus to take a comprehensive approach to empower young people to protect themselves from HIV/AIDS:

> By putting young people's leadership at the centre of national responses, providing rights-based sexual and reproductive health education and services and empowering young people to prevent sexual and other transmission of HIV infection among their peers. By ensuring access to HIV testing and prevention efforts with and for young people in the context of sexuality education. And by ensuring enabling legal environments, education and employment opportunities to reduce vulnerability to HIV.[80]

However, there are few examples of rigorously tested approaches concerning the effectiveness of social interventions that primarily aim to address HIV/AIDS among youth in developing countries by addressing the contextual circumstances of risk behavior such as poverty, marginalization, stigma, and discrimination. Although there have been some successes, such as increasing the enrollment of adolescent girls in schools,[81] it is not always clear what can be done to change the contextual determinants of youth's vulnerability—and for those interventions that have been implemented, the mechanisms of action are not clear and the evidence of their effectiveness remains weak.

Published studies on interventions and programs designed to reduce HIV/AIDS-related stigma in developing countries are particularly scarce.[82] A recent review identified 22 experimental or quasi-experimental studies that have evaluated interventions aimed at reducing AIDS stigma, most of them (16 out of 22) in developed countries.[83] Of the studies carried out in developing countries, only two focused on young adults.[84] These interventions were designed to reduce stigma at the community level by increasing the tolerance toward persons living with HIV/AIDS (PLHIV) through the provision of education and information about HIV/AIDS. The review concluded that the effectiveness of interventions carried out in developing countries was generally low, since they had achieved only small and short-lived improvements in attitudes and tolerance toward PLHIV from both the general population and health personnel.

The effectiveness of social interventions is also difficult to assess because they are seldom implemented in isolation from behavioral interventions. Comprehensive intervention programs inscribe behavioral interventions into the larger contextual changes sought by implementing social interventions, and these have been shown to be key for sustainable HIV prevention. The effectiveness of these comprehensive interventions is generally gauged indirectly, by evaluating the association at the macro level between HIV prevalence or incidence and existing national AIDS programs. Uganda and Namibia are the two success stories most often cited in this respect (see Box 7.1).

Box 7.1

UGANDA AND NAMIBIA FIGHT AIDS

Uganda's Ministry of Health adopted the ABC (Abstain, Be faithful to a single partner, and use Condoms) approach to fighting HIV/AIDS in 1987, and deployed it through a broad range of governmental and nongovernmental organizations. The reason for the success of Uganda's ABC strategy is its emphasis on more than behavioral change alone. Indeed, "the government focused on prevention among heterosexual couples through community mobilization and education, but also pioneered programs designed to combat stigma and taboos associated with discussion of sexuality and to promote abstinence, monogamy, and condom use as tools to protect oneself from contracting HIV. Programs aimed to involve HIV-infected people in public education, to persuade individuals and couples to be tested and counseled, and to improve the status of women, and involved many different sectors and actors such as religious organizations to traditional healers."[85] Most observers agree that this strategy played an important role in battling the epidemic and reducing HIV infection rates in Uganda from 18% in 1992 to 6% in 2005.[86]

In recent years, the Government of Namibia has also become committed to strengthening the country's response to HIV/AIDS. Reducing HIV incidence is the ultimate goal of its most recent 5-year strategic plan, which has prompted the country to more than double its domestic spending on HIV programs and to mobilize external support. The government has enacted further legislation to sustain the HIV prevention effort in 2007, which includes prohibition of HIV as a basis for discrimination. Recent data indicate that these programs have already been effective in improving HIV/AIDS-related knowledge (79% of secondary schools now include skill-based HIV education in their curriculum), increasing HIV testing uptake (now the highest among the 38 countries surveyed by the Demographic and Health Survey), and reducing risk behaviors such as early sexual initiation and condom use. HIV prevalence among women attending antenatal clinics has also declined from 18% in 2003 to 14% in 2007.[87]

THE GAPS IN THE AVAILABLE EVIDENCE

Under the terms of the Declaration of Commitment on HIV/AIDS, success in the AIDS response is measured by the achievement of concrete, time-bound targets. In keeping with these mandates, in 2002, the UNAIDS Secretariat collaborated with national AIDS committees, UNAIDS cosponsors, and other partners to develop a series of core indicators to measure progress in implementing the Declaration of Commitment.[88] Analyzing data provided by countries with respect to these indicators, the UN General Assembly (UNGA) last reviewed progress in implementing the Declaration of Commitment during its High-Level Meeting on AIDS, held in June 2006.[89] The UNGA stressed that progress had been made, but that "HIV prevention efforts remain notably inadequate for young people."[90] The UNGA indicated that this was because of three main reasons: existing interventions were not comprehensive enough (thus failing to address some of the key determinants of youth's vulnerability), not all sectors were involved to implement them, and young people were not sufficiently involved in the prevention effort. In addition, the UNGA stressed that "stigma and discrimination remain key barriers to HIV prevention, treatment and support programs," especially for young women.[91]

Existing studies on youth HIV interventions form a large body of literature that has enabled us to know what programs work best and what needs to be done to scale up HIV prevention efforts among youth. We presented the key findings of this literature in the previous section. We stressed in more than one instance that assessing the effectiveness of behavioral and social HIV interventions among youth poses, however, delicate problems of definitions and faces important limitations of available evaluation methods, which we illustrate in this section.

Evaluating the effectiveness of complex areas of program development and delivery such as the prevention of HIV among young people is not a straightforward task, for two main reasons. First, interventions and programs differ widely, insofar as each emphasizes a unique approach to risk reduction, and varies along multiple dimensions, including underlying theoretical frameworks, targeted risk factors, specific individuals involved, and outcomes measured. Second, and perhaps most importantly, youth interventions implemented so far have been seldom designed for robust evaluation, and evaluation data have been rarely analyzed and disseminated, especially in developing countries. Both issues contribute to the paucity and low quality of existing evaluations, as several authors have indicated.[92]

We review these problems and limitations of existing studies about the effectiveness of HIV interventions among youth by focusing on two issues: the limitations of existing studies and the "gray areas" that have received only limited attention.

Does "What We Know Works" Really Work?
The Limitations of Existing Studies

We argue that this assessment disregards an inherent limitation of existing HIV prevention efforts: the gaps in the empirical evidence that is necessary to correctly monitor and evaluate progress toward stated goals. Particularly, two main lacunae hamper our knowledge of the effectiveness of youth HIV interventions: first, existing indicators to monitor progress toward the goals set by the Declaration of Commitment are inadequate to properly do so; second, there are no specified guidelines to determine how changes in core indicators can be linked to existing interventions.

GAP 1: AVAILABLE INDICATORS TO MONITOR PROGRESS TOWARD THE GOALS SET BY THE DECLARATION OF COMMITMENT ARE INADEQUATE

Few core indicators are available to monitor progress toward the goals set by the Declaration of Commitment that refer specifically to youth.[93] These are: the percentage of young women and men aged 15–24 who both correctly identify ways of preventing the sexual transmission of HIV and who reject major misconceptions about HIV transmission, the percentage of young women and men aged 15–24 who have had sexual intercourse before the age of 15, and the percentage of young women and men aged 15–24 who are infected with HIV. Other key indicators to monitor changes in risk behaviors with respect to multiple sexual partnerships and condom use are to be collected for all adults aged 15–49,[94] although UNAIDS recommends that they should be disaggregated by sex and age. This is also the case for indicators to evaluate national HIV programs,[95] as well as national programs for HIV-infected individuals and for orphans.[96] Yet, this recommendation clashes with the reality that age and sex differences in key indicators are not adequately monitored in most countries, although there has been some improvement in the latest round of reporting.[97]

It is also not possible to track with available indicators the number and proportion of young adults who are orphaned or made vulnerable by HIV/AIDS because estimates for orphans and vulnerable children are generally presented for all children less than 15 years of age, and they do not distinguish parental deaths due to HIV/AIDS from those due to other causes. The lack of this information is critical to permit tracking of the situation of orphaned and vulnerable youth, since improved access to ARVs increases the chance that a child will become an adolescent before becoming an orphan because the former translates into longer survival for his or her parents.

GAP 2: LINKING CHANGES IN CORE INDICATORS TO AVAILABLE INTERVENTIONS IS DIFFICULT

Several authors have stressed the difficulties of definition and measurement associated with evaluating the effectiveness of youth HIV interventions.[98] This is mainly because only a few published *experimental* studies test the effectiveness of an intervention to reduce behavioral risk among youth using both behavioral and biomedical endpoints (incidence of STIs including HIV). As we have indicated earlier, these studies have generally reached mixed conclusions about the link between interventions and changes in sexual behavior and HIV incidence in developing countries.[99]

At the same time, if we look at *observational* studies from countries and communities that have documented behavioral change, it is difficult to ascertain exactly what produced the change; this is especially true for specific behavioral interventions. Even for the "success stories" of Uganda and Namibia (see Box 7.1), the actual interventions (scientifically tested or otherwise) that produced the observed behavioral changes have seldom been specified in published studies.[100] Without an established methodology to link changes in core indicators to available interventions, our capability to understand how to achieve stated goals and reproduce effective interventions is limited.

Ross et al. have recently proposed a method for reviewing evidence on the effectiveness of interventions that aim to contribute to reaching the global goals related to

HIV prevention among young people in developing countries.[101] However, this method relies on an evaluation ex post of published studies, and does not draw from intervention data that have been collected in a standardized fashion to allow for comparisons over time and across countries.

What Do We Still Not Know?

The Declaration of Commitment has focused most prevention efforts among youth in developing countries around behavioral interventions targeted at improving HIV/ AIDS knowledge and education and, to a more limited extent, access to health services. Attention to other core areas of action, most notably social interventions for youth, is recent, and the evidence about the effectiveness of comprehensive programs for HIV prevention in developing countries is limited. Indeed, we are not aware of any comprehensive review of the effectiveness of social interventions targeting youth in developing countries.

We argue that, without a full understanding of the effectiveness of behavioral and social interventions, we do not have enough evidence to really know what works for HIV prevention among youth in developing countries. Indeed, we believe that this is one of the keys to understanding why we are failing to reach the targets of the Declaration of Commitment, and why progress toward these goals has been relatively slow.

RECOMMENDED ACTIONS AND INTERVENTIONS

To address the gaps that we have identified above, we make three main recommendations.

- *Recommendation 1: Improve and expand available indicators.*
  We recommend that actions be taken to improve available indicators to monitor progress toward the goals set by the Declaration of Commitment. To do so, the set of core indicators to monitor progress toward these goals should be expanded to monitor changes in risk behaviors among youth with respect to multiple and concurrent sexual partnerships as well condom use. In addition, we suggest developing and monitoring new indicators with respect to AIDS-related stigma and the situation of orphaned youth.
- *Recommendation 2: Standardize intervention evaluation procedures.*
  We recommend that a standard methodology be developed to design, plan, and evaluate the effectiveness of interventions implemented to achieve the goals of the Declaration of Commitment on HIV/AIDS. The methodology should be included ex ante in the intervention design, and should differ for experimental and observational studies.
- *Recommendation 3: Systematically review existing knowledge about social interventions and comprehensive approaches to HIV prevention.*
  We recommend that a comprehensive review of existing social interventions for youth in developing countries be undertaken using a standardized

evaluation procedure (as suggested above), to identify what programs work best in different contexts.

CONCLUSION

In the context of the HIV/AIDS epidemic, young people have unique and multifaceted needs, and are vulnerable to risky sexual behaviors and HIV infection insofar as these needs are not met. An essential package of HIV prevention, treatment, care, and support interventions is now in place in many countries as part of efforts to ensure universal access. Although recent trends seem to indicate some improvement, the situation of youth in the context of the HIV/AIDS epidemic remains critical, especially in sub-Saharan Africa.

We have argued that one of the critical factors that hampers our progress toward the goals of the Declaration of Commitment is the gaps in the available evidence. Existing indicators to monitor progress toward the goals set by the Declaration of Commitment are inadequate, there are no specified guidelines to determine how trends in core indicators can be linked to existing interventions, and there is surprisingly little empirical evidence about the effectiveness of social interventions. We thus recommend improving and expanding the core indicators for youth and standardizing intervention evaluation procedures to better tackle and monitor the situation of young adults in the context of the HIV/AIDS epidemic.

NOTE

1. UNAIDS. (2004). *Report on the global HIV/AIDS epidemic 2004.* Geneva, Switzerland: UNAIDS; (p. 97).
2. United Nations General Assembly. (2004). *Resolution adopted by the General Assembly: Declaration of commitment on HIV/AIDS.* New York: United Nations General Assembly. Retrieved May 7, 2010, http://www.un.org/ga/aids/docs/aress262.pdf
3. United Nations General Assembly. (2006). *Resolution adopted by the General Assembly on June 15, 2006: Political declaration on HIV/AIDS.* New York: United Nations General Assembly. Retrieved May 7, 2010, http://data.unaids.org/pub/Report/2006/ 20060615_hlm_politicaldeclaration_ares60262_en.pdf
4. UNAIDS. (2010). *Joint action for results: Outcome framework 2009–2011.* Geneva, Switzerland: UNAIDS. Retrieved September 10, 2010, http://data.unaids.org/pub/Report/2010/jc1713_joint_action_en.pdf
5. UNICEF. (2009). *Children and AIDS, fourth stocktaking report, 2009.,* Table 1. New York: UNICEF.
6. UNAIDS. (2010). *Outlook report 2010.* Geneva, Switzerland: UNAIDS. Retrieved September 10, 2010, from http://data.unaids.org/pub/Outlook/2010/20100713_outlook_report_web_en.pdf
7. UNICEF. (2009). *Children and AIDS.*
8. These surveys were carried out between 2005 and 2010 in Cameroon, Ethiopia, Guinea, Lesotho, Liberia, Mali, Niger, Rwanda, Senegal, Swaziland, Uganda, and Zimbabwe.
9. UNFPA. (2006). *State of world population 2005.* New York: UNFPA.
10. UNAIDS. (2010). *Outlook.*

11. Dick, B., Ferguson, J., & Ross, D.A. (2006). Introduction and rationale. In UNAIDS Inter-agency Task Team on HIV and Young People (Eds.), *Preventing HIV/AIDS in young people* (pp. 1–14). Geneva, Switzerland: World Health Organization; UNAIDS, *Outlook*, 2010.

12. UNAIDS. (2008). *Report on the global HIV/AIDS epidemic 2008*. Geneva, Switzerland: UNAIDS. UNICEF. (2009). *Children and AIDS*.

13. UNAIDS IATT/YP. (2004). *At the crossroads: Accelerating youth's access to HIV/ AIDS interventions*. New York: UNAIDS IATT/YP, p. 5. Retrieved May 6, 2010, http://www.unfpa.org/upload/lib_pub_file/316_filename_UNFPA_ Crossroads.pdf

14. UNAIDS IATT/YP. (2004). *At the crossroads*, p. 5; Ruland, C. D., et al. (2005). *Adolescents: Orphaned and vulnerable in the time of HIV/AIDS*. Family Health International, YouthNet Program, Youth Issues Paper 6, p. 4. Arlington, Virginia: Family Health International.

15. Kirby, D. B., Laris, B. A., & Rolleri, L. A. (2007). Sex and HIV education programs: Their impact on sexual behaviors of young people throughout the world. *Journal of Adolescent Health, 40*, 206–217; UNAIDS IATT/YP. (2008). *Guidance brief: Overview of HIV interventions for young people*. New York: UNFPA.

16. UNAIDS. (1997). *Impact of HIV and sexual health education on the sexual behavior of young people: A review update*. Geneva, Switzerland: UNAIDS; Kirby, Laris, & Rolleri (2007). Sex and HIV; UNAIDS IATT/YP. (2008). *Guidance brief.*

17. Global Coalition on Women and AIDS. (2006). *Keeping the promise: An agenda for action on women and AIDS*. Geneva, Switzerland: UNAIDS.

18. UNAIDS IATT/YP. (2004). *At the crossroads*, pp. 3, 5; UNAIDS IATT/YP. (2008). *Guidance brief.*

19. Varga, C.A. (1999). South African young people's sexual dynamics: implications for behavioral responses to HIV/AIDS. In J. Caldwell, et al. (Eds.), *Resistances to behavioral change to reduce HIV/AIDS infection in predominantly heterosexual epidemics in Third World countries* (pp. 13–34). Canberra, Australia: Health Transition Center, National Center for Epidemiology and Population Health, Australian National University; Andersson, N., et al. (2007). Risk factors for domestic physical violence: National cross-sectionals household surveys in eight Southern African countries. *BMC Women's Health, 7*, 11–20; Khobotlo, M., et al. (2009). *Lesotho: HIV prevention response and modes of transmission analysis*. Maseru, Lesotho: National AIDS Commission; UNAIDS. (2008). *Report on the Global HIV/AIDS Epidemic 2008.*

20. UNAIDS/IATT/YP. (2004). *At the crossroads*; National Research Council and Institute of Medicine. (2005). *Growing up global: The changing transitions to adulthood in developing countries. Panel on Transitions to Adulthood in Developing Countries*. Washington, DC: The National Academies Press; UNAIDS IATT/YP. *Guidance brief*, 2008.

21. National Research Council and Institute of Medicine. (2005). *Growing up global.*

22. Hargreaves, J. R., et al. (2008). Systematic review exploring time trends in the association between educational attainment and risk of HIV infection in sub-Saharan Africa. *AIDS, 22*, 403–414.

23. Hargreaves, J. R., & Boler, T. (2006). *Girl power: The impact of girls' education on HIV and sexual behaviour*. London: ActionAid International.

24. International Labor Organization. (2006). *HIV/AIDS and work: Global estimates, impact on children and youth, and response.* Geneva, Switzerland: International Labor Organization.

25. Jemmott, J. B. Jammott, L. S. & Fong, G. T. (1992). Sexual behaviors among black male adolescents: Effect of an AIDS prevention intervention. *American Journal of Public Health, 82,* 372–377; Pronyk, P. M., et al. (2008). A combined microfinance and training intervention can reduce HIV risk behavior in young female participants. *AIDS, 22,* 1659–1665.

26. UNAIDS IATT/YP. (2004). *At the crossroads,* p. 5;; UNAIDS IATT/YP. (2008). *Guidance brief.*

27. Blum, R. W., & Ireland, M. (2004). Reducing risk, increasing protective factors: Findings from the Caribbean Youth Health Survey. *Journal of Adolescent Health, 35,* 493–500.

28. Guiella, G., & Bignami-Van Assche, S. (2010, April). *Determinants of HIV risk perception among adolescents in four sub-Saharan African countries.* Paper presented at the annual meeting of the Population Association of America, Dallas, Texas.

29. Ruland et al. (2005). *Adolescents.*

30. Brown, L., Macintyre, K., & Trujillo, L. (2003). Interventions to reduce HIV/AIDS stigma: What have we learnt? *AIDS Education and Prevention, 15,* 49–69; MacPhall, C. L., et al. (2008). 'You must do the test to know your status': Attitudes to HIV voluntary counseling and testing for adolescents among South African youth and parents. *Health Education & Behavior, 35,* 87–104; Nyblade, L., et al. (2003). *Disentangling HIV and AIDS stigma in Ethiopia, Tanzania and Zambia.* Washington DC: International Center for Research on Women; Mahajan, A. P., et al. (2008). Stigma in the HIV/AIDS epidemic: A review of the literature and recommendations for the way forward. *AIDS, 22,* S67–S79.

31. UNAIDS IATT/YP. (2008). *Guidance brief,* p. 5.

32. Brown, L. K., et al. (2000). Children and adolescents living with HIV and AIDS: A review. *Journal of Child Psychology and Psychiatry, 41,* 81–96; UNAIDS. (2008). *Report*; UNAIDS. (2010). *Key populations: Young people.* Geneva, Switzerland: UNAIDS.

33. Nyblade et al. (2003). *Disentangling.*

34. Campbell, C., et al. (2005). 'I have an evil child at my house': Stigma and HIV/AIDS management in a South African community. *American Journal of Public Health, 95,* 808–815.

35. Pugatch, D., Bennett L., & Patterson, D. (2005). HIV medication adherence in adolescents: A qualitative study. *Journal of HIV/AIDS Prevention & Education for Adolescents and Children, 5,* 9–29; Brown et al. (2000). *Interventions*; Nyblade et al. (2003). *Disentangling*; Rao, D., et al. (2007). Stigma and social barriers to medication adherence with urban youth living with HIV. *AIDS Care, 19,* 28–33; Mahajan et al. (2008). Stigma.

36. Engender Health. (2003). *No missed opportunities: Engender Health response to HIV/AIDS* (pp. 1–4). New York: Engender Health.

37. UNAIDS, UNICEF & USAID. (2004). *Children on the brink 2004: A joint report of new orphans estimates and a framework for action.* Geneva, Switzerland: UNAIDS, UNICEF, USAID.

38. Mishra, V., & Bignami-Van Assche, S. (2008). *Orphans and vulnerable children in high HIV-prevalence countries in sub-Saharan Africa.* DHS Analytical Studies

no.15 (p. 26, Table 10). Calverton, MD: Macro International. These figures overestimate the burden of AIDS-related orphanhood insofar as all these studies classify as orphans children and young adults who have lost one or both parents, and generally cannot establish with certainty whether parental death was due to AIDS.

39. Hallman, K. (2006). *Orphanhood and adolescent HIV risk behaviors in KwaZulu-Natal, South Africa.* Paper presented at the Annual Meeting of Population Association of America, Los Angeles, California, April 30–May 1; Thurman, T. R., et al. (2006). Sexual risk behavior among South African adolescents: Is orphan status a factor? *AIDS and Behavior, 10,* 627–635; Juma, M., Askew I., & Ferguson, A. (2007). *Situation analysis of the sexual and reproductive health and HIV risks and prevention needs of older orphaned and vulnerable children in Nyanza Province, Kenya.* Nairobi, Kenya: Department of Children's Services, Government of Kenya; Campbell, P., & Handa, S. (2008). *A situation analysis of orphans in 11 eastern and southern African countries.* Nairobi, Kenya: UNICEF-ESARO; Mishra & Bignami-Van Assche, *Orphans,* 2008; Nyamukapa, C., et al. (2008). HIV-associated orphanhood and children's psychosocial distress: Theoretical framework tested with data from Zimbabwe. *American Journal of Public Health, 98,* 133–41; Palermo, T., & Peterman, A. (2008). Orphanhood as a risk factor for child marriage, sexual debut and teen pregnancy in sub-Saharan Africa. Nairobi, Kenya: UNICEF-ESARO.

40. Hallman. (2006). *Orphanhood*; Operario, D., et al. (2007). Prevalence of parental death among young people in South Africa and risk for HIV infection, *Journal of Acquired Immune Deficiency Syndromes, 44,* 93–8.

41. Hallman. (2006). *Orphanhood*; Juma et al. (2007). *Situation.*

42. Gregson, S., et al. (2005). HIV infection and reproductive health in teenage women orphaned and made vulnerable by AIDS in Zimbabwe. *AIDS Care, 17,* 785–794.

43. Ibid.; Kissin, D., et al. (2007). HIV seroprevalence in street youth, St. Petersburg, Russia, *AIDS, 21,* 2333–40; Operario et al. (2007). Prevalence; Birdthistle, I. J., et al. (2008). From affected to infected? Orphanhood and HIV risk among female adolescents in urban Zimbabwe. *AIDS, 22,* 759–766.

44. UNAIDS, UNICEF & USAID. (2004). *Children on the brink*; Ruland et al. (2005). *Adolescents.*

45. Mishra & Bignami-Van Assche. (2008). *Orphans.*

46. UNAIDS, UNICEF, & USAID. (2004). *Children on the brink.* (2005). Ruland et al. *Adolescents*; Thurman, T. R., et al. (2006). Psychosocial support and marginalization of youth-headed households in Rwanda. *AIDS Care, 18,* 220–229; Cluver, L., Gardner, F., & Operario, D. (2007). Psychological distress among AIDS-orphaned children in urban South Africa. *Journal of Child Psychology and Psychiatry, 48,* 755–63; Boris, N. W., et al. (2008). Depressive symptoms in youths head of households in Rwanda: Correlates and implications for interventions. *Archive of Pediatric and Adolescent Medicine, 162,* 836–843.

47. Hosek, S., Harper, G., & Domanico, R. (2005). Predictors of medication adherence among HIV-infected youth. *Psychology, Health, and Medicine, 10,* 166–79.

48. Cluver, L., Gardner, F., & Operario, D. (2008). Effects of stigma on the mental health of adolescents orphaned by AIDS. *Journal of Adolescent Health, 42,* 410–417; Cluver, L., & Orkin, M. (2009). Cumulative risk and AIDS-orphanhood:

Interactions of stigma, bullying and poverty on child mental health in South Africa. *Social Science and Medicine, 69,* 1186–1193.

49. United Nations General Assembly. (2004). *Declaration of commitment.*
50. United Nations General Assembly. (2004). *Declaration of commitment* (pp. 7–8). Note that four of the targets outlined in the *Declaration of Commitment* are also indicators for measuring the implementation of the Millennium Development Goals. These are to improve knowledge about HIV/AIDS among young people, to increase condom use among young people, to increase current school attendance among orphans, and to reduce HIV prevalence among young people aged 15–24.
51. United Nations General Assembly. (2006). *Political declaration,* p. 4.
52. UNAIDS. (2010). *Joint action.*
53. United Nations General Assembly. (2004). *Declaration of commitment,* pp. 1, 3.
54. United Nations Population Fund. (2011). "HIV and Young People", Retrieved January 30, 2011, from http://www.unfpa.org/public/iattyp
55. WHO. (2006). *Preventing HIV in young people: A systematic review of the evidence from developing countries* Geneva, Switzerland: WHO and UNAIDS Inter-Agency Task Team on HIV and Young People.
56. UNAIDS IATT/YP. (2008). *Guidance brief;* UNAIDS IATT/YP. (2008). *Community-based HIV interventions for young people.* New York: UNFPA; UNAIDS IATT/YP. (2008). *HIV interventions for young people in the education sector.* New York: UNFPA; UNAIDS IATT/YP. (2008). *HIV Interventions for young people in the workplace.* New York: UNFPA; UNAIDS IATT/YP. (2008). *HIV Interventions in the health sector for young people.* New York: UNFPA.
57. UNAIDS IATT/YP. (2008). *Guidance brief,* p. 1.
58. UNAIDS IATT/YP. (2008). *Guidance brief.*
59. Ibid.
60. UNAIDS. (1997). *Impact,* p. 3; Monasch, R., & Mahy, M. (2006). Young people: The center of the HIV epidemic. In UNAIDS Inter-agency Task Team on HIV and Young People (Eds.), *Preventing HIV/AIDS in young people* (pp. 15–42). Geneva, Switzerland: World Health Organization; UNAIDS, *Report,* 2008, p. 2.
61. Monasch & Mahy. (2006). Young people.
62. For a detailed typology of interventions available to increase young people's access and use of health services, see Dick et al. (2006), Introduction and rationale.
63. Maticka-Tyndale, E., & Brouillard-Coyle, C. (2006). The effectiveness of community interventions targeting HIV and AIDS prevention at young people in developing countries. In UNAIDS Inter-agency Task Team on HIV and Young People (Eds.), *Preventing HIV/AIDS in young people* (pp. 103–150). Geneva, Switzerland: World Health Organization.
64. Dick et al. (2006). Introduction and rationale.
65. UNAIDS. (1999). *Sex and youth: Contextual factors affecting risk for HIV.* Geneva, Switzerland: UNAIDS.
66. Dick et al. (2006). Introduction and rationale, p. 2.
67. Coyle, S. L., Boruch, R. F., & Turner, C. F. (1991). *Evaluating AIDS prevention programs* (Expanded Ed.). Washington, DC: National Academy Press.
68. Donenberg, G. R., Paikoff R., & Pequegnat, W. (2006). Introduction to the special section on families, youth and HIV: Family-based intervention studies. *Journal of Pediatric Psychology, 31,* 869–873.

69. Gallant, M., & Maticka-Tyndale, E. (2004). School-based HIV prevention pro-grammes for African youth. *Social Science and Medicine, 58*, 1337–1351; Kirby, Laris, & Rolleri. (2007). Sex and HIV.

70. Bertrand J. T., & Anhang, R. (2006). The effectiveness of mass media in chang-ing HIV/AIDS-related behaviour among young people in developing countries. In: UNAIDS Inter-agency Task Team on HIV and Young People (Eds.), *Preventing HIV/AIDS in young people* (pp. 103–150). Geneva, Switzerland: World Health Organization.

71. UNICEF. (2009). *Children and AIDS.*

72. Gallant & Maticka-Tyndale. (2004). School-based HIV prevention programmes; Speizer, I. S., Magnani R. J., & Colvin, C. E. (2003). The effectiveness of adoles-cent reproductive health interventions in developing countries: A review of the evidence. *Journal of Adolescent Health, 33*, 324–348.

73. UNAIDS. (2008). *Report.*

74. Dick et al. (2006). Introduction and rationale; UNAIDS IATT/YP. (2008). *Community.*

75. McCauley, A.P. (2004). *Equitable access to HIV counseling and testing for youth in developing countries: A review of current practice,* Horizons report (p. 2). Washington, DC: Population Council; MacPhall et al. (2008). 'You must.'

76. Weinhardt, L., et al. (1999). Effects of HIV counseling and testing on sexual risk behavior: A meta-analytic review of published research, 1985–1997. *American Journal of Public Health, 89*, 1397–1405; Voluntary HIV Counseling and Testing Efficacy Study Group. (2000). Efficacy of voluntary HIV-1 counseling and test-ing in individuals and couples in Kenya, Tanzania, and Trinidad: A randomized trial. *Lancet, 356*, 103–112; UNAIDS. (2001). *The impact of voluntary counsel-ing and testing: A global review of the benefits and challenges.* Geneva, Switzerland: UNAIDS.

77. Sherr, L., et al. (2007). Voluntary counselling and testing: Uptake, impact on sexual behaviour, and HIV incidence in a rural Zimbabwean cohort. *AIDS, 21*, 851–860; Kennedy, C., et al. (2007). The impact of HIV treatment on risk behaviour in developing countries: A systematic review. *AIDS Care, 19*, 707–720.

78. Crepaz, N., et al. (2006). Do prevention interventions reduce HIV risk behav-iours among people living with HIV? A meta-analytic review of controlled trials. *AIDS, 20*, 143–157.

79. Perrino, T., et al. (2000). The role of families in adolescent HIV prevention: A review. *Clinical Child and Family Psychology Review, 3*, 81–96; Pequegnat, W., & Szapocznik, J. (2000). The role of families in preventing and adapting to HIV/AIDS: Issues and answers. In W. Pequegnat, & J. Szapocznik (Eds.), *Working with families in the era of HIV/AIDS.* Thousand Oaks, CA: Sage Publications; Crosby, R. A., & Miller, K. S. (2002). Family influences on adolescent females' sexual health. In G. Wingood, & R. DiClemente (Eds.), *Handbook of women's sexual and reproductive health* (pp. 113–127). New York: Kluwer Academic/Plenum; Donenberg et al. (2006). Introduction.

80. UNAIDS. (2010). *Joint action*, p. 8.

81. National Research Council and Institute of Medicine. (2005). *Growing up global.*

82. Brown et al. (2003). Interventions; Mahajan et al. (2008). Stigma.

83. Brown et al. (2003). Interventions.

84. Kuhn, L., Steinberg M., & Mathews, C. (1994). Participation of the school community in AIDS education: An evaluation of a high school programme in South Africa. *AIDS Care, 6,* 161–171; Fawole, I. O., et al. (1999). A school-based AIDS education programme for secondary school students in Nigeria: A review of effectiveness. *Health Education Research, 14,* 675–683.

85. Cohen, S. A. (2003). *Beyond slogans: Lessons from Uganda's experience with ABC and HIV/AIDS.* New York: Alan Guttmacher Institute; Darabi, L., et al. (2008). *Protecting the next generation in Uganda.* New York : Alan Guttmacher Institute.

86. Kirungi, W. L., et al. (2006). Trends in antenatal HIV prevalence in urban Uganda associated with uptake of preventive sexual behaviour. *Sexually Transmitted Diseases, 82,* i36–i41; Murphy, E. M., et al. (2006). Was the 'ABC' approach (abstinence, being faithful, using condoms) responsible for Uganda's decline in HIV? *PLoS Medicine, 3,* e379; Singh, S., Darroch, J. E., & Bankole, A. (2003). *A, B and C in Uganda: The roles of abstinence, monogamy and condom use in HIV decline in Uganda.* New York: Alan Guttmacher Institute.

87. UNAIDS. (2008). *Report.*

88. UNAIDS. (2009). *Declaration of commitment on HIV/AIDS: Guidelines on construction of core indicators: 2010 reporting.* Geneva, Switzerland: UNAIDS.

89. The next review of the progress achieved in realizing the commitments set in the *Political Declaration* is scheduled for 2011.

90. United Nations General Assembly. (2006). *Declaration of commitment on HIV/ AIDS: Five years later. Report of the Secretary General to the United Nations General Assembly, March 24, 2006* (p. 8). New York: United Nations.

91. Ibid.

92. Speizer, Magnani, & Colvin. (2003). Effectiveness, p. 12; Ross, D. A., et al. (2006). The weight of evidence: A method for assessing the strength of evidence on the effectiveness of HIV prevention interventions among young people. In UNAIDS Inter-agency Task Team on HIV and Young People (Eds.), *Preventing HIV/AIDS in Young People* (pp. 79–102). Geneva, Switzerland: World Health Organization; Magnussen, L., Ehiri, J. E., & Jolly, P. E. (2004). Interventions to prevent HIV/AIDS among adolescents in less developed countries: Are they effective? *International Journal of Adolescent Medicine and Health, 16,* 303–323; Michielsen, R., et al. (2010). Effectiveness of HIV prevention for youth in sub-Saharan Africa: Systematic review and meta-analysis of randomized and nonrandomized trials. *AIDS, 24,* 1193–1202.

93. UNAIDS. (2009). *Guidelines.*

94. These indicators are the percentage of adults aged 15–49 who have had sexual intercourse with more than one partner in the last 12 months, and the percentage of adults aged 15–49 who had more than one sexual partner in the last 12 months who reported using a condom during their last intercourse.

95. These indicators are the percentage of schools that provided life skills-based HIV education within the last academic year, and the percentage of women and men aged 15–49 who received an HIV test in the last 12 months and who know the results.

96. The indicators to evaluate national programs for HIV-positive individuals are the percentage of adults and children with advanced HIV infection receiving antiretroviral therapy; the percentage of HIV-positive pregnant women who receive antiretroviral medicines to reduce the risk of mother-to-child

transmission; the percentage of estimated HIV-positive incident tuberculosis (TB) cases that received treatment for TB and HIV; and the percentage of HIV-positive adults and children known to be on treatment 12 months after initiation of antiretroviral therapy. The indicator to evaluate national programs for orphans is the percentage of orphans and vulnerable children whose households received free basic external support in caring for the child.

97. UNAIDS. (2009). *Guidelines.*

98. Speizer, Magnani, & Colvin. (2003). Effectiveness; Ross et al. (2006). Weight; Magnussen, Ehiri, & Jolly. (2004). Interventions; Michielsen et al. (2010). Effectiveness.

99. Bertrand & Anhang. (2006). Effectiveness; Gallant & Maticka-Tyndale. (2004). School-based programmes; Speizer, Magnani, & Colvin. (2003). Effectiveness.

100. UNAIDS. (2009). *Guidelines.*

101. Ross et al. (2006). Weight.

PART THREE

Meeting Health Care Needs

8

Effective HIV Prevention and Treatment for Pregnant Mothers and Their Children

HOOSEN M. COOVADIA AND MARIE-LOUISE NEWELL ■

The HIV pandemic has dramatically altered the lives of mothers and children in many countries, especially those of sub-Saharan Africa, where the HIV prevalence is highest. The impact of this epidemic on the individual, social, political, and economic lives of societies over the past quarter century has been enormous. In this chapter, we describe the impact of the HIV epidemic on the children born to women infected with HIV from a medical perspective and show how this plays a key role in the holistic needs of children.

HIV in children, unlike in adults, is transmitted during pregnancy, during birth, or through breast milk. Transmission can occur across the maternal placenta during pregnancy, from maternal blood during delivery, and postnatally through breast milk. Illness related to HIV appears to be more severe and rapidly progressing in young infants, especially those infected before or during birth. Moreover, in resource-poor settings, complications among children often reflect the background health problems that are regional causes of childhood illness and death. Finally, the choice of anti-HIV drugs suitable for children is limited.

As this chapter discusses, the unique transmission patterns, progression of disease, and treatment constraints in young children require prevention and treatment options tailored to this population. In preventing infants from acquiring HIV from mothers, it is as essential to prevent men from transmitting the virus to women as it is to prevent women from transmitting the virus perinatally. We briefly discuss this, then turn our focus to the latter stage of perinatal transmission and to postnatal transmission of HIV from mother to child. The most relevant data for developing countries on diagnosis and treatment of infants who become HIV infected are briefly described. Finally, there are significant consequences to children born to HIV-infected mothers but who remain HIV uninfected—HIV-exposed children—and this often-neglected aspect is covered in some depth.

BACKGROUND

The priority interventions for HIV in pregnant women, and those necessary to reduce mother-to-child transmission of HIV while simultaneously improving child survival, need to be determined in the light of contextual social and development factors. Midway assessment of progress toward achieving the Millennium Development Goals (MDGs) by 2015 is probably the most acceptable and reliable indicator of the overall change in environmental factors critical to child health.[1] The MDGs (listed here) have served as both incentive and lodestar to all countries, but especially to those that are economically fragile, to reach quantitative benchmarks in health.

Millennium Development Goals

1. Eradicate extreme poverty and hunger.
2. Achieve universal primary education.
3. Promote gender equality and empower women.
4. Reduce child mortality.
5. Improve maternal health.
6. Combat HIV/AIDS, malaria, and other diseases.
7. Ensure environmental sustainability.
8. Develop a global partnership for development.

It is evident from this list of goals that individually, together, and cumulatively, they have direct (MDGs 3, 4, 5) and indirect effects on maternal and child health. However, current trends in child nutrition, gender equality, and employment predict a likely failure to meet MDGs by 2015.[2] According to the Countdown 2008 Report,[3] the key problems in terms of MDGs 4 and 5 were increasing under-5 mortality rates and very high maternal mortality rates. Every year, 4.5 million African children die, including 1.2 million newborns (MDG 4); 1.5 million Africans die from AIDS, including 290,000 children under 5 years of age (MDG 5); and 276,000 African mothers die of causes related to their pregnancies (MDG 6).

HIV IN PREGNANT WOMEN

In 2008, 60% of HIV infections in women were in sub-Saharan Africa, amounting to 12.3 million women.[4] By December 2008, UNAIDS estimated that, globally, about 1.4 million HIV-infected women had become pregnant and required antiretrovirals (ARVs) for prevention of mother-to-child-transmission (PMTCT) of HIV; only 45% (628,400) of them actually received PMTCT treatment.[5]

Counseling on a range of issues is central to the management of HIV in pregnancy. Primary among these issues are advice on the use of ARVs for either a woman's own health or for PMTCT,[6] and the use of elective caesarean section. HIV in pregnancy can worsen outcomes for infants and mothers.[7] In a recent study, rural African women in South Africa were enrolled during pregnancy and followed-up for 24 months postdelivery. Mothers with HIV-1 experienced more morbidity and mortality than did HIV-uninfected women; this was predicted by the mother's immune status and by various socioeconomic factors.[8] The current World Health Organization (WHO) recommendations are to initiate highly active antiretroviral treatment (HAART) for the pregnant woman's own health. The standard indicator for such treatment relates to the mother's immune status as indicated by CD4 level readings. The current medical standard is that women should commence treatment at a CD4 threshold of 350 cells/µL. A recent study from Zimbabwe suggests that although there is a steep decline in the risk of death as CD4 counts rise above this threshold of 350 cells/µL, there remains a six times higher mortality over 24 months in those with the higher levels of CD4 (mean 803 cells/µL) compared to HIV-negative women.[9] This finding reignites the unresolved debate about universal HAART during pregnancy, which is based on the putative benefit of a low transmission rate with HAART versus the potentially serious adverse consequences, particularly when HAART is discontinued after delivery. The evidence base on treatment regimes and their outcomes is the subject of constantly updated research. It is important that this evolving knowledge be integrated into updated treatment plans. The current evidence does not prove that maternal HAART is superior in terms of prevention to antenatal dual therapy and postnatal single-drug therapy given to the breastfeeding baby. Moreover, there are issues around the cost of HAART, implementation difficulties, adverse effects, and the real danger of longer-term complications when HAART is discontinued in women who had been prescribed the drugs for PMTCT rather than for their own health. The recent WHO guidelines to expand eligibility for HAART should benefit about half of pregnant women, but do not support universal HAART.[10]

Another key decision related to maternal health is whether to perform a caesarean section. A caesarean section substantially reduces transmission to the infant, but in developing countries may be associated with serious adverse consequences, including infant and maternal morbidity and mortality.[11] With the new combination ARV treatment regimes (which include more than one medication), transmission rates of HIV to the newborn are extremely low and may not be improved much by caesarean section; thus, in the United States, elective caesarean section is recommended only for HIV pregnant women with detectable viral loads that indicate an elevated chance of transmission. The current guidance suggests elective caesarean section when the viral load reading is greater than 1,000 copies/mL.[12] During delivery, additional precautions should be taken to avoid any possible exposure of the infant to the virus. This means specific attention should be paid to avoiding prolonged labor after the membranes have ruptured, preventing any tears in infant skin, and limiting the use of medical monitoring equipment that may pierce the skin and thereby create a portal of infection, such as the use of scalp electrodes during vaginal delivery.

HIV IN CHILDREN

In 2008, there were approximately 2.1 million (1.2–2.9 million) HIV-infected children under 15 years of age in the world; 370,000 of these had become newly infected and 280,000 (150,000–410,000) had died of AIDS related diseases in that year. Ninety-one percent of the new HIV infections in children were in sub-Saharan Africa, and about 95% of these infections were due to mother-to-child-transmission.

PREVENTION OF MOTHER-TO-CHILD TRANSMISSION OF HIV

The effectiveness of PMTCT interventions against HIV-1 is one of the great successes in the basket of prevention strategies used to control the HIV epidemic. Transmission of HIV-1 can occur in utero, during delivery, and postnatally during breastfeeding. The benefits of intervention programs directed at all three routes of transmission have been clearly evident in industrialized countries, where transmission rates have fallen from about 25% to under 2%, and survival of infants has increased.[13]

However, in resource-poor settings, PMTCT services are often unavailable or inaccessible to large proportions of those in need, health personnel and facilities are inadequate, and the quality of services is low. The use of artificial milk formulas instead of breast milk to prevent postnatal HIV transmission, especially in the critical first 6 months of life, is associated with growth failure, high morbidity, protein-energy malnutrition, and death[14] because of the inability to afford an adequate supply of formula and the poor quality of water with which it is often mixed.

To utilize available PMTCT services, pregnant women have to both be tested for HIV and attend antenatal clinics; these services have expanded in recent years. Overcoming the well-documented loss of mothers in the PMTCT "cascade" requires dealing effectively with a rapid decline in the numbers of pregnant women attending antenatal care early or at all in pregnancy, of women seeking counseling on HIV testing or infant feeding, of women having CD4 counts done and the results obtained, of women taking ARVs themselves and administering ARVs to their infant, of women delivering within health facilities, and of women seeking postnatal care.

Globally, the Joint United Nations Program on HIV and AIDS (UNAIDS) reports that 21% of pregnant women received an HIV test in 2008, up from 15% in 2007,[15] although still leaving the majority of women untested. The recent WHO program to undertake mass HIV counseling and testing in affected countries, vigorous implementation of these recommendations by governments, and community mobilization should improve testing of women. In 2008, 45% of HIV-positive pregnant women in low- and middle-income countries received ARVs for PMTCT, up from 35% in 2007.

A COMPREHENSIVE SET OF INTERVENTIONS TO PREVENT MOTHER-TO-CHILD TRANSMISSION

PMTCT has focused mainly on the prophylaxis of perinatal transmission, but more recently also on breastfeeding transmission. A broader conceptualization of PMTCT, introduced by the WHO,[16] is gaining ground. This conceptualization views the issue throughout the reproductive cycle, from preconception through to the first few postnatal years for both mother and child.

Prevention of HIV-1 and of Unintended Pregnancies

The first phase aims at preventing the acquisition of HIV in women of childbearing age and preventing unwanted pregnancy and delivery in those already HIV infected.

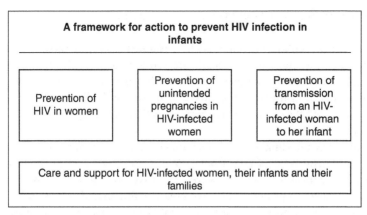

Figure 8.1 A framework for action to prevent HIV infection in infants.

In generalized HIV epidemics, it is appropriate to target prevention messages to those women most at risk and their partners; in many southern African countries, young women between the ages of 15 and 24 years have a three- to four-fold higher risk of becoming HIV infected than their male counterparts in the same age group. However, men become infected on average 5 years later, and the cumulative figures by 50 years of age are similar in women and men.[17]

Recent evidence from Zimbabwe[18] and from Thailand[19] suggests that primary prevention works. In Thailand, the prevalence of HIV infection in pregnant women fell between 1994 and 2007; the number of pediatric HIV infections also decreased.[20] In Zimbabwe,[21] mother-to-child transmission of HIV decreased from 8.2% in 2000 to 6.2% in 2005, predominantly attributable to declining maternal HIV prevalence rather than to the PMTCT program.

Infection with HIV immediately prior to or during pregnancy can be particularly risky. It has been noted that between 1.3% and 10.7% women who are found to be HIV uninfected when first tested in an antenatal clinic subsequently seroconvert;[22] these women are at great risk of transmitting because of high viral loads during the acute phase of HIV infection. This is probably as a result of the fact that the antibody test during early pregnancy may have been carried out during the "window period," while the virus was replicating but not yet registering on the screening test. Repeat testing later in pregnancy or at delivery has been suggested in settings with high HIV incidence. This strategy would pick up those women who were in fact newly infected but tested HIV negative due to the limitations of the antibody tests in picking up new infection.

Family planning and provision of contraceptives have been proven effective in reducing the risk of mother-to-child transmission.[23] For example, a 1.25% reduction in new HIV infections in women and a 16% increase in prevention of unintended pregnancies has been estimated to result in reductions in mother-to-child transmission equivalent to those achieved with prevention using ARVs in the peripartum period. The percentage of HIV-infected women who have unintended pregnancies is very high: worldwide, unintended pregnancy is a common outcome every year for more than 200 million women;[24] the prevalences for HIV-positive women are 51% in Cote d'Ivoire,[25] 84% in South Africa,[26] and 93% in Uganda.[27]

Prevention of Transmission from an HIV-infected Mother to Her Infant

A number of prevention measures, such as planned ARVs, caesarean section, safe delivery with minimum instrumental intervention, and avoidance of delays (>4 hours) in rupture of membranes have been shown to be successful in reducing mother-to-child transmission. These have been extensively discussed in recent publications and, with the exception of caesarean section, are of importance for developing countries.[28]

Exclusive breastfeeding, which is recommended for all infants for 6 months, can reduce the transmission of HIV from HIV-infected mothers compared to mixing breastfeeding with other food. However, exclusive breastfeeding is not the norm globally. Measures to promote exclusive breastfeeding include community promotion; community engagement; early antenatal visits; counseling by trained feeding counselors antenatally and postnatally, especially during the difficult first weeks after delivery; regular clinic visits for immunization and nutrition support; home-based care for infant nutrition; and monitoring of appropriate feeding. There is good evidence that such measures can work to increase the rates of exclusive breastfeeding by all women, including HIV-positive women.

Antiretrovirals given to breastfeeding infants or lactating mothers can greatly reduce breastfeeding transmission and improve infant survival. In 2006, the WHO recommended that ARVs be provided to HIV-positive pregnant women in the third trimester (beginning at 28 weeks) to prevent mother-to-child transmission of HIV. At the time, there was insufficient evidence on the protective effect of ARVs during breastfeeding. To reduce the risk of HIV transmission and improve the infant's chance of survival, the WHO now recommends that breastfeeding continue until the infant is 12 months of age, provided the HIV-positive mother or baby is taking ARVs during that period. The 2009 recommendations, reflecting new data from clinical trials, promote the use of ARVs earlier in pregnancy, starting at 14 weeks and continuing during the first year postpartum to cover the breastfeeding period.[29]

The interventions to reduce breastfeeding transmission of HIV have been studied in a number of recently conducted trials, all of which showed the efficacy of either maternal or infant ARVs given during breastfeeding. These have been reviewed recently[30] and are presented in Tables 8.1, 8.2, and 8.3. The choice of a specific maternal or infant prophylactic regimen to prevent breastfeeding transmission will be a matter determined by a number of different factors such as efficacy, effectiveness, cost, feasibility, incorporation into existing health services, and others.

Box 8.1

WORLD HEALTH ORGANIZATION (WHO) RECOMMENDATIONS ON INFANT FEEDING

1. Ensuring mothers receive the care they need
   Mothers known to be HIV-infected should be provided with lifelong antiretroviral therapy (ART) or antiretroviral (ARV) prophylaxis interventions to reduce HIV transmission through breastfeeding conforming to WHO recommendations.

2. Which breastfeeding practices and for how long?

Mothers known to be HIV infected (and whose infants are HIV uninfected or of unknown HIV status) and who choose to initiate breastfeeding should exclusively breastfeed their infants for the first 6 months of life, introducing appropriate complementary foods thereafter, and continue breastfeeding for the first 12 months of life. After this time, breastfeeding should only stop once a nutritionally adequate and safe diet without breast milk can be provided.

3. When mothers decide to stop breastfeeding

Mothers known to be HIV infected who decide to stop breastfeeding at any time should stop gradually, within 1 month. Mothers or infants who have been receiving ARV prophylaxis should continue prophylaxis for 1 week after breastfeeding is fully stopped. Stopping breastfeeding abruptly is not advisable.

4. What to feed infants when mothers stop breastfeeding

When mothers known to be HIV infected decide to stop breastfeeding at any time, infants should be provided with safe and adequate replacement feeds to enable normal growth and development.

5. Conditions needed to safely formula feed

Mothers known to be HIV infected should only give commercial infant formula milk as a replacement feed to their HIV-uninfected infants or infants who are of unknown HIV status when specific conditions are met—referred to as AFASS for affordable, feasible, acceptable, sustainable, and safe, in the 2006 WHO recommendations on HIV and Infant Feeding:

a. Safe water and sanitation are assured at the household level and in the community, and,

b. the mother, or another caregiver, can reliably provide sufficient infant formula milk to support normal growth and development of the infant, and,

c. the mother or caregiver can prepare it cleanly and frequently enough so that it is safe and carries a low risk of diarrhoea and malnutrition, and,

d. the mother or caregiver can, in the first 6 months, exclusively give infant formula milk, and,

e. the family is supportive of this practice, and,

f. the mother or caregiver can access health care that offers comprehensive child health services.

6. When the infant is HIV-infected

If infants and young children are known to be HIV infected, mothers are strongly encouraged to exclusively breastfeed for the first 6 months of life and continue breastfeeding as per the recommendations for the general population, that is, up to 2 years or beyond.

The 2010 South African guidelines now suggest HAART be given to pregnant women with a CD4 count at or less than 350 cells (for life), which would also offer protection against transmission during breastfeeding. Further, for infants born to women with higher CD4 counts, the recommendation includes administering oral nevirapine (NVP) during the first year of life, while breastfeeding continues.

Clearly, any good-quality service must be set up with adequate provision in terms of medical interventions and the ability to update and respond as the knowledge base is refined. The current understanding of maternal HAART for the prevention of

Table 8.1 MATERNAL HIGHLY ACTIVE ANTIRETROVIRAL THERAPY (HAART) FOR THE PREVENTION OF POSTNATAL TRANSMISSION THROUGH BREASTFEEDING

Study	Median Maternal CD4 cells/μL	Mother-to-child transmission at 4–6 weeks	Mother-to-child transmission at 6 months; cumulative; and incremental	Reference[31]
DREAM (ARVs 26.8 weeks to 6 months)	489	3.8% at 6 weeks; no birth data	5.3% at 6 months (1.7% 4 weeks–6 months)	Marazzi et al. (2009)
DREAM (ARVs 28 weeks to 6 months)	Not specified	Formula fed: 0.9% at 6 weeks; breastfed: 1.2% at 6 weeks; no birth data	Formula fed: 2.7% at 6 months Breastfed: 2.2% at 6 months and (0.8% 4 weeks–6 months)	Palombi et al. (2007)
Kibs (ARVs 34 weeks to 6 months)	394 (23% <250)	3.9% at 6 weeks; 2.4% at birth; 1.5% day 1–6 weeks	5.0% at 6 months (2.6% 6 weeks–6 months)	Thomas et al. (2008)
MITRA-Plus (ARVs 34 weeks to 6 months)	460 (14% <200)	4.1% at 6-week; no birth data	5.0% (range 2.9–7.1) at 6 months (0.9% 6 weeks–6 months)	Kilewo et al. (2009)
AMATA (ARVs 28 weeks to 6 months)	Not specified	1.1% at birth; no 6-week data	Breast fed: 1.6% (range 0.7–4.8) at 7 months (0.5% day 1–6 months)	Arendt et al. (2007)
Cote d'Ivoire (ARVs 24 week to 6 months)	Only CD4 <200	1.0% at birth; no 6-week data	3.3% at 6 months (1.9% 4 weeks–6 months)	Tonwe-Gold et al. (2007)
Kesho Bora (ARVs 34–36 weeks to 6 months)	Only CD4 <200	No birth or 6-week data	Breast fed 8% at 6 months formula fed 11% at 12 months	De Vincenzi & Group KBS (2008)

postnatal transmission through breastfeeding is summarized in Table 8.1. The table breaks down the studies (together with references) and gives the measures used.

Usually CD4 cells/µL are measured and then mother-to-child transmission rates at 4–6 weeks and again at 6 months are recorded. Five trials are under way studying infant ARV prophylaxis for the prevention of postnatal infection. These are the MASHI, MITRA, SIMBA, SWEN, and PEPI trials. These medical trials compare different regimes in a highly controlled way and report on outcomes in terms of transmission rates in the infant. The data from these trials are summarized in Table 8.2.

Another set of trials examines the outcomes for the infant of compounds given to the mother. Two such trials are summarized in Table 8.3 (MMA BANA and BAN). All centers need to be updated and informed of these ongoing trials as the information base emerges, results are published, and evidence-based policies are implemented.

The development of resistance to ARVs used in PMTCT programs is an important issue for the subsequent management of an HIV-infected infant or mother. In the studies described in the tables that used prophylactic infant NVP or maternal HAART, there was a high incidence of resistance to NVP. The resistance following extended doses of NVP is much higher and persists for longer periods than with single-dose nevirapine (sdNVP).[32] HIV-infected infants who are infected during the course of extended NVP have greater frequency of resistance than do those who are infected after NVP has been discontinued.[33] Infants who are HIV infected during breastfeeding while exposed to preventive ART can also develop resistance.[34] The subsequent ARV management of children and women who had developed resistance to these drugs during participation in PMTCT programs is being investigated. There is a suggestion that the longer the duration between exposure to the prophylactic ARV employed in PMTCT and initiation of HAART for the children's or women's own health, the better the response;[35] and perinatal use of other ARVs reduces resistance in the women.[36]

In 2008, about 31% of HIV-positive pregnant women in 97 reporting countries, compared to 49% in 2007, continued to receive a single-dose drug. Single-dose nevirapine has been shown to be effective in reducing mother-to-child transmission by about 40%; however, it greatly increases drug resistance in the mother, and in the infant if he or she acquires infection despite PMTCT prophylaxis. Drug resistance interferes with effective treatment when this becomes necessary at a later stage.

Postnatal Care

Although the postnatal period is important for the care and monitoring of HIV-positive mothers and their infants, such care was reported unavailable or insufficient in most of the 68 Countdown for the Millennium Development Goals countries.[37] Important aspects of infant and child care for all infants born to HIV-positive mothers include testing for HIV, management of ART and of the illnesses associated with HIV infection (known as opportunistic infections), medical treatment to prevent some illnesses developing in the first place (e.g., prophylaxis with co-trimoxazole), case-management of malnourished children, and support for psychosocial health. Routine child health protection and promotion of services for immunization, micronutrients, nutrition and growth monitoring, and community outreach are also essential to the health and survival of all infants and children irrespective of HIV

Table 8.2 Infant Antiretroviral Prophylaxis for the Prevention of Postnatal Acquisition of HIV Infection

Study	Median Maternal CD4 cells/μL	Mother-to-child transmission at 4–6 weeks	Mother-to-child transmission at 6 months: cumulative; incremental	Reference[38]
MASHI: 6-month AZT: Antepartum (34- week delivery); at delivery AZT +-single dose (sd) NVP	366	Cumulative: 4.6% Incremental: 3.3% at birth; 1.3% day 1–6 weeks	Cumulative AZT in breastfed babies: 9.0% at 7 months Incremental: 4.4% 4 weeks–7 months	Thior et al. (2006)
MITRA: 6-month 3TC AP (36 week to 1 week postpartum): postpartum AZT + 3TC	459 (9% <200)	Cumulative: 3.8% No birth data	Cumulative: 4.9% Incremental: 1.2% 6 weeks–6 months	Kilewo et al. (2008)
SIMBA: 6-month 3TC vs. NVP; Antepartum 36 weeks to 1 week: AZT + ddI	423	Cumulative: 6.9% Incremental: 5.3% at birth 1.6% birth–4 weeks	Cumulative: 7.7% Incremental: 0.8% 4 weeks–6 months	Vyankandondera et al. (2008)
SWEN: 6-week NVP No antepartum ARVs	316–463	Cumulative: 7.2% Incremental: 4.7% at birth 2.5% day 1–6 weeks	Cumulative: 14.3% Incremental: 4.4% 6 weeks–6 months	SWEN Study Team (2008)
PEPI: 14-week NVP or NVP/AZT No antepartum ARVs	379–401	Cumulative: 8.8% at14 weeks NVP Incremental 7.1% birth 1.7% day 1–6 weeks NVP/AZT not significantly different	Cumulative: 11.1% Incremental: 2.3% 6 week–6 months NVP	Kumwenda et al. (2008)

Table 8.3 Infant and Maternal Antiretroviral Prophylaxis for the Prevention of Postnatal Transmission of HIV Infection

Study	Inclusion Criteria for Maternal CD4 cells/μL	Mother-to-child transmission at 6 months (cumulative; incremental)	Reference[39]
MMA BANA Trial, Maternal: Two HAART regimens: triple nucleoside or protease inhibitor regimen Antepartum 26–34 weeks Postpartum 6 months Infant sdNVP+ 4 weeks AZT	<200 cells	1% (range: 0.5%– 2.0%) No difference between two HAART groups	Shapiro et al. (2010)
BAN: 1. Control: Maternal and Infant: sdNVP+ 1 week AZT/3TC 2. Control regimen + Maternal HAART; 1 week to 6 months postpartum 3. Control regimen + daily infant NVP; 1 week to 6 months postpartum	>250 cells	Mother-to-child transmission in those uninfected at birth (comparisons: groups 2:1 and 3:1) 1. 6.4% 2. 3.0% ($p = 0.003$) 3. 1.8% ($p = 0.0001$)	Chasela et al. (2010)

status, and HIV services for mothers and children are best integrated with overall maternal and child health services.

The integration of HIV testing in infants into national immunization programs would be a useful and simple start. Postnatal follow-up for HIV-positive mothers and their infants should be integrated into treatment services for HIV, as well as within treatment services for opportunistic infections such as tuberculosis. Health monitoring of children born to HIV-positive women and of the women themselves should be closely tied to programs to prevent mother-to-child transmission; such integration can be effective and more cost-efficient than separate programs. Complications of pregnancy, postnatal mental health problems, and monitoring of progression of HIV are some of the features of a potential PMTCT services program for mothers after delivery.

Further progress in the prevention and management of HIV in infants and children and their mothers will require substantial adjustments to national health policies, resource allocations, and the quality of health services and personnel.

HIV-INFECTED CHILDREN

Early Diagnosis

Diagnosis after about 18 months of age can be made by detection of specific HIV antibodies. During infancy, passively transferred maternal antibodies obscure detection of HIV. Thus, other, more elaborate tests are required to diagnose infection in young infants. Knowledge of the mother's HIV status or exposure to risky sexual encounters can alert the health professional to the need for testing both mother and infant. See Box 8.2 on WHO guidelines on testing.

Box 8.2

Pediatric HIV/ART Care Guidelines[40]

Recommendations on When to Test Infants

1. Infants known to be exposed to HIV should have a virological test (HIV nucleic acid test) at 4–6 weeks of age or at the earliest opportunity for infants seen after 4–6 weeks.
2. Urgent HIV testing is recommended for any infant that comes to a health facility showing signs, symptoms, or medical conditions that could indicate HIV.
3. All infants should have their HIV exposure status established at their first contact with the health system, ideally before 6 weeks of age.
4. Infants under 6 weeks of age, of unknown HIV exposure status and in settings where local or national antenatal HIV seroprevalence is greater than 1%, should be offered maternal or infant HIV antibody testing and counseling to establish exposure status.

Early Treatment

Children have faster progression of disease than do adults, so delays in diagnosis may result in death.[41] This is especially important for diagnosis of newborns and infants because, without appropriate ARV treatment, as many as a third of infected babies will die within a year, and most of these within a few months of birth. New WHO recommendations concerning treatment of children, shown in Box 8.3, provide practical information. Given how rapidly treatment recommendations evolve, readers should check for updated WHO recommendations.

Early Referral of Infants and Children to Antiretroviral Treatment Programs

It is essential that, once the diagnosis of HIV is made in infants and children, they be referred to an appropriate medical team for preparation and initiation of ART. Integration of prevention and treatment clinic services, as discussed above, will reduce the dangers of delayed or missed treatment. In the CHER Trial, 6- to 12-week-old HIV-infected infants were randomized to immediate or deferred ARV therapy. After a median of 40 weeks, 16% of infants in the deferred group and 4% in the immediate group had died (HR 0.24 95%; confidence interval [CI] 0.11–0.51).

Overall, early diagnosis and treatment with ARVs reduced early infant mortality by 76% and HIV progression by 75%.[42]

Box 8.3

RECOMMENDATIONS ON WHEN TO INITIATE ANTIRETROVIRAL THERAPY

1. All infants under 24 months of age with confirmed HIV infection should be started on ART, irrespective of clinical or immunological stage.
2. Where virological testing is not available, infants under 12 months of age with clinically diagnosed presumptive severe HIV should start ART. Confirmation of HIV infection should be obtained as soon as possible.
3. For children age 24 months or older, clinical and immunological thresholds should be used to identify those who need to start ART.
4. For HIV-infected infants with no exposure to maternal or infant non-nucleoside reverse transcriptase inhibitors, or whose exposure to maternal or infant ARVs is unknown, standard nevirapine-containing triple therapy should be started.
5. For HIV-infected infants with a history of exposure to single-dose nevirapine or non-nucleoside reverse transcriptase inhibitor containing maternal ART or preventive ARV regimens, a protease inhibitor-based triple ART regimen should be started. Where protease inhibitors are not available, affordable, or feasible, nevirapine-based therapy should be used. The availability and optimal use of ARVs is a rapidly developing field, and specialist advice often has to be obtained for issues of resistance and serious complications of HIV. However, the availability of multiple sources of information for use by generalists allows them to keep abreast with progress.

CHALLENGES OF THE HEALTH SYSTEM

The major success of controlling HIV/AIDS in industrialized countries and in some middle-income countries was due to a combination of: a sociopolitical milieu that supports human research and responds to scientific evidence with appropriate policies; a health services infrastructure that can rapidly incorporate reliable research findings into practical programs; a convincing trial of the efficacy of maternal ARVs in reducing perinatal mother-to-child transmission; safe vaginal and caesarean section deliveries; and a socioeconomic environment that meets basic needs, thereby allowing avoidance of breastfeeding to reduce postnatal transmission without incurring the costs of increased infections, malnutrition, and death. Many of these supportive elements are missing in developing countries.

Infrastructural deficiencies in poor countries remain a barrier to delivery of health services.[43] There is an estimated global shortage of 4 million trained health workers, and an urgent need for transferring responsibilities to less specialized health workers and professionals. Worldwide, about 53% of countries had such "task-shifting" policies in place in 2008; in sub-Saharan Africa the figure was 63%.

An emerging literature is beginning to address in greater detail the delivery of optimum health services for PMTCT through more effective use of resources—more health for less cost.[44] The use of childhood immunization clinics to detect and treat early HIV infection has been tested in a study from KwaZulu-Natal, South Africa.[45] Universal HIV testing of 646 mothers of 6-week-old infants attending immunization clinics showed that 584 (90.4%) agreed to HIV testing of their infant and 332 (56.8%) subsequently returned for results. Three hundred and thirty-two of 646 (51.4%) mothers and infants thereby had their HIV status confirmed or reaffirmed by the time the infant was 3 months of age. The majority of mothers interviewed said they were comfortable with testing their infant at immunization clinics and would recommend it to others. The authors conclude that screening of all infants at immunization clinics is acceptable and feasible as a means for early identification of HIV-infected infants and referral for ART.

HIV-EXPOSED BUT UNINFECTED CHILDREN

In the coming years, as the risk of transmission decreases, the uninfected millions born to HIV-positive mothers will dwarf the numbers who are infected. The risk of transmission is already very low in the industrialized world; it has fallen to about 1%–2% from a figure of roughly 25%. In some middle-income countries with broad coverage of PMTCT programs, the risk has fallen to about 4%–6%.[46] In other words, more than 90%–95% of infants born to HIV-positive mothers can now be expected to remain uninfected by HIV. A key question is whether these HIV-uninfected children are similar to children born to HIV-uninfected women. There is some suggestion that, in some aspects, they may deviate from a "normal range," although there are limitations to the strength of this evidence and more research is required.

Regardless of their own status, children exposed to HIV-infected mothers often live in circumstances that make them vulnerable and put them at risk of illness and death. These circumstances include recurring illness and loss of productive capacity of parents, increased health costs, decreased income, and increased risk of poverty, starvation, and destitution.[47] Moreover, these children may have less access to health services such as immunization.[48] Orphaned children (both HIV-uninfected and HIV-infected) and other children in the household suffer greatly from malnutrition, disease, homelessness, depression, fear, guilt, and shame. Children are often forced to assume headship of the family and home; there are limited resources for shelter, food, education, hygiene, and personal needs, and even less for comfort and enjoyment. Poverty increases exposure to child abuse and sexual coercion.[49] Premature death of a parent and dislocation of children from a stable family to others, as well as stigma and discrimination, cumulatively create an inhospitable internal household environment for growth and development of all children and adults (Figure 8.2).[50]

Survival and Mortality

The relative importance of HIV-exposed but uninfected children is increasing as the number of infected children diminishes with the widespread implementation of PMTCT programs. A recent UNAIDS pooled analysis of data for 12,112 infants born to HIV-infected mothers from 12 trials in Western, Eastern, and Southern Africa

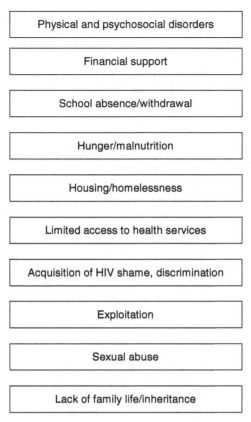

Figure 8.2 Problems among children and families affected by HIV and AIDS

reported the mortality rate was higher in children born to HIV-infected mothers, regardless of the infant's own HIV status,[51] confirming and extending a similar analysis undertaken in 2004.[52] Further, infant mortality rates climbed even higher if their mother died within the 2-year observation period. The most important findings from this UNAIDS study are summarized here:

1. All children born to HIV-infected mothers, regardless of whether they are HIV infected or not, are at higher risk of disease and death than are children born to HIV-uninfected mothers.
2. Mortality, in the absence of appropriate management, especially ARVs, is extremely high in HIV-infected infants, with more than 50% dead by 2 years of age.
3. The mortality rate per 1,000 child-years of follow-up was about nine- to tenfold higher in HIV-infected compared to HIV-uninfected infants.
4. Mortality is lower in infants who acquired HIV through breastfeeding than perinatally; at 18 months of age, the mortality risks are 36% and 60%, respectively.
5. The mortality rate over the 24 months of observation was about twice as high in the children whose mothers had died compared to the children whose mothers were alive.

6. Low maternal CD4 count (maternal CD4 <350 cells/µL) increased mortality in the children by about 36%.
7. Exposure to maternal ARVs for PMTCT reduced child mortality almost threefold, and exposure to infant ARVs about twofold.
8. Low birth weight was an important contributor to child mortality, whereas breastfeeding had only a marginal effect, and background mortality had none.

Whether HIV-exposed children have higher rates of mortality may depend on context. In Zimbabwe, HIV-exposed but uninfected children were shown to have higher mortality than children born to uninfected mothers.[53] Over a period of about 2 years, Marinda et al. demonstrated that the death rate in exposed children was three times higher than in unexposed children. HIV-exposed children had a steady but increasing death rate; the percentage of deaths in the HIV-exposed group increased from 1.9% at 30 days to 9.2% at 730 days. However, in a recent review comparing mortality rates in HIV-exposed and -unexposed children in six African countries,[54] rates varied markedly by country. Mortality was significantly higher in the HIV-exposed group in only three of the six countries (Botswana, Uganda, Zimbabwe). Another two reports from Malawi, in 1995 and 1999, showed no significant differences in mortality after the first year of life between HIV-exposed and -unexposed children.[55]

Reasons for differences in results from different settings may reflect differences in maternal circumstances and the stage of the HIV epidemic. Severity of maternal disease is associated with an increase in mortality in HIV-exposed children.[56] In an individual data analysis from seven randomised intervention trials in sub-Saharan Africa, which included 3,468 children, the mortality risks in HIV-uninfected children were dependent on the location of the sample (West/East Africa worse than South Africa), maternal death (adjusted odds ratio 3.65), and low maternal CD4 count (<200 cells/µL).[57] Risk factors for death in HIV-exposed children, obtained from the above and other studies[58] include maternal death, maternal health status, maternal socioeconomic status, low birth weight, and avoidance of breastfeeding.

What are the long-term prospects for HIV-exposed children? This is unclear. In a Rwandan study[59] with a 5-year period of follow-up and <12% loss to follow-up, there was no apparent difference in mortality between HIV-exposed and -unexposed children. However, the mortality rate of 0.04 (CI 95% 0.02–0.07) was extremely low for a developing country; 96% of the cohort of HIV-exposed, uninfected children survived, which may reflect the research setting. In an interesting account from a population-based survey in Karonga District in Malawi, individuals were identified as HIV positive in the 1980s and these individuals, their spouses, and offspring were traced in 1998–2000; they were matched for age and sex with HIV-negative individuals.[60] The HIV status of the mothers at the birth of their infants in the 1980s correlated with the death of their offspring in 1998–2000: 41.3% of the offspring of HIV-positive mothers were dead, compared with 15.1% of the offspring of HIV-uninfected mothers.

Growth and Development

It has been suggested that the growth of HIV-exposed children may be impaired, but whether this is due to exposure to family or social environments or to other factors is unclear. In a Zambian study, HIV-infected mothers were randomly assigned to exclusive breastfeeding for 4 months followed by rapid weaning to replacement foods or exclusive breastfeeding for 6 months followed by introduction of complementary foods and continued breastfeeding for a duration of the mother's choice. In the HIV-exposed group, weight-for-age z scores, but not length-for-age z scores, fell sharply between 4.5 months (when the experimental group weaned rapidly) and 15 months; this decline was slower in breastfeeding infants. There was no effect of breastfeeding on weight gain after 15 months; after adjustment, breastfeeding continued to have a beneficial effect on growth.[61] Growth between 1 week and 4 months of age was negatively associated, after adjustment, with not breastfeeding, female gender, twin births, maternal death, high viral load, and body mass.[62]

Other studies in Africa have shown variable effects on weight gain and increased height, usually suggesting failure of early growth.[63] However, in a well-conducted study in KwaZulu-Natal with breastfeeding support for all mothers, there were no significant differences in growth in early life between HIV-uninfected children born to HIV-positive mothers and children born to HIV-negative mothers,[64] although the growth of infected children was consistently below that of their uninfected counterparts. These results suggest that optimal early feeding practices ameliorate the effect of being born to an HIV-infected mother and strengthen the recommendation of exclusive breastfeeding for HIV-infected women in terms of long-term child health. The lack of precise data from many studies has led to variable results and differences in health outcomes reported from other studies;[65] this may have been due to the lack of support received by the mother in the study and inappropriate selection of the unexposed population.[66]

Morbidity

Exposed but uninfected children are at risk for a number of medical conditions as well as psychosocial and developmental challenges. These include acute respiratory infection, diarrhoea, and malnutrition, especially if not breastfeeding.[67] In a study in Zimbabwe, causes of death were similar in HIV-exposed and -unexposed children; the causes were those commonly found in poor children, such as pneumonia, acute diarrhoea, meningitis, sepsis, chronic diarrhoea, tuberculosis, dysentery, and malaria.[68] In the 5-year follow-up in Rwanda,[69] there was an increase in severe pneumonia, generalized dermatitis, chronic parotitis, and hospitalizations in HIV-exposed children. Similar findings have been reported by Read et al.[70]

In Botswana, morbidity and mortality were higher in HIV-exposed than in unexposed children.[71] Overall, HIV-exposed children may be at high risk for early infant mortality and severe morbidity, especially if not breastfeeding and if maternal HIV infection is advanced.[72]

Mental Health

There are very good reasons, a priori, to expect cognitive and behavioural problems in HIV-exposed children. Rotheram-Borus et al.[73] have shown that adolescents who suffer the death of an HIV-positive parent show impaired psychosocial adjustment compared to adolescents with living parents. However, Forehand et al.[74] did not find such an effect on 6- to 11-year-old children.

In the United States, children of HIV-infected African American mothers have more behavioural problems, greater levels of depression, and less social competence than do children of HIV-uninfected mothers.[75] Pelton and Forehand[76] found that a higher percentage of children whose mothers had died of AIDS had clinically significant internalizing (depression) and externalizing (aggression, noncompliance) problems than those whose mothers were alive. These behavioural problems were detected before and after maternal death. In 6- to 11-year-old children (39 HIV exposed and 78 unexposed), the exposed children displayed significantly more problems related to psychosocial adjustment, attention, and externalizing symptoms; they also displayed more anxiety, depression, and difficulties in verbal recall.[77]

However, a number of studies also demonstrate that the neurodevelopmental outcomes of HIV-exposed children are similar to those of unexposed children.[78]

Immune Responses

A growing set of studies examines the immune responses for HIV-exposed and HIV-infected children. The general literature shows some immune changes among HIV-exposed children. The medical details are summarized below. In terms of policy, this shows the importance of updated study and understanding, and the need for medical knowledge to be integrated into management policies. It also highlights the importance of detailed monitoring of potential problems.

Immune responses to HIV antigens and to nonspecific stimulants have been demonstrated in a number of studies in HIV-exposed children,[79] showing that a number of cytokines are different in HIV-exposed compared to HIV-infected newborns: Interleukin (IL) 2, IL4, IL7, IL10, and interferon (IF) gamma are increased, whereas IL12 is decreased. Similar findings have been shown by Kuhn et al.,[80] who also detected high levels of cytotoxic T cells and CD8 cells. In another study, Kuhn et al. showed that lymphocyte responses to specific and nonspecific stimuli were present in HIV-exposed children and were similar to those in HIV-infected children.[81] More importantly, they demonstrated that T-helper cell responses to HIV envelope peptides in cord blood correlated with protection against subsequent HIV infection to 6 months. Hygino et al. showed that IL10 was decreased significantly in exposed children whose mothers had detectable viral loads compared to normal[82] and that IF-gamma and tumor necrosis factor-gamma were also increased, although the proportion and number of CD4 cells and CD8 cells did not differ between exposed and unexposed children. Breast milk from HIV-infected and -uninfected mothers had detectable levels of immune factors, with some of these (total IgM, IgG, and IgA; SLPI and IgG to H influenza) being higher in HIV-infected mothers.[83]

In brief, these findings imply exposure of the fetus to peptides/antigens of HIV in utero, in the absence of HIV infection. At least one study[84] suggests that a helper T-cell response to HIV envelope peptides correlates with protection against postnatal HIV infection in the first few months of life. The effects on the immune response in the infant show an increase in the function and number of both helper and cytotoxic T cells and factors that are proinflammatory (IF gamma); promote T lymphocyte growth, development, and differentiation (IL2, IL7); and enhance immunoregulation (IL10) and humoral immunity. The implications of these changes are not clear.

CONCLUSION

Interventions Targeting HIV-exposed Children

The health status and diseases associated with HIV exposure in early life as described above show increased mortality and morbidity. The interventions to deal with these involve the delivery of high quality primary health care (PHC) designed to treat acute diseases and manage chronic disorders.[85] Those aspects of PHC relevant, but not specific, to HIV-exposed children include: perinatal care; immunization, especially against infections causing pneumonia and diarrhoea; early exclusive breastfeeding; nutrition support and food security for the infant and family; careful growth monitoring; psychosocial support for mothers and babies; and school programs. Maternal antiretrovirals, when indicated, preferably when CD4 counts are less than 350 cells/µL, are critical to maintain low viral loads and normal CD4 counts, to keep the mother alive, and to prevent mother-to-child transmission. Antiretrovirals, when indicated, and co-trimoxazole, when given to all affected members of the household, reduce opportunistic infections, tuberculosis, and other infectious agents. It is also essential to scale up and improve the quality and efficiency of health services, including the introduction of community-based programs and home-based care, institute the appropriate use of nonmedical health professionals and workers, and attend to the social determinants of health, including antipoverty measures.

NOTES
1. Countdown Coverage Writing Group. (2008). Countdown to 2015 for maternal, newborn and child survival: The 2008 report on tracking coverage of interventions. *Lancet, 371*(9620), 1247–1258.
2. United Nations. (2009). *The millennium development goals report.* New York: UN.
3. Countdown Coverage Writing Group. (2008). Countdown to 2015.
4. UNAIDS. (2009). *AIDS Epidemic update.* Geneva, Switzerland: UNAIDS & WHO.
5. UNAIDS, WHO & UNICEF. (2009). *Towards universal access: Scaling up priority HIV/AIDS interventions in the health sector.* Geneva, Switzerland: World Health Organization
6. McIntyre, J. (2010). Use of antiretrovirals during pregnancy and breastfeeding in low-income and middle-income countries. *Current Opinion in HIV and AIDS, 5*(1), 48–53.
7. Chersich, M. F., et al. (2008). Morbidity in the first year postpartum among HIV-infected women in Kenya. *International Journal of Gynaecology and Obstetrics, 100*(1), 45–51; Mataka, E. (2007). Maternal health and HIV: Bridging the gap. *Lancet, 370*(9595), 1290–1291; Ziraba, A. K., et al. (2009). Maternal mortality in the informal settlements of Nairobi city: What do we know? *Reproductive Health, 6*(6), doi:10.1186/1742-4755-6-6.

8. Coutsoudis, A., et al. (2010). Women's morbidity and mortality in the first 2 years post-delivery, according to HIV-status and infant feeding practices: The Vertical Transmission Study, South Africa. *AIDS, 24*(18), 2859–2866.

9. Hargrove, J. W., & Humphrey, J. H. (2010). Mortality among HIV-positive postpartum women with high CD4 cell counts in Zimbabwe." *AIDS, 24*(3), F11–14.

10. Becquet, R. et al. (2009). Universal antiretroviral therapy for pregnant and breast-feeding HIV-1-infected women: Towards the elimination of mother-to-child transmission of HIV-1 in resource-limited settings. *Clinical Infectious Diseases, 49*(12), 1936–1945.

11. Bulterys, M., et al. (1996). Fatal complications after Cesarian section in HIV-infected women. *AIDS,* 10(8), 923–924.

12. American College of Obstetricians and Gynecologists Committee Opinion. (2000). Scheduled cesarean delivery and prevention of vertical transmission of HIV infection. *International Journal of Gynecology and Obstetrics,* 73(3), 279–281.

13. Townsend, C. L., et al. (2008). Low rates of mother-to-child transmission of HIV following effective pregnancy interventions in the United Kingdom and Ireland, 2000–2006. *AIDS, 22*(11), 973–981.

14. Coovadia, H. M., & Bland, R. M. (2007). Preserving breastfeeding practice through the HIV pandemic. *Tropical Medicine and International Health, 12*(9), 1116–1133.

15. UNAIDS, WHO & UNICEF. (2009). *Towards universal access.*

16. WHO. (2002). *Strategic approaches to the prevention of HIV infection in infants.* Geneva, Switzerland: WHO.

17. UNAIDS, WHO & UNICEF. (2009). *Towards universal access.*

18. Dube, S., et al. (2008). Estimating vertically acquired HIV infections and the impact of the prevention of mother-to-child transmission program in Zimbabwe: Insights from decision analysis models. *Journal of Acquired Immune Deficiency Syndromes, 48*(1), 72–81.

19. WHO. (2002). *Strategic approaches.*

20. Ibid.

21. Dube et al. (2008). Estimating vertically acquired HIV infections.

22. Gray, R. H., et al. (2005). Increased risk of incident HIV during pregnancy in Rakai, Uganda: A prospective study. *Lancet, 366*(9492), 1182–1188; Lu, L., et al. (2009). *HIV incidence in pregnancy and the first post-partum year and implications for PMTCT programs, Francistown, Botswana, 2008.* 16th Conference on Retroviruses and Opportunistic Infections, Montreal, Canada; Moodley, D., et al. (2009). High HIV incidence during pregnancy: Compelling reason for repeat HIV testing. *AIDS, 23*(10), 1255–1259; Morrison, C. S., et al. (2007). Pregnancy and the risk of HIV-1 acquisition among women in Uganda and Zimbabwe. *AIDS, 21*(8), 1027–1034; Rehle, T., et al. (2007). National HIV incidence measures—new insights into the South African epidemic. *South African Medical Journal, 97*(3), 194–199.

23. Reynolds, H. W., et al. (2006). The value of contraception to prevent perinatal HIV transmission. *Sexually Transmitted Diseases, 33*(6), 350–356; Stover, J., et al. (2003). *Costs and benefits of adding family planning to services to prevent mother-to-child transmission of HIV (PMTCT).* Retrieved from http://www.k4health.org/system/files/FP_at_PMTCT_sites_Oct_1%5B1%5D.pdf; Sweat,

M. D., et al. (2004). Cost-effectiveness of nevirapine to prevent mother-to-child HIV transmission in eight African countries. *AIDS, 18*(12), 1661–1671.

24. Mesce, D., & Sines, E. (2006). *Unsafe abortion: Facts and Figures 2006.* Washington, D.C.: Population Reference Bureau.

25. Desgrees-Du-Lou, A., et al. (2002). Contraceptive use, protected sexual intercourse and incidence of pregnancies among African HIV-infected women. DITRAME ANRS 049 Project, Abidjan 1995–2000. *International Journal of STD and AIDS, 13*(7), 462–468.

26. Rochat, T. J., et al. (2006). Depression among pregnant rural South African women undergoing HIV testing. *JAMA: Journal of the American Medical Association, 295*(12), 1376–1378.

27. Homsy, J., et al. (2009). Reproductive intentions and outcomes among women on antiretroviral therapy in rural Uganda: A prospective cohort study. *PLoS One, 4*(1), e4149.

28. Coovadia, H. M. (2000). Prevention and treatment of perinatal HIV-1 infection in the developing world. *Current Opinion in Infectious Diseases, 13*(3), 247–251.

29. WHO. Recent documents by WHO on PMTCT (and on infant feeding). Retrieved from http://www.who.int/hiv/en/

30. Mofensen, L. (2009). Prevention of breast milk transmission of HIV: The time is now. *Journal of Acquired Immune Deficiency Syndromes, 52*, 305–308.

31. Marazzi, C. M., et al. (2007). Implementing anti-retroviral triple therapy to prevent HIV mother-to-child transmission: a public health approach in resource-limited settings. *European Journal of Pediatrics, 166*(12), 1305–1307; Palombi, L., et al. (2007). Treatment acceleration program and the experience of the DREAM program in prevention of mother-to-child transmission of HIV. *AIDS, 21*(Suppl 4), S65–71; Thomas, T., et al. (Eds.). (2008). *PMTCT of HIV-1 among breastfeeding women using HAART: The Kisumu Breastfeeding Study. Kisumu Kenya. 2003–2007 (45aLB).* 15th Conference on Retroviruses and Opportunistic Infections, Boston, MA; Kilewo, C., et al. (2009). Prevention of mother-to-child transmission of HIV-1 through breastfeeding by treating mothers with triple antiretroviral therapy in Dar es Salaam, Tanzania: The Mitra Plus study. *Journal of Acquired Immune Deficiency Syndromes, 52*(3), 406–416; Tonwe-Gold, B., et al. (2007). Antiretroviral treatment and prevention of peripartum and postnatal HIV transmission in West Africa: Evaluation of a two-tiered approach. *PLoS Med, 4*(8), e257; De Vincenzi, & Group KBS (Eds.). (2008). *HIV-free survival at 12 months among children born to HIV-infected women receiving antiretrovirals from 34 to 36 weeks of pregnancy (638).* 15th Conference on Retroviruses and Opportunistic Infections, Boston, MA.

32. Church, J. D., et al. (2008). Analysis of nevirapine (NVP) resistance in Ugandan infants who were HIV infected despite receiving single-Dose (SD) NVP versus SD NVP plus daily NVP up to 6 weeks of age to prevent HIV vertical transmission. *Journal of Infectious Diseases, 198*(7), 1075–1082.

33. Moorthy, A., et al. (2009). Nevirapine resistance and breast-milk HIV transmission: Effects of single and extended-dose nevirapine prophylaxis in subtype C HIV-infected infants. *PLoS One, 4*(1), e4096.

34. Zeh, C., et al. (2008.) *Emergence of HIV-1 drug resistance among breastfeeding infants born to HIV-infected mothers taking antiretrovirals for prevention of mother-to-child transmission of HIV: The Kisumu Breastfeeding Study, Kenya (84LB).* 15th Conference on Retroviruses and Opportunistic Infections, Boston, MA.

35. Lockman, S., et al. (2007). Response to antiretroviral therapy after a single, peripartum dose of nevirapine. *New England Journal of Medicine, 356*(2), 135–147.

36. Chi, B. H., et al. (2007). Single-dose tenofovir and emtricitabine for reduction of viral resistance to non-nucleoside reverse transcriptase inhibitor drugs in women given intrapartum nevirapine for perinatal HIV prevention: An open-label randomised trial. *Lancet, 370*(9600), 1698–1705.

37. Countdown Coverage Writing Group. (2008). Countdown to 2015; Horton, R. (2008). Countdown to 2015: A report card on maternal, newborn, and child survival. *Lancet, 371*(9620), 1217–1219.

38. Thior, I., et al. (2006). Breastfeeding plus infant zidovudine prophylaxis for 6 months vs. formula feeding plus infant zidovudine for 1 month to reduce mother-to-child HIV transmission in Botswana: A randomized trial: The Mashi Study. *JAMA: Journal of the American Medical Association, 296*(7), 794–805; Kilewo, C., et al. (2008). Prevention of mother-to-child transmission of HIV-1 through breast-feeding by treating infants prophylactically with lamivudine in Dar es Salaam, Tanzania: The Mitra Study. *Journal of Acquired Immune Deficiency Syndromes, 48*(3), 315–323; Vyankandondera,J., et al. (Eds.). (2003). *Reducing risk of HIV-1 transmission from mother to infant through breastfeeding using antiretroviral prophylaxis in infants (SIMBASTUDY).* 2nd IAS Conference on HIV Pathogenesis and Treatment, Paris, France; SWEN Study Team. (2008). Extended-dose nevirapine to 6 weeks of age for infants to prevent HIV transmission via breastfeeding in Ethiopia, India, and Uganda: An analysis of three randomized controlled trials. *Lancet, 372*(9635), 300–313; Kumwenda, N. I., et al. (2008). Extended antiretroviral prophylaxis to reduce breast-milk HIV-1 transmission. *New England Journal of Medicine, 359*(2), 119–129.

39. Shapiro, R. L., et al. (2010). Antiretroviral regimens in pregnancy and breast-feeding in Botswana. *New England Journal of Medicine, 362*(24), 2282–2294; Chasela, C., et al. (2010). Both maternal HAART and daily infant nevirapine (NVP) are effective in reducing HIV-1 transmission during breastfeeding in a randomized trial in Malawi: 28 week results of the Breastfeeding, Antiretroviral and Nutrition (BAN) Study (WeLB C103). *New England Journal of Medicine, 362*(24), 2271–2281.

40. WHO. (2008). *Report of the WHO Technical Reference Group.* Paediatric HIV/ART Care Guideline Group Meeting, WHO Headquarters, Geneva, Switzerland.

41. Violari, A., et al. (2008). Early antiretroviral therapy and mortality among HIV-infected infants. *New England Journal of Medicine, 359*(21), 2233–2244.

42. Ibid.

43. UNAIDS, WHO & UNICEF. (2009). *Towards universal access.*

44. Ekouevi, D. K., et al. (2004). Acceptability and uptake of a package to prevent mother-to-child transmission using rapid HIV testing in Abidjan, Cote d'Ivoire. *AIDS, 18*(4), 697–700; Fowler, M. G., et al. (2007). Reducing the risk of mother-to-child human immunodeficiency virus transmission: Past successes, current progress and challenges, and future directions. *American Journal of Obstetrics and Gynecology, 197*(Suppl. 3), S3–9; International Center for AIDS Care & Treatment Programs (Ed.). (2008). *Leveraging HIV scale-up to strengthen health systems in Africa.* Bellagio Conference Report, Mailman School of Public Health, Columbia University, New York; Lehmann, U., & Sanders, D. (2007).

Community health workers: What do we know about them? The state of the evidence on programmes, activities, costs and impact on health outcomes of using community health workers. Geneva, Switzerland: World Health Organization Evidence and Information for Policy, Department of Human Resources for Health; Megazzini, K. M., et al. (2009). Predictors of rapid HIV testing acceptance and successful nevirapine administration in Zambian labor wards *Journal of Acquired Deficiency Syndromes, 52*(2), 273–279; Stringer, E. M., et al. (2008). Monitoring effectiveness of programmes to prevent mother-to-child HIV transmission in lower-income countries. *Bulletin of the World Health Organization, 86*(1), 57–62; WHO Maximizing Positive Synergies Collaborative Group. (2009). An assessment of interactions between global health initiatives and country health systems. *Lancet, 373*, 2137–2169.

45. Rollins, N., et al. (2009). Universal HIV testing of infants at immunization clinics: An acceptable and feasible approach for early infant diagnosis in high HIV prevalence settings. *AIDS, 23*(14), 1851–1857.

46. Townsend et al. (2008). Low rates of mother-to-child transmission of HIV.

47. Barnett, T., & Whiteside, A. (2006). *AIDS in the twenty-first century: Disease and globalisation.* New York: Palgrave MacMillan.

48. Ndirangu, J., et al. (2009). Levels of childhood vaccination coverage and the impact of maternal HIV status on child vaccination status in rural KwaZulu-Natal, South Africa. *Tropical Medicine and International Health, 14*(11), 1383–1393.

49. Nyirenda, M., McGrath, N., & Newell, M. L. (2010). Gender differentials in the impact of parental death: Adolescent's sexual behaviour and risk of HIV infection in rural South Africa. *Vulnerable Children and Youth Studies, 5*, 284–296.

50. Chopra, M., et al. (2009). Saving the lives of South Africa's mothers, babies, and children: Can the health system deliver? *Lancet, 374*(9692), 835–846; Ford, K., & Hosegood, V. (2005). AIDS mortality and the mobility of children in KwaZulu Natal, South Africa. *Demography, 42*(4), 757–768; Hosegood V., & Timaeus, I. M. (2001). Household composition and dynamics in Kwazulu-Natal, South Africa: Mirroring social reality in longitudinal data collection. In E. Van der Walle (Ed.), *African households: An exploration of census data* (pp. 58–77). New York: ME Sharpe Inc.; M. U. Rompel, R. Gronemeyer, & G. A. Rakelmann (Eds.). (2002). *The social impact of AIDS on families in Botswana and Namibia* (abstract no E11467). International Conference on AIDS, Barcelona, Spain; Williamson, J. (Ed.). (2004). *A family is for a lifetime.* Washington, DC: The Synergy Project.

51. UNAIDS. (2010). *Survival of children HIV infected perinatally and through breastfeeding: A pooled analysis of individual data from resource constrained settings.* (UNAIDS report on survival of HIV infected children in Africa, final report). Geneva, Switzerland: UNAIDS.

52. Newell, M. L., et al. (2004). Mortality of infected and uninfected infants born to HIV-infected mothers in Africa: A pooled analysis. *Lancet, 364*(9441), 1236–1243.

53. Marinda, et al. (2007). Child mortality according to maternal and infant HIV status in Zimbabwe. *Pediatric Infectious Disease Journal, 26*(6), 519–526.

54. Filteau, S. (2009). The HIV-exposed, uninfected African child. *Tropical Medicine and International Health, 14*(3), 276–287.

55. Read, J. S., et al. (2009). Primary HIV-1 infection among infants in sub-Saharan Africa: HPTN 024. *Journal of Acquired Immune Deficiency Syndromes, 51*(3), 317–322; Taha, T. E., et al. (1995). The effect of human immunodeficiency virus

infection on birthweight, and infant and child mortality in urban Malawi. *International Journal of Epidemiology, 24*(5), 1022–1029.

56. Newell et al. (2004). Mortality of infected and uninfected infants; Marinda et al. (2007). Child mortality according to maternal and infant HIV status.

57. Newell et al. (2004). Mortality of infected and uninfected infants.

58. Ibid.; Marinda et al. (2007). Child mortality according to maternal and infant HIV status; Filteau. (2009). The HIV-exposed, uninfected African child; Read et al. (2009). Primary HIV-1 infection among infants in sub-Saharan Africa; Taha et al. (1995). The effect of human immunodeficiency virus infection on birthweight; Arpadi, S., et al. (2009). Growth faltering due to breastfeeding cessation in uninfected children born to HIV-infected mothers in Zambia. *American Journal of Clinical Nutrition, 90*(2), 344–353; Becquet, R., et al. (2007). Two-year morbidity-mortality and alternatives to prolonged breast-feeding among children born to HIV-infected mothers in Cote d'Ivoire. *PLoS Med, 4*(1), e17; Kagaayi, J., et al. (2008). Survival of infants born to HIV-positive mothers, by feeding modality, in Rakai, Uganda. *PLoS One, 3*(12), e3877; Kuhn, L., et al. (2005). Does severity of HIV disease in HIV-infected mothers affect mortality and morbidity among their uninfected infants? *Clinical Infectious Diseases, 41*(11), 1654–1661; Shapiro, R. L., et al. (2007). Infant morbidity, mortality, and breast milk immunologic profiles among breast-feeding HIV-infected and HIV-uninfected women in Botswana. *Journal of Infectious Diseases, 196*(4), 562–569.

59. Crampin, A.C., et al. (2002). Long term follow up of HIV positive and HIV negative individuals in rural Malawi. *AIDS, 16*(11), 1545–1550.

60. Kuhn et al. (2005). Does severity of HIV disease in HIV-infected mothers affect mortality?

61. Arpadi et al. (2009). Growth faltering.

62. Kuhn et al. (2005). Does severity of HIV disease in HIV-infected mothers affect mortality?

63. Bailey, R. C., et al. (1999). Growth of children according to maternal and child HIV, immunological and disease characteristics: A prospective cohort study in Kinshasa, Democratic Republic of Congo. *International Journal of Epidemiology, 28*(3), 532–540; Lepage, P., et al. (1996). Growth of human immunodeficiency type 1-infected and uninfected children: A prospective cohort study in Kigali, Rwanda, 1988 to 1993. *Pediatric Infectious Disease Journal, 15*(6), 479–485; Makasa, M., et al. (2007). Early growth of infants of HIV-infected and uninfected Zambian women. *Tropical Medicine and International Health, 12*(5), 594–602.

64. Patel, D., et al. (2010). Breastfeeding, HIV status and weights in South African children: A comparison of HIV-exposed and unexposed children. *AIDS, 24*(3), 437–445.

65. Makasa et al. (2007). Early growth of infants; Patel et al. (2010). Breastfeeding, HIV status and weights; Aylward, E. H., et al. (1992). Cognitive and motor development in infants at risk for human immunodeficiency virus. *American Journal of Diseases of Childhood, 146*(2), 218–222; Bagenda, D., et al. (2006). Health, neurologic, and cognitive status of HIV-infected, long-surviving, and antiretroviral-naive Ugandan children. *Pediatrics, 117*(3), 729–740; Fair, C. D., et al. (1995). Healthy children in families affected by AIDS: Epidemiological and psychological considerations. *Child & Adolescent Social Work Journal, 12*,

165–181; Mellins C. A., & Ehrhardt, A. A. (1994). Families affected by pediatric acquired immunodeficiency syndrome: Sources of stress and coping. *Journal of Developmental and Behavioral Pediatrics, 15*(3 Suppl.), S54–60.

66. Agostoni, C., et al. (1998). Growth in the first two years of uninfected children born to HIV-1 seropositive mothers. *Archives of Disease in Childhood, 79*(2), 175–178; Berhane, R., et al. (1997). Growth failure as a prognostic indicator of mortality in pediatric HIV infection. *Pediatrics, 100*(1), E7; Briand, N., et al. (2006). Growth of human immunodeficiency virus-uninfected children exposed to perinatal zidovudine for the prevention of mother-to-child human immunodeficiency virus transmission. *Pediatric Infectious Disease Journal, 25*(4), 325–332; Henderson, R. A., et al. (1996). Longitudinal growth during the first 2 years of life in children born to HIV-infected mothers in Malawi, Africa. *Pediatric AIDS and HIV Infection, 7*(2), 91–97; Moye, J., et al. (1996). Natural history of somatic growth in infants born to women infected by human immunodeficiency virus. Women and Infants Transmission Study Group. *Journal of Pediatrics, 128*(1), 58–69; Newell, M. L., Cortina-Borja, M., & Peckham, C. (2003). Height, weight, and growth in children born to mothers with HIV-1 infection in Europe. *Pediatrics, 111*(1), e52–60.

67. Becquet et al. (2007). Two-year morbidity-mortality.

68. Marinda et al. (2007). Child mortality.

69. Spira et al. (1999). Natural history of human immunodeficiency virus.

70. Read et al. (2009). Primary HIV-1 infection.

71. Shapiro et al. (2007). Infant morbidity, mortality.

72. McNally, L.M., et al. (2007). Effect of age, polymicrobial disease, and maternal HIV status on treatment response and cause of severe pneumonia in South African children: A prospective descriptive study. *Lancet, 369*(9571), 1440–1451; Otieno, R. O., et al. (2006). Increased severe anemia in HIV-1-exposed and HIV-1-positive infants and children during acute malaria. *AIDS, 20*(2), 275–280; Thea, D. M., et al. (1993). A prospective study of diarrhea and HIV-1 infection among 429 Zairian infants. *New England Journal of Medicine, 329*(23), 1696–1702.

73. Rotheram-Borus, M. J., Stein J. A., & Lin, Y. Y. (2001). Impact of parent death and an intervention on the adjustment of adolescents whose parents have HIV/AIDS. *Journal of Consulting and Clinical Psychology, 69*(5), 763–773.

74. Forehand, R., et al. (1999). Orphans of the AIDS epidemic in the United States: Transition-related characteristics and psychosocial adjustment at 6 months after mother's death. *AIDS Care, 11*(6), 715–722.

75. Forehand, R., et al. (1998). The Family Health Project: Psychosocial adjustment of children whose mothers are HIV infected. *Journal of Consulting and Clinical Psychology, 66*(3), 513–520.

76. Pelton, J., & Forehand, R. (2005). Orphans of the AIDS epidemic: An examination of clinical level problems of children. *Journal of the American Academy of Child and Adolescent Psychiatry, 44*(6), 585–591.

77. Esposito, S., et al. (1999). Behavioral and psychological disorders in uninfected children aged 6 to 11 years born to human immunodeficiency virus-seropositive mothers. *Journal of Developmental and Behavioral Pediatrics, 20*(6), 411–417.

78. Bagenda et al. (2006). Health, neurologic, and cognitive status; Drotar, D., et al. (1997). Neurodevelopmental outcomes of Ugandan infants with human immunodeficiency virus type 1 infection. *Pediatrics, 100*(1), E5; Msellati, P., et al. (1993).

Neurodevelopmental testing of children born to human immunodeficiency virus type 1 seropositive and seronegative mothers: A prospective cohort study in Kigali, Rwanda. *Pediatrics, 92*(6), 843–848.

79. Filteau. (2009). The HIV-exposed, uninfected African child.
80. Kuhn, L., et al. (2002). Human immunodeficiency virus (HIV)-specific cellular immune responses in newborns exposed to HIV in utero. *Clinical Infectious Diseases, 34*(2), 267–276.
81. Kuhn, L., et al. (2001). T-helper cell responses to HIV envelope peptides in cord blood: protection against intrapartum and breast-feeding transmission. *AIDS, 15*(1), 1–9.
82. Hygino, J., et al. (2008). Altered immunological reactivity in HIV-1-exposed uninfected neonates. *Clinical Immunology, 127*(3), 340–347.
83. Shapiro et al. (2007). Infant morbidity, mortality.
84. Kuhn et al. (2005). Does severity of HIV disease in HIV-infected mothers affect mortality?
85. Sepulveda, J., et al. (2006). Improvement of child survival in Mexico: The diagonal approach. *Lancet, 368*(9551), 2017–2027.

9

Breaking the Cycle

Challenges and Solutions in Pediatric HIV Policy

LIEZL SMIT, ANGELA DRAMOWSKI, KEVIN CLARKE,
JANINE CLAYTON, ANNEMADELEIN SCHERER,
AMY SLOGROVE, HAPPYSON MUSVOSVI,
MARINA RIFKIN, AND MARK COTTON ■

Children are one-third of our population and all of our future.
—SELECT PANEL FOR THE PROMOTION OF CHILD HEALTH, 1981

Talk is downhill. Do is uphill.
—PROVERB, OVERBERG DISTRICT, SOUTH AFRICA

Pediatric HIV, usually transmitted vertically, is a preventable disease. Although commonly referred to as mother-to-child transmission (MTCT), we prefer the term "vertical transmission" since both parents may play a role. In many developed countries, antiretroviral (ARV) drugs for vertical transmission prevention (VTP) have virtually eliminated childhood infection and have improved maternal survival.[1] Without any intervention, the risk of transmission ranges from 20% to 45%. With specific interventions, the risk can be reduced to below 5%.

HIV-infected children under 1 year of age are among the most vulnerable. Without treatment, one-third will die in the first year of life and half by 2 years of age.[2] However, with access to antiretroviral therapy (ART), good outcomes have been documented, with probability of survival 1 year after the start of ART ranging from 84% to 97%.[3] Although provision of ART to HIV-infected children is critical, maternal health is equally important for child survival. Children born to HIV-infected mothers are three to six times more likely to die, irrespective of their own HIV status.[4]

Progress in addressing the needs of children infected and affected by HIV/AIDS has been made in the last decade through improved evidence and accelerated action. Governments have displayed political will, endorsing progressive policies around

HIV prevention, care, and treatment services. Substantial external funding from the U.S. President's Emergency Plan for AIDS Relief (PEPFAR), the Global Fund, and others has supported national HIV programs. Treatment guidelines, policy documents, and HIV conferences and workshops are regularly developed.

Despite these global efforts, more than 1,000 HIV-infected babies were born on each day of 2009. HIV/AIDS remains one of the leading causes of under-5 mortality in low- and middle-income countries, reversing previous gains made in child survival. An estimated 260,000 children under the age of 15 died due to AIDS in 2009, and only 28% of eligible children under 15 actually received ART. HIV is also the leading cause of mortality among women of reproductive age.[5] As the response to HIV/AIDS moves forward, policy-makers, funders, and program leaders must reflect on why policies and guidelines are not being translated into more effective implementation and program outcomes.

Knowledge of the "ideal" medical intervention is insufficient to eliminate pediatric HIV infection. Many practical and social barriers prevent the implementation of policy guidelines. Understanding these barriers and developing locally appropriate solutions are critical to successfully addressing the needs of HIV-infected and -affected children and their families.

This chapter describes the current situation, policies and recommendations, and main medical barriers to implementation and highlights potential ways forward to address pediatric HIV/AIDS. Strategies are discussed from the perspectives of prevention, HIV detection, care and treatment, and high-risk groups, focusing on both health system and client factors.

PREVENTION OF PEDIATRIC HIV INFECTION

Vertical transmission prevention is a critical element of pediatric HIV services. Reduction to below 5% is an achievable goal. An estimated 53% of HIV-infected pregnant women in low- and middle-income countries received at least some ARVs for VTP in 2009, up from 35% in 2007 and 10% in 2004.[6] Several countries in Eastern and Southern Africa, Latin America, East Asia, and Central and Eastern Europe have achieved the United Nations General Assembly Special Session (UNGASS) goal of 80% coverage.

Despite progress in VTP coverage, some low- and middle-income countries' programs face considerable challenges related to the quality of services provided and, consequently, are making limited progress against HIV transmission. In 2009, only 26% of pregnant women received an HIV test. Of those tested, an estimated 51% testing positive were assessed for eligibility to receive ART for their own health, and 53% received ARVs for VTP. Only 35% of infants received ARV prophylaxis, and only 15% had an HIV test within the first 2 months of life.

Revised World Health Organization (WHO) guidelines on VTP, infant feeding, and ART were released in 2010. More efficacious ART regimens were recommended, including provisions for pregnant women requiring treatment for their own health and maternal or infant prophylaxis during breastfeeding. The effectiveness of these recommendations will depend on the implementation of key components that address both health system and client barriers: early booking, identification of HIV status, a robust ARV component, strategies to maintain target women in care, structured follow-up of the HIV-exposed infant, and appropriate infant feeding practices.

Early Access of Antenatal Services for Timely Testing and Treatment Initiation

Key to the elimination of VTP is the identification of maternal HIV status early in pregnancy. Focusing exclusively on the women who access antenatal care (ANC) without reaching all women in the community reduces the effectiveness of VTP programs. Infants born to mothers who have not received ANC have an HIV transmission risk of 25%.[7]

Many pregnant women access antenatal services when in utero transmission may have already occurred. In Ethiopia, only 6% of pregnant women had their first ANC visit before the fourth month of pregnancy. In South Africa, more than 50% of pregnant women attend antenatal care for the first time after 20 weeks gestation.[8] Lack of understanding and empowerment of women, exclusion of male partners, and poor knowledge and understanding by health care providers and communities have been documented as main barriers to early ANC access and HIV testing.

An example of a program that has addressed the above-mentioned barriers is the Family Health International's (FHI) Zambia Prevention, Care, and Treatment Partnership (ZPCT). HIV and VTP health education were implemented at community and health facility levels, with a focus on information programs for both women and men to foster understanding, reduce stigma, and involve male partners. Community leaders were engaged in sensitization and mobilization, in which all males were encouraged to accompany their spouses for their first ANC visit. This led to increased uptake of HIV counseling and testing from 45% to 99%.[9]

A proven strategy[10] to increase HIV testing uptake is to routinely recommend HIV testing following a group information session at the first ANC booking visit, with the possibility of opting out. HIV testing in the labor unit improves uptake by capturing unbooked women, women who did not have third-trimester retesting, and those who report a result different from the documented result.

Poor and unclear documentation of test results on maternal and child health records is a barrier to communication between health care workers when women move between different points of care. In South Africa, documentation tools such as the maternal care record and child health booklet now capture HIV test results and VTP interventions clearly.

Access to Antiretroviral Drugs

Traditionally, VTP and HIV care programs have been implemented in parallel with weak linkages; two-thirds of HIV-infected pregnant women fail to access ART interventions.[11] Health system barriers include high transport costs to clinics, inadequate referral information, long clinic wait times, unreliable access to laboratory diagnostics, lack of health care worker knowledge, problems with stock management, and overcrowding of ART clinics, with concomitant lack of privacy. Client factors include competing life priorities, such as earning income, seeking food and shelter, and stigma associated with HIV. The implementation of simple referral forms is effective in linking patients with ART clinics in rural Tanzania.[12] Innovative organizational changes, including nurse visits and pharmacy-only visits, have successfully decreased wait times in Ugandan clinics.[13] VTP psychosocial support groups promote health-seeking behavior and combat HIV-related stigma.[14]

Decentralization of HIV care and treatment services to primary clinic level, including CD4 testing, has significantly improved ART access in some settings. Effective models that use outreach teams to provide care and build capacity in rural clinics have shown success (see Box 9.1). With too few doctors in the public sector, nurses must be provided with proper training and support to initiate ART in primary care clinics. In settings with high antenatal care and maternity coverage, integrating VTP into basic antenatal care is cost-effective, utilizing existing infrastructure and human resources.[15]

Box 9.1

ART Outreach Teams Provide Support and Mentoring to Ensure ART for PMTCT Mothers in Rural Primary Health Care Clinics[16]

Location: Uthungulu District, KwaZulu-Natal, South Africa

Partners: KwaZulu-Natal Provincial Department of Health, Health Care Improvement Project/University Research Co. LLC (HCI/URC)

The problem: Uthungulu District experienced major challenges in initiating antiretroviral therapy (ART) for vertical transmission prevention (VTP) clients owing to human resource constraints and lack of integration of services. There were problems identifying eligible clients and long waiting lists for initiation.

The intervention: Geographic clustering of ART outreach teams consisting of a doctor, two professional nurses, a pharmacy assistant, a nutrition assistant, a lay counselor, and a data capturer covered all district primary health facilities. Data from each cluster were captured and discussed weekly to identify and address challenges. Onsite training and mentoring was provided to facility staff for data analysis and interpretation. Monthly meetings with district management were held for feedback, discussing issues of integration, and addressing challenges as a team.

Results: Early HIV transmission rates decreased from 23% to 4.5% in 2009. The program resulted in good integration of services at all levels, improvement in HIV testing rates in pregnancy (97%) since July 2009, and increases in pregnant women initiating ART from 524 in 2007 to 1,104 in 2009.

Maintaining Women in Care

One of the biggest challenges is patient attrition at each step of the VTP cascade. Recent research from Africa showed actual coverage rates at around 50%, despite the availability of services in more than two-thirds of antenatal facilities.

If the issue of health system performance is not addressed, adding more effective prevention of mother-to-child transmission (PMTCT) drug regimens and raising

CD4 thresholds for lifelong maternal ART will not eliminate HIV transmission to infants.[17] Each step of the cascade (counseling, HIV testing, CD4 testing, dispensing of ARVs at ANC and labor wards, testing of infants) must be delivered with greater than 90% reliability. Quality improvement methods and task shifting can yield benefits relatively quickly.[18] Reasons for attrition include human resource and infrastructure inadequacies, fractured services resulting in multiple clinic visits and high user costs for patients, poor health information, and lack of community-based support services.[19]

Vertical transmission prevention programs must address dropout rates among clients who undergo initial HIV testing early in pregnancy. Women testing negative early in pregnancy may still acquire infection during pregnancy. The high viral load associated with recent infection presents a much greater risk of transmission to their infants. Women who test positive may fail to return for follow-up for various reasons, such as negative experiences in the health care facility, inadequate counseling and poor understanding of the need for follow-up care, stigma, and fear of disclosure. There are additional barriers to ARV adherence. HIV-infected women may fail to take the ARVs, and those eligible for lifelong ART (to preserve their own health) may fail to register with and attend the treatment clinic. Strategies to facilitate access and retention in care include bundling laboratory tests into one visit, accompanying the patient to a referral point of care if within the same facility, and using referral forms with a feedback portion to help document successful referrals.

Initiating lifelong ART or a VTP prophylaxis regimen within the antenatal clinic reduces waiting times and allows the antenatal clinic staff to support adherence. Paper-based clinic registers of women enrolled in antenatal/VTP care facilitate tracking and defaulter tracing. Clients are entered into the register upon enrollment into care, and essential clinical interventions are documented longitudinally, including follow-up visits, on the same row in the register. Failed clinic appointments are detected by inspection of the register, and the clients are traced though a telephone call or home visit. Community health workers and other primary care support staff should be tasked with patient tracking when clinic visits are missed.

Follow-up of the HIV-exposed Infant

Early initiation of ART in HIV-infected children leads to a substantial reduction in mortality,[20] highlighting the critical importance of follow-up and early infant diagnosis of HIV infection. Globally, follow-up of HIV-exposed infants remains poor, with low uptake of HIV testing and co-trimoxazole prophylaxis. Lack of clarity around the roles and responsibilities of health care workers in postnatal care for HIV-exposed infants and their mothers is commonly reported. Service fragmentation, when VTP care and routine child health services are delivered in separate clinic areas and by different health care workers, is a major barrier to follow-up care.[21] PMTCT services are frequently not available at routine well-child clinics, and there is poor recording of PMTCT interventions and HIV testing results on child records. Fear of stigmatization after unintended disclosure when bringing infants for follow-up care[22] results in missed opportunities for diagnosis and early intervention.

The 6-week immunization visit provides an excellent opportunity for follow-up and testing of HIV-exposed infants within routine primary health services. Infants of mothers with no record of VTP interventions or who were tested early in pregnancy, or infants with signs and symptoms suggestive of HIV, should be screened for HIV exposure and if necessary, undergo HIV DNA polymerase chain reaction (PCR) testing.[23] Training of all levels of nurses in VTP and the care package for HIV-exposed infants will facilitate integration of VTP into routine well-child services.

Early infant HIV diagnosis uptake is enhanced through dedicated mother–baby clinics that link maternal postnatal care to infant testing and care in the same clinic room15 (see Box 9.2). Postnatal registers documenting maternal HIV status may identify infants needing HIV testing. Mother–infant pairs failing to attend their scheduled postnatal appointment can be easily identified for tracing. Longitudinal registers of HIV-exposed infants also facilitate the tracking and tracing of infants who drop out of care.

Box 9.2

SUPPORTING THE VULNERABLE MOTHER–INFANT PAIR[24]

Location: Durban, KwaZulu-Natal, South Africa

Partners: McCord Hospital PMTCT program, KwaZulu-Natal Provincial Department of Health

The problem: Linking vertical transmission prevention (VTP) mothers on antiretroviral therapy (ART) into routine chronic care after 6-week post-delivery visit with retention in care <50%.

The intervention: Establishment of a postnatal clinic for VTP mothers and their babies in the same venue as the antenatal clinic, staffed by the same counselors and clinicians, but held on a different day of the week. Patients graduated to the general ART clinic after the final 18-month HIV test for infants.

Services provided to the mother/child pair:

Baby: HIV testing at 6 weeks and 18 months, health promotion services (growth monitoring and nutritional advice, immunization, co-trimoxazole prophylaxis), and primary health care for infants.

Mother: Postnatal monitoring and care, general and HIV-related clinical support services including ART, psychosocial support.

Results: Retention in care improved to >80%, with an increasing number graduating at the end of 18 months, both mother and child being healthy.

Appropriate Infant Feeding Practices

HIV transmission via infant feeding is frequently overlooked and can undo prevention gains achieved earlier during pregnancy and delivery. The 2010 WHO principles and recommendations for HIV and infant feeding are based on accumulated programmatic and research outcomes within African countries. Considering the experiences of countries in implementing previous infant feeding guidelines and the difficulty in providing high-quality counseling to assist HIV-infected mothers to make appropriate infant feeding choices, it is recommended that countries decide on a single national infant feeding strategy estimated to give the greatest chance of HIV-free survival in that setting; either breastfeeding with ARV interventions or avoiding all breastfeeding. Evidence clearly shows an increased mortality associated with formula feeding in various VTP research studies from countries with high rates of malnutrition and a large infectious disease burden.[25] Strategies to reduce postnatal transmission that include free infant formula milk are two to six times more costly than ARV prophylaxis.[26]

In South Africa, with its sociodemographic pattern and urban–rural inequities, the majority of the population does not meet the WHO AFASS (Acceptable, Feasible, Affordable, Sustainable, and Safe) criteria for formula feeding. Until recently, the National Infant feeding policy advocated for both exclusive breastfeeding with prophylaxis and the continued provision of free commercial infant formula through public health facilities. The latter may have influenced feeding choices without taking WHO AFASS into account, leading to avoidable infant HIV transmission and death,[27] as well as sending mixed messages on infant feeding practices, and confusing both health care workers (who need to counsel and support their clients) and the mothers obliged to make difficult feeding decisions. Since August 2011 a single clear and consistent infant feeding policy, supporting breastfeeding with prophylaxis as the best practice, has been developed which should facilitate the implementation of appropriate feeding practices in South Africa.

PEDIATRIC HIV DETECTION, CARE, AND TREATMENT

Identification of HIV in children is vital to ensure timely access to care. Many of the children dying each day have either not received an HIV diagnosis or have not been initiated on ART.[28] Opportunities abound—but are often missed—for testing and diagnosing HIV in children who attend under-5 primary health clinics or TB services, in children who are pediatric in- and outpatients, and in the children of adults attending VCT services or HIV care and treatment programs (especially nutritional).[29]

The scale-up of pediatric ART at primary and secondary care facilities is further hampered by limited human resources, the perceived complexity of treating children, inadequate pediatric clinical skills, and weak referral and communication linkages. Successful and sustainable delivery of pediatric HIV/AIDS care and treatment services in resource-limited settings requires significant investment in transitioning from an acute health care system to a community-level chronic care framework. This transition poses significant leadership, financial, and human resource challenges, yet also offers an opportunity to strengthen primary health care services. There are also secondary benefits for health outcomes beyond those directly related to HIV/AIDS. Frequently, pediatric care is seen as an "add-on" service to already established adult care and treatment programs.

Globally, pediatric HIV care and treatment services have expanded rapidly in recent years, with multiple guidance documents developed by international health agencies and nongovernmental organization (NGO) stakeholders.[30] Essential to the launch of service delivery is thorough planning and preparation to be undertaken by governments, major implementing partner organizations, and communities. Key issues to be addressed include:

- Performance of a situational analysis, both at national and district level, to identify pediatric HIV service delivery gaps and resources available for mobilization.
- Policy and guideline development to support active case finding, close treatment gaps, and address necessary components for ART program expansion. The WHO 2010 Antiretroviral Therapy for HIV Infection in Infants and Children: Towards Universal Access guidelines incorporate many excellent evidence-based best practices. Policies must also ensure:
  - HIV testing consent laws are youth-friendly.
  - User fees are eliminated when feasible.
  - Any duties that shift the tasks of health care workers are outlined and authorized by relevant regulatory bodies.
  - The procurement of pediatric drug formulations and fixed-dose combination (FDC) preparations is prioritized.
  - Competencies form the foundation of human resource training and the standard to which mentorship and performance evaluations are measured.
- Establishment of a district-level framework for family-focused HIV/AIDS care incorporating the unique needs of children; this must be paired with ongoing supportive supervision and quality improvement review using established health program indicators.
- Community education and mobilization on expanding pediatric HIV services.

Task Shifting

A major challenge for rapid scale-up of ART provision to infants and children is the shortage of health personnel, especially in rural locations. Models estimate that the increase in human resources needed to achieve and sustain universal ART coverage in South Africa by 2017 equals two to three times the currently available resources.[31] In many low- and middle-income countries, such as South Africa, with its relatively recent access to ART, most children are started on ART in hospitals under the care of a physician or specialist.[32] Once established on ART, care is sometimes devolved to community-based ART programs.[33]

Task shifting, the delegation of tasks traditionally held by one cadre to another, has become an accepted and necessary public health strategy in the delivery of HIV/AIDS services in severely resource-constrained settings. Success is influenced by the confidence and competence of health care workers in the diagnosis and management of HIV-infected infants and children. Several reports have confirmed the success of nurse-led and community-based HIV care programs, with patient outcomes comparable to that of traditional, physician-led ART programs.[34] In Kigali, Rwanda, pediatric ART care was decentralized to nurse providers at the primary health care level with good clinical and virologic outcomes.[35] Important to this program and others is the task shifting of traditional nursing duties to other support staff or expert patients, inclusion of practicum training, mentorship, and physician referral support (see Box 9.3).

Box 9.3

Task Shifting ART Delivery to Nurse Providers: The South African Nurse Initiation and Management of ART (NIMART) Initiative[36]

Location: South Africa

Partners: Department of Health and various implementing partners

Intervention: On December 1, 2009, President Jacob Zuma declared bold new initiatives in the expansion of HIV testing and treatment services, including the expansion of ART services to every primary health care facility in the country. To achieve this goal, primary health care nurses were authorized to prescribe ART care on April 1, 2010, whereas historically pediatric ART care was physician- and often specialist-dependent.

Results: A number of barriers have surfaced that inform future planning:

1) Policy and legal conflicts exist between laws impacting health care workers; these require harmonization to establish a comfortable practice environment for nurse prescribers.

2) An effort to standardize nurse prescriber training curriculum lacks enforcement to uniformity by government and funder organizations, resulting in a myriad of nongovernmental organization-led training, often neglecting the unique needs of pediatric antiretroviral therapy (ART) management.

3) A framework for applied mentorship requires development and has highlighted the need to revisit physician job expectations to include greater support for nurse prescribers.

4) As more clinics provide ART services, a greater demand for effective referral network procedures and communication develops. District-level technical working groups consisting of local health authorities and implementation stakeholders are a possible forum to design, evaluate, and refine HIV care referral networks.

Pediatric HIV Testing and Case Detection

Testing children for HIV is the gateway to life-saving health interventions, whether through early infant diagnosis of the HIV-exposed infant or through diagnosis of any youth with concerning clinical findings or risk behavior. Globally, only 6% of infants in need are receiving early diagnosis.[37] Frequently, HIV testing is offered in counseling rooms far removed from areas of child health delivery, such as immunization clinics, integrated management of childhood illnesses (IMCI) focal points, and inpatient wards. A survey of nurses providing routine child health services in South African primary health care facilities found that "nurses were frequently unwilling to check for HIV in all children, believing it was unnecessary, unacceptable to mothers, and that they lack skills to implement HIV care."[38] This is despite findings in this and other studies that guardians do, in fact, want routine HIV testing services for their children. Incorporation of HIV screening into IMCI protocols should offer health care workers the necessary core skills to provide this service. The large testing gap must be overcome.

One strategy, provider-initiated testing and counseling (PITC), has demonstrated that it dramatically increases rates of pediatric HIV testing in resource-limited settings (see Box 9.4).[39] The 2010 WHO Policy Requirements for HIV Testing and Counseling of Infants and Young Children in Health Facilities clearly outlines PITC principles and programmatic considerations for implementation. Entry points include immunization clinics, labor wards, postnatal clinics, pediatric wards, IMCI focal areas, and TB clinics, as well as the targeting of children of adults already in ART care.

Box 9.4

PROVIDER-INITIATED TESTING AND COUNSELING IN THE HOSPITAL SETTING[40]

Location: University Teaching Hospital Lusaka, Zambia, and Kamuzu Central Hospital, Lilongwe, Malawi

Partners: Zambian Ministry of Health, International Centre for AIDS Care and Treatment Programs (ICAP), U.S. Centers for Disease Control and Prevention (CDC), Boston University School of Medicine

The problem: Hospitalized children in HIV-prevalent regions represent a high risk group for HIV and related opportunistic infections. Lack of HIV test results may lead to misdiagnosis, inappropriate treatments, and increased mortality.

The intervention: At the University Teaching Hospital, Lusaka, Zambia, counselors were placed at the admissions area to the pediatric ward to offer HIV testing services. At Kamuzu Central Hospital in Lilongwe, a similar approach also incorporated "patient escorts" to assist counselors and clinical staff in ensuring all pediatric admissions and their mothers were offered HIV testing.

Results: Over 18 months, 13,239 guardians were offered testing with 84.5% accepting at the University Teaching Hospital, Lusaka. Of those tested, 29.2% were HIV-antibody positive and thus in need of further HIV-related care services that may have been overlooked without a PITC approach. At Kamuzu Central Hospital, Lilongwe, a total of 10,244 HIV antibody tests and 453 DNA polymerase chain reaction (PCR) tests were performed with 97.8% of guardians accepting testing; 19.6% of all mothers and 8.5% of all children were HIV-infected and thereafter linked to HIV care services.

Antiretroviral Therapy Delivery in Children

Following HIV case detection, the child must be evaluated by a trained health care worker to determine if he or she meets ART eligibility criteria based on age, clinical staging, or CD4 criteria. In locations of endemic poverty and regionalized pediatric

HIV care, simply making it to the clinic is often the first barrier. Transport costs, disclosure of the child's HIV status to relatives, school absenteeism, user fees at the clinic, long clinic queues, and other demands on the guardian, such as income-generating needs, caring for other children, or personal illness, all contribute to this challenge.

Once in a care program, HIV-infected children and their families must be supported financially, emotionally, and socially to ensure optimal ART adherence and retention in care (see Box 9.5). It is vital for clinicians and policy-makers to realize that the best way of promoting child health and survival is to ensure the well-being of their primary caregivers. Thus, inclusive family-based HIV clinics that treat parents and children concurrently as a cohesive unit may achieve better ART outcomes.[41] There are many barriers to family clinics, however. Often, children are treated on a specific morning in a busy general clinic, and clinics need to be open at convenient times for working parents. There remains a need for further operational research on the organization and implementation of family clinics in low- and middle-income countries. Community buy-in and support are also critical factors that influence the success of ART programs for individuals enrolled. In some settings, community support was the most important predictor of outcome.[42]

Box 9.5

INCREASED ART ACCESS[43]

Location: Chipini is a rural community of high HIV prevalence located in a valley of rural Zomba District, Malawi.

Partners: Malawi Ministry of Health, Chipini Rural Hospital, Dignitas International (Canada), Baylor International Pediatric AIDS Initiative, Clinton Foundation

The problem: Access to Chipini from the Central Hospital referral facility is by a rugged, dirt road down a steep escarpment that becomes difficult to use during the rainy season. The community is served by a rural mission hospital, which began antiretroviral therapy (ART) services in 2006 with the support of a Canadian non-governmental organization (NGO). However, children were not routinely considered, therefore requiring referral to the Central Hospital for evaluation. Those who made it often did so by being carried on their grandmothers' backs for up to 2 days, where the CD4 would be taken and the trip repeated in several days' time for the results. Frequently, the walk would result in disappointment when the CD4 machine was malfunctioning.

The intervention: In 2009, Chipini began a process of decentralized CD4 collection from the Central Hospital and transport using the existing ambulance and NGO network. This was paired with monthly outreach support from a mobile mentorship team focused on building pediatric ART capacity.

Results: Since implementation, Chipini has seen a decrease in the number of children started on ART due to World Health Organization (WHO) Stage 4 conditions, an increase in those initiated due to CD4 criteria, and an overall increased percentage of pediatric ART patients.

An HIV-infected child, once evaluated, will be classified as either in need of ART initiation or not yet eligible (i.e., pre-ART). Due to donor and government documentation requirements, ART patients are usually well documented and can be traced if they default on their treatment. However, pre-ART patients are frequently lost due to documentation gaps, crowded clinics, and a lack of consistent messaging regarding the frequency of clinical and laboratory monitoring required. This is of special concern in children because the disease progresses faster in children than in adults.[44] Pre-ART patients are often in need of co-trimoxazole preventative therapy (CPT) and require a chronic care model of follow-up. One possible solution widely used in South Africa is the establishment of wellness clinics that cater to newly diagnosed HIV-infected patients and perform routine follow-ups of those not yet eligible for ART. In 2010, the National Department of Health rolled out nationwide pre-ART registers for standardized and enhanced documentation. Such documentation can improve patient monitoring, reduce redundant laboratory testing, and offer enhanced source data on the identified HIV patient burden soon to need ART.

Chronic ART delivery to children and youth will largely hinge on the competence of the health care workers who deliver it. Again, task shifting is a key strategy. However, a framework whereby patient complexity is paired with level of care can be a helpful adjunct. For example, where should a child with HIV and chronic lung disease receive care, as opposed to a healthy child with good nutrition? The answer will vary with the specific locale; however, the presence of some structure informing referrals and care complexity can greatly aid the processes of task-shifting and care decentralization (see Box 9.6).

Box 9.6

Building a Provider Network[45]

Location: Tshwane District, Gauteng, South Africa

Partners: Tshwane District Department of Health leadership, South to South Program for Comprehensive Family HIV Care and Treatment (S2S), Kalafong Academic Hospital, District Hospital and Primary Clinic Staff, National Laboratory Services, Regional Pharmacist, Foundation for Professional Development (FPD)

The problem: Pediatric antiretroviral therapy (ART) care is concentrated at the tertiary care hospital level despite a recent rapid increase in the number of community ART facilities.

The intervention: A focus group of stakeholders was convened to explore the reasons behind the slow decentralization and to develop a district implementation plan for timely HIV testing and decentralizing pediatric care and treatment services.

Results: A main reason identified was that referring physicians who had built good relationships with their patients simply did not know to whom they were referring their patients and whether quality care would be available. Effective patient referrals were described as those in which the referring provider knew that the patient would receive good care and that any concerns would be reported back. Forums that increase health care worker interaction within the referral network and foster better understanding of the service delivery standards were identified as possible solutions. The focus group has since begun drafting patient clinical criteria that inform the most appropriate level of care within the network.

Retention in Care

A systematic review of adult patient retention among sub-Saharan African ART programs revealed wide variation, with an overall attrition of 40% after 2 years.[46] Limited data are available on the rates of retention in care for children in developing countries. Pooled data from the Kids' Antiretroviral Treatment in Lower-income countries (KIDS-ART-LINC) collaborators show loss to follow-up rates of 10.3% at 2 years. In the International Epidemiological Databases to Evaluate AIDS (IeDEA)-South Africa analysis of 6,078 children, attrition due to loss to follow-up or death after 3 years was 7.7%. Reasons are unclear, and further prospective research is needed to clarify risk factors in developing countries. Possible causes suggested by the ART-LINC study include unreported death, unreported move, death or disease of the caregiver, financial distress, stigmatization, and negative experiences of HIV services.[47]

Program managers should look to ART programs with higher retention rates to improve pediatric ART services. A further challenge will be ensuring that treatment adherence levels and retention rates are maintained in the face of rapid scale-up.

ORPHANS AND VULNERABLE CHILDREN

There are an estimated 12 million orphans due to HIV in sub-Saharan Africa. By 2015, one-third of children younger than 18 years of age in South Africa will have lost one or both parents due to HIV.[48] The impact of AIDS on children starts well before the death of their parents and is aggravated by stigma, discrimination, and isolation in the community. Without a protective home environment, orphans and vulnerable children (OVC) face increasing violence, exploitation, abuse, food insecurity, nutritional deficits, educational compromise, and engagement in risky sexual behavior.

Strategies to prevent vulnerability include universal access to maternal health services, universal birth registration, and social service provision to ensure access to health, nutrition, and adequate housing. Other important interventions are access to early childhood and formal education, and skills-building opportunities for new parents. Although some governments do offer social welfare grants, many parents or caregivers are unskilled and unable to cope with the simple paperwork required for processing these applications. In South Africa, only one-third of mothers or caregivers access the child care grant.[49]

The effects and cost of HIV can be catastrophic to a family. The loss of an economically active parent, which includes functional handicaps due to chronic illness, disability and death, results in many challenges for the affected child. These include the responsibility of caring for siblings and ill parents; loss of property and accommodation in the community; abuse; role-shifting, with children taking responsibility

"I struggle to listen in class. My mother is sick at home, and I am afraid that she will be dead when I come home. There is no one to look after her. Some days I do not go to school because she is too sick for me to leave her." (16-year-old girl)

"When your mother has HIV . . . and she dies and leaves that small baby also with HIV, then you have to go to school, but also look after the baby" (13-year-old)

"Once when my sister collapsed at school, the other children laughed at her and teased..." (17 year old)

for activities of daily life, such as household chores; responsibility of generating an income for the household; and school drop-out, often to save on school fees as well as to participate in income-generating activities and to take care of sick family members.[50]

In 2004, UNICEF[51] provided a framework for the protection, care, and support of OVC living in a world with HIV/AIDS. Strategies include:

- *Strengthening the capacity of families to cope with their problems.* Home-based care workers could support families with palliative home care to facilitate the children attending school.
- *Mobilizing and strengthening community-based responses,* such as adapting school hours to allow vulnerable children to partake in income-generating activities.
- *Strengthening the capacity of children and young people to meet their own needs,* such as child-friendly health clinics and retention in the educational system (see Box 9.8).
- *Ensuring that governments protect the most vulnerable children and provide essential services,* such as implementing national policies addressing child rights in local municipality plans.
- *Creating an enabling environment for affected children and families,* such as projects to reduce public stigmatization.

Box 9.7

Grandmothers Against Poverty and AIDS (GAPA)[52]

Location: Khayelitsha informal settlement, Cape Town, South Africa

Partners: Community, occupational therapist

The problem: Grandmothers looking after HIV-orphaned grandchildren often lack the financial means and knowledge to care for them.

The intervention: Life skills and income-generation activities through crafts.

Results: Grandmothers are empowered to teach their grandchildren the newly gained skills and to focus on supporting the education of the children.

Even though collaborative systems render good results (see Box 9.8), there are still challenges to overcome.[53] Well-intentioned programs and funds are often misdirected and lack robust outcome evaluation due to poor documentation of methodology and lack of research. A review of community interventions providing care and support to OVC concluded that community interventions were valuable and achieved measurable improvements in child and family well-being. However, the same review found that the quality and rigor of evidence varied, necessitating a strategic research agenda to inform resource allocation and program management.[54] In addition, none of the community interventions for improving the psychosocial well-being of HIV-affected children was adequate, highlighting the urgent need for operational research in this area.[55]

BOX 9.8

INTERSECTORAL COLLABORATION TO ADDRESS THE NEEDS OF HIV ORPHANS

Location: School in rural South Africa

Partners: Department of Social Services, Department of Health, Department of Education, community members

The problem: The headmaster realized that some of her pupils were sleeping on the school premises. On closer investigation she realized that they were HIV orphans.

The intervention: Intersectoral collaboration between government departments and community members.

Results: Accommodation was arranged for the children. The school became the hub for child-focused services: The clinic provides child-friendly health services once a week at the school; the appropriate government department regularly visits to assist with needed documentation; social services render weekly counseling and support for children on the school premises; and the school developed a vegetable garden, using the crop to provide lunch, with the remainder of the crop being sold. One of the main reasons this initiative was successful was close communication between three government departments and the community.

ADOLESCENTS

HIV-infected adolescents may be either long-term child survivors or newly infected. The calculation of HIV incidence among this group remains challenging due to their limited interaction with the health system and the delayed onset of HIV-related illnesses.

Early sexual debut, intergenerational sex, multiple sexual partners, and concurrency of sexual partners increase the risk of HIV infection during adolescence.[7] For adolescents enrolled in ART programs, problems of treatment adherence and retention in care are magnified. In developed nations, multidisciplinary teams, including social workers, psychologists, and peer counselors, support adolescent ART programs.[56] Such programs could provide a model of care for the development of adolescent services in low- and middle-income countries. Managing the transition of adolescent care from pediatric to adult services has also not been sufficiently explored in sub-Saharan Africa.

Programs that build on adolescents' primary need to belong to a social group and take into account their complex developmental needs are more likely to be effective in reaching this group, often lost between pediatric and adult health care services (see Box 9.9). Examples of adolescent- friendly initiatives are support groups, such as informal social or sports groups. These groups have had undocumented and unpublished successes in providing referral avenues for adolescent treatment. Several groups use organized team sports, such as soccer, to provide key HIV messaging and also as a source for detection and referrals to clinical services.

Box 9.9

ADOLESCENT CLINIC AT BOTSWANA-BAYLOR CHILDREN'S CLINICAL CENTRE OF EXCELLENCE[57]

Location: Botswana-Baylor Children's Clinic, Botswana

Partners: Baylor International Pediatric AIDS Initiative, Texas Children's Hospital, and Teen Club International

The problem: The complex developmental and societal challenges experienced by adolescents increases the vulnerability of teenagers living with HIV.

The intervention: In addition to the clinical HIV management, a program of appropriate psychosocial support interventions was prioritized. The focus on peer education groups in Teen Clubs provides safe spaces where adolescents, through a variety of activities including social events and themed interest groups, have opportunities to develop life skills necessary to live with the complexities of adolescence and an HIV-positive diagnosis.

Results: Although very little has been documented of these interventions, this center reports a significant increase in adolescents enrolled in their clinical program and the Teen Clubs. They also report improved adherence to treatment.

The national legal framework regarding consent for HIV testing and the provision of care and treatment is often a barrier. In many countries, these laws are criticized for their inconsistency, which contributes to the difficulties that health care workers experience when interacting with and providing care to children and adolescents in a lawful manner.[58] The capacity of children and adolescents to consent, as well as who should be able to grant consent when children lack that capacity, are often not clearly defined. The inability of health care workers to accurately interpret and implement these laws often results in missed health care opportunities for children and adolescents.

In Moretele, a rural South African district, nurses and lay counselors often communicate their difficulties and tensions in providing adequate care for adolescents. Lack of knowledge, problems of interpersonal understanding, and lack of training are identified as inhibiting factors (see Box 9.10). Attitudes of health care workers toward adolescents are often not conducive to providing adequate health care. These attitudes are often informed by societal and cultural beliefs about the place of adolescents within society. For HIV care, these negative attitudes are compounded by issues relating to sexuality, and are often considered taboo for discussion between adults and adolescents. The sexual debut of children in South Africa occurs at around 12 years of age.[59] Nevertheless, there is widespread neglect in managing the health of older children and adolescents as potentially active sexual beings. Furthermore, intricate issues relating to the management of child sexual abuse in health care settings complicates the engagement of health care workers with children and adolescents seeking medical intervention due to abuse.

Future research should focus on how best to target HIV-infected adolescents, modify risk behaviors, ensure treatment adherence, promote retention in care, and successfully transition to adult programs.

Box 9.10

TRAINING OF LAY COUNSELORS[60]

Location: Moretele sub-District, North West Province, South Africa

Partners: Department of Health, South to South Program for Comprehensive Family HIV Care and Treatment (S2S)

The problem: Attitudes and perceptions of health care workers regarding children and adolescents may act as barriers to implementation of HIV prevention, care, and treatment.

The intervention: Psychosocial support training with lay counselors was initiated. The curriculum includes exploration of personal values and attitudes impacting on practice, as well as theoretical input on psychosocial support needs of individuals living with and affected by HIV.

Results: Although further work still is required with the lay counselors, the initial exploration through experiential learning methodologies facilitates further corrective action. A comment from a workshop participant after a training session is "I can see now that my attitude was not helping the client, I did not think that my attitude was making my work difficult."

PROGRAM MONITORING AND EVALUATION

Although programmatic efforts to reach targets are under way, major challenges in obtaining accurate data from clinical sites to track progress have been reported.[61] National health systems rely on data for national reports and planning of resource allocation, thus impacting on programs and patient management. The success of any program hinges on the ability of health care workers to evaluate patient and program outcomes easily and to intervene when needed. For both clinic staff and health system managers, access to reliable data that reflect the process of care and clinical outcomes is the first step to ensuring effective service delivery.

This can be partially achieved through simplification of the collecting and reporting process. However, data will only attain significant value if used by clinic staff in an ongoing process to manage patients and populations. Lack of unique patient identification numbers complicates patient tracking and causes confusion

Table 9.1 Vulnerable, Hard-to-Reach Populations

Target Populations and ideal interventions	Barriers to Achieving Interventions	Possible Solutions
Pregnant Women		
Early access of antenatal services for timely testing	Lack of understanding and empowerment of women	Health education at community and health facility levels for both women and men
		Engage community leaders in sensitization and mobilization
Access to Antiretroviral Drugs	Exclusion of male partners	Encourage disclosure and testing of father
		Encourage males to accompany their spouses for their first ANC visit
Maintaining women in care	Inefficiencies within the health care system, weak linkages between VTP and HIV care programs	Effective referral forms to link patients with ART clinics
		Routine HIV testing following a group information session at the first ANC booking visit, with the option to opt-out
		Quality improvement methods (i.e., bundling laboratory tests into one visit and task shifting)
		Initiating lifelong ART or the VTP prophylaxis regimen within the antenatal clinic
		Accompanying the patient to a referral point of care if within the same facility.
		Use of referral forms with a feedback portion to help document successful referrals
		Paper-based clinic registers of women enrolled into antenatal/VTP care facilitate tracking and defaulter tracing
	Problems in health care access, infrastructure, and human resources	Decentralize HIV care and treatment services to primary clinic level
		Integrate VTP into basic antenatal care, utilizing existing infrastructure and human resources
		Nurse-initiated ART
		Clinic organizational changes including nurse visits and pharmacy-only visits
		ART outreach teams to provide support and mentoring to ensure ART for PMTCT mothers
		Human resource training with competencies as outcome

	Competing life priorities for patients, such as earning income, seeking food and shelter, and stigma	VTP psychosocial support and income-generating groups
		Access to social grants
		Community health workers and other primary care support staff to track patient when clinic visits are missed
	Lack of community-based support services	Health education at community and health facility levels
		Engage community leaders
HIV-exposed Infant	VTP and child health services fragmentation, lack of clarity around health care worker roles and responsibilities in postnatal care for HIV-exposed infants and their mothers	Integration of services: 6-week immunization visit for follow-up and testing of HIV-exposed infants within routine primary health services
Early infant diagnosis of HIV infection		Dedicated mother–baby clinics that link maternal postnatal care to infant testing and care in the same clinic room
Access to follow-up care and prophylaxis		Training of all levels of nurses in VTP and the care package for HIV-exposed infant
Appropriate infant feeding practices		Human resource training with competencies as outcome
Early initiation of ART in HIV-infected infants	Poor and unclear documentation of maternal test results with missed opportunities to identify exposed infants	Documentation tools such as maternal care record, child health booklet, postnatal registers with maternal HIV status, longitudinal registers of HIV-exposed infants
	Inadequate counseling of adult provider	Counseling and (re)testing of all mothers with unknown or early pregnancy HIV-negative status
		Health education; inform adults including parents and grandparents of need to establish HIV status
		Clear and consistent evidence-based infant feeding policy
	Fear of stigmatization	Psychosocial support groups
		Health education at community and health facility levels

(continued)

Table 9.1 (CONTINUED)

Target Populations and ideal interventions	Barriers to Achieving Interventions	Possible Solutions
HIV-infected child Active case finding ART eligibility assessment Pre-ART care Early access to ARV drugs if eligible Maintaining children in care Ensure well-being of primary caregivers	Service fragmentation with treatment and routine child health services delivered in separate clinics; weak referral and communication linkages	Wellness clinics catering to newly diagnosed HIV-infected patients and the routine follow-up of those not yet eligible for ART Nurse-led and community-based HIV care programs Longitudinal pre-ART and ART registers Accompanying the patient to a referral point of care if within the same facility Use of referral forms with a feedback portion to help document successful referrals Incorporation of HIV screening into integrated management of childhood illnesses (IMCI) protocols Provider initiated testing and counseling (PITC) Testing and diagnosing HIV in children at all health entry points: primary health clinics, immunization clinics, TB services, pediatric in- and outpatients, children of adults attending VCT services or HIV care and treatment programs, orphans, cases of sexual abuse
	Poor understanding by communities	Community education and mobilization
	Problems in health care access, infrastructure, and human resources	Scale-up of pediatric ART access at primary and secondary care facilities Decentralized provider network, access to laboratory and health care services. Inclusive family-based HIV clinics that treat parents and children concurrently, as a cohesive unit Nurse initiation of ART Task shifting of traditional nursing duties to other support staff or expert patients with referral support and patient complexity paired with level of care Outreach support from a mobile mentorship team building pediatric ART capacity

		Procurement of pediatric drug formulations and fixed-dose combination (FDC) preparations
	Competing life priorities such as earning income, caring for other children, and personal illness	Competencies-based human resource training with mentorship and performance evaluations
		Psychosocial support and income-generating groups, including access to social grants
		Health education at community and health facility levels
	Disclosure of the child's HIV status	Parental support groups
Orphans and Vulnerable Children (OVC)	Stigma, discrimination, and isolation in the community, food insecurity, nutritional consequences, educational compromise, and engagement in risky sexual behavior	Social service provision, including welfare grants, to ensure access to health, nutrition, and adequate housing
Protective home and community environment		Access to early childhood and formal education
Physical and psychosocial well-being		Home-based care workers to support families with palliative home care to facilitate the children attending school
		Mobilizing and strengthening community-based responses such as adapting school hours to allow vulnerable children to partake in income-generating activities
		Strengthening the capacity of children and young people to meet their own needs
		Skills-building and income-generation opportunities for guardians
		Intersectoral collaboration between government departments and community members
	Lack of outcomes evaluation of community process	Needs further research

(continued)

Table 9.1 (CONTINUED)

Target Populations and ideal interventions	Barriers to Achieving Interventions	Possible Solutions
Adolescents Accessible health services for testing and information Address complex developmental and societal challenges Behavioral risk reduction Treatment adherence and retention in care	Adolescents' lack information about disease	Health education at community (school) and health facility levels Engage community leaders in sensitization and mobilization Peer education groups in Teen Clubs provide safe spaces where adolescents, through a variety of activities including social events and themed interest groups, have opportunities to develop life skills necessary to live with the complexities of adolescence and an HIV-positive diagnosis
	Adolescents have poor interaction with the health care system (health care worker attitudes toward adolescents, societal position, structural constraints)	Adolescent-friendly initiatives prioritizing clinical HIV management and psychosocial support interventions. Multidisciplinary teams, including social workers, psychologists and peer counselors to support the adolescent ART programs Clinic organizational changes including extended clinic hours (after school and over weekends) Psychosocial support training of health care workers, in which the curriculum includes exploration of personal values and attitudes impacting on practice, as well as theoretical input on psychosocial support needs of individuals living with and affected by HIV
	Weak implementation of national legal framework regarding consent for testing and care and treatment	Health education at community (school) and health facility levels Engage community leaders in sensitization and mobilization
	Lack of outcomes evaluation	Needs further research

ANC, antenatal clinics; ART, antiretroviral therapy; PMTCT, prevention of mother-to-child transmission; VTP, vertical transmission prevention with patient files and laboratory results. Clinic staff require support and supervision in performing data management tasks.

CONCLUSION

A concerted and multipronged approach is needed to eliminate pediatric HIV infections and to improve maternal, newborn, and child health and survival in the context of HIV.[62] The future of children and families infected and affected by HIV will depend on the abilities of policy-makers, funders, and program leaders to translate policies, research, and guidelines into more effective implementation and program outcomes. We need to get this right; lives depend on our actions.

Key points in the chapter are summarized in Table 9.1.

ACKNOWLEDGMENTS

We thank Drs. Helena Rabie, Steve Innes, and Helen Weber, and Makabongwe Ngxota for additional thoughts and inputs into the chapter.

DISCLAIMER

The South to South Program for Comprehensive Family HIV Care & Treatment (S2S) is funded by United States Agency for International Development (USAID) and US President's Emergency Plan for AIDS Relief (PEPFAR). The content expressed herein does not necessarily reflect the views of the USAID.

NOTES

1. Paintsil, E. & Andiman, W. A. (2009). Update on successes and challenges regarding mother-to-child transmission of HIV. *Current Opinion in Pediatrics, 21*(1), 94–101.
2. Paediatric HIV Prognostic Markers Collaborative Study Group. (2003). Short-term risk of disease progression in HIV-1-infected children receiving no antiretroviral therapy or zidovudine monotherapy: A meta-analysis. *Lancet, 362*(9396), 1605–1611; Dabis, F., et al. (2001). 18-month mortality and perinatal exposure to zidovudine in West Africa. *AIDS, 15*(6), 771–779; Spira, R., et al. (1999). Natural history of human immunodeficiency virus type 1 infection in children: A five-year prospective study in Rwanda. Mother-to-Child HIV-1 Transmission Study Group. *Pediatrics, 104*(5), e56; Newell, M. L., et al. (2004). Mortality of infected and uninfected infants born to HIV-infected mothers in Africa: A pooled analysis. *Lancet, 364*(9441), 1236–1243.
3. Eley, B. J., et al. (2004). Initial experience of a public sector antiretroviral treatment programme for HIV-infected children and their infected parents. *South African Medical Journal, 94*(8), 643–646; Reddi, A., et al. (2007). Preliminary outcomes of a paediatric highly active antiretroviral therapy cohort from Kwazulu-Natal, South Africa. *BMC Pediatrics, 7*, 13; Wamalwa, D. C., et al. (2007). Early response to highly active antiretroviral therapy in HIV-1-infected Kenyan children. *Journal of Acquired Immune Deficiency Syndromes, 45*(3), 311–317.

4. Kuhn, L., et al. (2005). Does severity of HIV disease in HIV-infected mothers affect mortality and morbidity among their uninfected infants? *Clinical Infectious Diseases, 41*(11), 1654–1661.

5. WHO, UNAIDS & UNICEF. (2010). *Towards universal access: Scaling up priority HIV/AIDS interventions in the health sector: Progress report 2010.* Geneva, Switzerland: WHO, UNAIDS, UNICEF. Retrieved December 12, 2010, http://www.who.int/hiv/pub/2010progressreport/report/en/index.html

6. Ibid.

7. Barker, P. M., Mphatswe, W., & Rollins, N. (2011). Antiretroviral drugs in the cupboard are not enough: The impact of health systems' performance on mother-to-child transmission of HIV. *Journal of Acquired Immune Deficiency Syndromes, 56*(2), e45–48.

8. Shisana, O., et al. (2009). *South African national HIV prevalence, incidence, behaviour and communication survey, 2008: A turning tide among teenagers.* Cape Town, South Africa: HSRC Press. Retrieved December 16, 2010, http://www.mrc.ac.za/pressreleases/2009/sanat.pdf

9. Torpey, K., et al. (2010). Increasing the uptake of prevention of mother-to-child transmission of HIV services in a resource-limited setting. *BMC Health Services Research, 10,* 29.

10. Perez, F., et al. (2006). Acceptability of routine HIV testing ('opt-out') in antenatal services in two rural districts of Zimbabwe. *Journal of Acquired Immune Deficiency Syndromes, 41*(4), 514–520.

11. Muchedzi, A., et al. (2010). Factors associated with access to HIV care and treatment in a prevention of mother to child transmission programme in urban Zimbabwe. *Journal of the International AIDS Society, 13,* 38; Posse, M., et al. (2008). Barriers to access to antiretroviral treatment in developing countries: A review. *Tropical Medicine and International Health, 13*(7), 904–913.

12. Nsigaye, R., et al. (2009). From HIV diagnosis to treatment: Evaluation of a referral system to promote and monitor access to antiretroviral therapy in rural Tanzania. *Journal of the International AIDS Society, 12*(1), 31.

13. Castelnuovo, B., et al. (2009). Improvement of the patient flow in a large urban clinic with high HIV seroprevalence in Kampala, Uganda. *International Journal of STD and AIDS, 20*(2), 123–124.

14. Lyttleton, C., Beesey, A., & Sitthikriengkrai, M. (2007). Expanding community through ARV provision in Thailand. *AIDS Care, 19*(Suppl. 1), S44–53.

15. Agadjanian, V., & Hayford, S. R. (2009). PMTCT, HAART, and childbearing in Mozambique: An institutional perspective. *AIDS and Behavior, 13*(Suppl 1), 103–112; G. Mazia, G., et al. (2009). Integrating quality postnatal care into PMTCT in Swaziland. *Global Public Health, 4*(3), 253–270.

16. Youngleson, M. (2010). Tried & tested: Models for the scale up of HIV prevention, treatment and care from South Africa and beyond. Pretoria, South Africa: South African National Department of Health.

17. Nkonki, L., et al. (2007). Missed opportunities for participation in prevention of mother to child transmission programmes: Simplicity of nevirapine does not necessarily lead to optimal uptake, a qualitative study. *AIDS Research and Therapy, 4,* 27.

18. Barker, P. M., et al. (2007). Strategies for the scale-up of antiretroviral therapy in South Africa through health system optimization. *Journal of Infectious Diseases, 196*(Suppl. 3), S457–463; Zachariah, R., et al. (2009). Task shifting in

HIV/AIDS: Opportunities, challenges and proposed actions for sub-Saharan Africa. *Transactions of the Royal Society of Tropical Medicine and Hygiene, 103*(6), 549–558.

19. Coetzee, D., Stringer E. M., & Chi, B. H. (2009, July). *Evaluation of PMTCT coverage in four African countries: The PEARL Study.* Report presented at the 5th IAS Conference on HIV Pathogenesis, Treatment and Prevention, Cape Town, South Africa.

20. Violari, A., et al. (2008). Early antiretroviral therapy and mortality among HIV-infected infants. *New England Journal of Medicine, 359*(21), 2233–2244.

21. Doherty, T. M., McCoy D., & Donohue, S. (2005). Health system constraints to optimal coverage of the prevention of mother-to-child HIV transmission programme in South Africa: Lessons from the implementation of the National Pilot Programme. *African Health Sciences, 5*(3), 213–218.

22. Varga, C. A., Sherman G. G., & Jones, S. A. (2006). HIV-disclosure in the context of vertical transmission: HIV-positive mothers in Johannesburg, South Africa. *AIDS Care, 18*(8), 952–960.

23. Nkonki et al. (2007). Missed opportunities; Barker et al. (2007). Strategies for the scale-up of antiretroviral therapy.

24. Youngleson, M. (2010). Tried & tested: Models for the scale up of HIV prevention, treatment and care from South Africa and beyond. Pretoria, South Africa: South African National Department of Health.

25. Lockman, S., Smeaton L. M., & Shapiro, R. L. (2006, August). Morbidity and mortality among infants born to HIV infected mothers and randomized to breastfeeding versus formula feeding in Botswana (MASHI Study). Report presented at The International AIDS Conference, Toronto, Canada; Mbori-Ngacha, D., et al. (2001). Morbidity and mortality in breastfed and formula-fed infants of HIV-1-infected women: A randomized clinical trial. JAMA: Journal of the American Medical Association, 286(19), 2413–2420.

26. WHO. (2010). Guidelines on HIV and infant feeding 2010: Principles and recommendations for infant feeding in the context of HIV and a summary of evidence. Geneva, Switzerland: WHO. Retrieved December 12, 2010, http://www.who.int/child_adolescent_health/documents/9789241599535/en/index.html

27. Doherty, T., et al. (2011). Implications of the new WHO guidelines on HIV and infant feeding for child survival in South Africa. *Bulletin of the World Health Organisation, 89*, 62–67; Doherty, T., et al. (2007). Effectiveness of the WHO/UNICEF guidelines on infant feeding for HIV-positive women: Results from a prospective cohort study in South Africa. *AIDS, 21*(13), 1791–1797.

28. WHO. (2008). *Mortality profiles.* Geneva, Switzerland: WHO. Retrieved September 12, 2001, http://www.who.int/whosis/mort/profiles/en

29. Krug, A., Pattinson, R. C., & Power, D. J. (2004). Why children die: An under-5 health care survey in Mafikeng Region. *South African Medical Journal, 94*(3), 202–206.

30. USAID. (2010). *USAID paediatric HIV toolkit.* Retrieved November 30, 2010, http://www.aidstar-one.com; WHO & UNAIDS. (2010). *WHO and UNAIDS resource kit for writing global fund proposals.* Geneva, Switzerland: WHO/UNAIDS. Retrieved June 12, 2010, http://www.who.int/hiv/pub/toolkits/GF-Resourcekit/en/; Baylor International Pediatric AIDS Initiative. (2010). *BIPAI toolkit: Providing care and treatment for children with HIV/AIDS in*

resource-limited settings. Retrieved December 8, 2010, http://www.bayloraids. org/toolkit; R. G. Marlink, & S. J. Teitelman (Eds.). (2009). *From the ground up: Building comprehensive HIV/AIDS care programs in resource-limited setting.* Washington, D.C.: Elizabeth Glaser Pediatric AIDS Foundation. Retrieved December 12, 2010, http://www.pedaids.org/Publications/From-the-Ground-Up

31. Barnighausen, T., et al. (2007). Human resources for treating HIV/AIDS: Needs, capacities, and gaps. *AIDS Patient Care and STDS, 21,* 799–812.

32. Meyers, T., et al. (2007). Challenges to pediatric HIV care and treatment in South Africa. *Journal of Infectious Diseases, 196*(Suppl 3), S474–81.

33. Eley, B., et al. (2006). Antiretroviral treatment for children. *South African Medical Journal, 96,* 988–993.

34. Callaghan, M., Ford N., & Schneider, H. (2010). A systematic review of task-shifting for HIV treatment and care in Africa. *Human Resources for Health, 8,* 8.

35. van Griensven, J., et al. (2008). Success with antiretroviral treatment for children in Kigali, Rwanda: Experience with health center/nurse-based care. *BMC Pediatrics, 8,* 39.

36. Dohrn, J., et al. (2009). The impact of HIV scale-up on the role of nurses in South Africa: Time for a new approach. *Journal of Acquired Immune Deficiency Syndromes, 52*(1), S27–29.

37. UNICEF. (2010). *Children and AIDS: 5th stocktaking report.* New York: UNICEF. Retrieved November 12, 2010, http://www.unicef.org/aids/index_57031.html

38. Horwood, C., et al. (2010). Routine checks for HIV in children attending primary health care facilities in South Africa: Attitudes of nurses and child caregivers. *Social Science & Medicine, 70*(2), 313–320.

39. Rollins, N., et al. (2009). Universal HIV testing of infants at immunization clinics: An acceptable and feasible approach for early infant diagnosis in high HIV prevalence settings. *AIDS, 23*(14), 1851–1857; Kankasa, C., et al. (2009). Routine offering of HIV testing to hospitalized pediatric patients at University Teaching Hospital, Lusaka, Zambia: Acceptability and feasibility. *Journal of Acquired Immune Deficiency Syndromes, 51*(2), 202–208; McCollum, E. D., et al. (2010). Task shifting routine inpatient pediatric HIV testing improves program outcomes in Urban Malawi: A retrospective observational study. *PLoS One, 5*(3), e9626.

40. Kankasa et al. (2009). Routine offering of HIV testing to hospitalized pediatric patients.

41. Leeper, A., et al. (2010). Lessons learned from family-centred models of treatment for children living with HIV: current approaches and future directions. *Journal of the International AIDS Society, 13*(Suppl 2), S3.

42. Torpey et al. (2010). Increasing the uptake of prevention.

43. Chan, A. K., et al. (2010). Outcome assessment of decentralization of antiretroviral therapy provision in a rural district of Malawi using an integrated primary care model. *Tropical Medicine and International Health, 15* (Suppl 1), 90–97.

44. Charlebois, E. D., et al. (2010). Short-term risk of HIV disease progression and death in Ugandan children not eligible for antiretroviral therapy. *Journal of Acquired Immune Deficiency Syndromes, 55*(3), 330–335.

45. South to South (S2S). *South to South Partnership for Comprehensive Family HIV Care & Treatment Program.* Faculty of Health Sciences, Stellenbosch University. Stellenbosch, South Africa: South to South. Retrieved January 12, 2011, http://www.sun.ac.za/southtosouth

46. Rosen, S., Fox, M. P., & Gill, C. J. (2007). Patient retention in antiretroviral therapy programs in sub-Saharan Africa: A systematic review. *PLoS Med, 4*(10), e298.

47. KIDS-ART-LINC Collaboration. (2008). Low risk of death, but substantial program attrition, in pediatric HIV treatment cohorts in sub-Saharan Africa. *Journal of Acquired Immune Deficiency Syndromes, 49*, 523–531.

48. University of Cape Town, Children's Institute. *Orphans and other children made vulnerable by HIV/AIDS in South Africa- A fact sheet for members of parliament.* Retrieved October 12, 2010, http://www.ci.org.za/depts/ci/pubs/pdf/hiv/resource/ovcfactsheet.pdf

49. Marais, B. J., et al. (2008). Poverty and human immunodeficiency virus in children: A view from the Western Cape, South Africa. *Annals of the New York Academy of Sciences, 1136*, 21–27.

50. Berry, L., & Guthrie, T. (2003). *Rapid assessment: The situation of children in South Africa* (pp. 25–28). Cape Town, South Africa: Children's Institute, University of Cape Town.

51. UNICEF. (2004). *Children on the brink 2004: A joint report of new orphan estimates and a framework for action.* Washington DC: USAID. Retrieved November 8, 2010, http://www.unicef.org/publications/index_22212.html

52. Grandmothers Against Poverty and Aids (GAPA). Retrieved November 30, 2010, http://www.gapa.org.za

53. Osher, D. M. (2002). Creating comprehensive and collaborative systems. *Journal of Child and Family Studies, 11*, 91–99.

54. Schenk, K. D. (2009). Community interventions providing care and support to orphans and vulnerable children: A review of evaluation evidence. *AIDS Care, 21*(7), 918–942.

55. King, E., et al. (2009). Interventions for improving the psychosocial well-being of children affected by HIV and AIDS. *Cochrane Database of Systematic Reviews, 2*, Art. No: CD006733. doi: 10.1002/14651858.

56. Foster, C., et al. (2009). Young people in the United Kingdom and Ireland with perinatally acquired HIV: The pediatric legacy for adult services. *AIDS Patient Care and STDs, 23*, 159–166.

57. Baylor International Paediatric AIDS Initiative (BIPAI), Botswana Teen Club. Retrieved December 8, 2010, http://botswanateenclub.wordpress.com

58. Strode, A., Slack C., & Essack, Z. (2010). Child consent in South African law: Implications for researchers, service providers and policy-makers. *South African Medical Journal, 100*(4), 247–249.

59. Shisana, O., et al. (2009) *South African national HIV prevalence.*

60. South to South (S2S). *South to South Partnership.*

61. Mate, K. S., et al. (2009). Challenges for routine health system data management in a large public programme to prevent mother-to-child HIV transmission in South Africa. *PLoS One, 4*(5), e5483; Garrib, A., et al. (2008). An evaluation of the district health information system in rural South Africa. *South African Medical Journal, 98*(7), 549–552.

62. WHO. (2010). PMTCT strategic vision 2010–2015: Preventing mother to child transmission of HIV to reach the UNGASS and millennium development goals. Geneva, Switzerland: WHO. Retrieved December 2, 2010, http://www.who.int/hiv/pub/mtct/strategic_vision/en/index.html

Getting Delivery Done Well

10

Choices and Consequences

Should Resources Be Directed Toward AIDS-affected Children or Poor Families? Targeting Choices, Methods, and Evidence

MICHELLE ADATO ∎

Targeting refers to the directing of resources to a particular group of people, often those who are believed to need them most—for example, the extremely poor—or those who are believed to be the best channel for reaching another group—for example, targeting grandparents to reach children. It rests on two principal assumptions. The first is that resources are insufficient to reach a larger population, or there is insufficient political consensus to cover a larger group. The second is that a mechanism is needed to systematically identify the desired group. This chapter examines targeting of social protection, particularly social assistance programs,[1] addressing the technical, ethical, and political questions involved with targeting social protection for families and children affected by HIV and AIDS. It considers the question of whether to target, explains the types of targeting methods available and their pros and cons, and then faces the question of who to target in high HIV prevalence countries, reviewing the evidence, arguments, and dilemmas surrounding the decision of whether to target poor families, AIDS-affected families, or orphans. Finally, it considers how to reach all these groups simultaneously, looking at case studies of targeted programs that are attempting to do this. Throughout this chapter, we refer to AIDS-affected families more often than children, based on strong evidence that the best way of reaching children is normally through their families.[2] The need to support families in order to reach children is particularly true for social protection programs involving economic support (child protection and support for children living outside of families require other methods). Although this chapter focuses primarily on economic support, it also addresses the issue of targeting services for children affected by AIDS.

TARGETING SOCIAL PROTECTION: METHODS, EVIDENCE, AND POLICY DEBATES

Targeting of social assistance programs refers to the provision of resources to a particular group that has been determined to be the highest priority for such assistance.

This group can be defined by their poverty status, age, disability, ethnicity, gender, where they live, or another priority characteristic.

The question of whether to target social assistance is a political-economic and ideological one. With social assistance, the question of whether to target counterposes universal benefits with targeted benefits. Universal systems are more desirable if a state has the financial resources and political will to guarantee them. In poor countries, this is unlikely to be the case. Even in South Africa, which has over 14 million beneficiaries in its various cash transfer programs, these programs are targeted. Universal price subsidies (as opposed to targeted subsidies) are the best example of a universal program, but given that these take considerable resources, the outcome is that the poor get proportionately less compared to those better off than they would in a targeted program.[3] Although a universal program could in theory reach all children affected by HIV and AIDS, in practice, poor countries like Zambia and Malawi are not likely to institute social assistance programs for 100% of the population and need to make some choices.

Social assistance targeting has a long history: food, fuel, or other subsidies; public works programs; food transfers; and cash transfers have all been targeted. Whether and how programs are targeted is driven by political economy, ideology, mobilization, social characteristics of communities, technical capacities, and priorities of institutions such as governments and donors. Most targeting is focused on socioeconomic characteristics of target groups, with poverty reduction a main goal. In the 1980s and 1990s, targeting gained new momentum against a global backdrop of economic downturns, a growing neo-liberal movement focused on efficiency of government expenditures and resultant reductions in poverty alleviation budgets, and a substantial body of evidence that universal programs such as general food subsidies were benefiting middle classes more than the poor. Social programs were re-examined for how to best allocate resources among a smaller group of beneficiaries, and the "extreme poor" became a new subset of "the poor." In Mexico in the 1990s, for example, the conditional cash transfer (CCT) program PROGRESA was targeted to the 20% of the population living in "extreme poverty," although government recognized a 40% poverty rate.[4] In the early 1990s, Besley and Kanbur observed that targeting had come to be seen as a panacea in poverty alleviation, where policy-makers thought that improved targeting meant they could alleviate poverty with less expenditure.[5] The political-economic determinants of social expenditure and targeting in turn affect subgroups among the poor, such as families affected by HIV/AIDS. However, issues confronted in poverty targeting are articulated with AIDS-specific issues to pose new dilemmas and designs to address them.

TARGETING CASH TRANSFERS TO POOR AND VULNERABLE OR AIDS-AFFECTED FAMILIES: CONCEPTUAL DILEMMAS, EVIDENCE, AND ARGUMENTS

A number of global initiatives and forums have coalesced around support for vulnerable children affected by AIDS, and many have taken up the cause of orphans. These include, among others, the United Nations General Assembly Special Session (UNGASS) Declaration of Commitment (2001); the U.S. President's Emergency Plan for AIDS Relief (PEPFAR)'s Orphans and Other Vulnerable Children Category; the

U.S. Assistance for Orphans and Other Vulnerable Children in Developing Countries Act of 2005; the Global Partners Forum on Children Affected by HIV and AIDS; the UN Inter-Agency Task Team on Children and HIV/AIDS; and the Joint Learning Initiative on Children and HIV/AIDS (JLICA). There are also regional forums, such as the National Plans of Action for Orphans and Vulnerable Children (NPAs), and the South Asian Association for Regional Cooperation (SAARC) Draft Framework for the Protection, Care, and Support of Children Affected by HIV/AIDS, among others. Apart and collectively, these initiatives have provided powerful opportunities for mobilizing strategies, resources, and action on behalf of children affected by HIV and AIDS. Although these allow room for "other vulnerable children," they vary with respect to their focus on HIV/AIDS versus children vulnerable from other causes.

A central targeting dilemma raised here is whether to target the directly AIDS-affected, such as orphans or families with ill members or recent deaths, or to target the most extremely poor households. This raises (1) questions about targeting accuracy—whether AIDS-affected households or orphans are always the poorest, and thus whether targeting them will reach those most in need; (2) as a corollary of (1), directly related implications for equity and fairness: non–AIDS-affected families and nonorphaned children may be equally in need of resources due to chronic poverty, illness and death from other causes, war, or other forms of shocks or discrimination; and (3) concerns about stigma—the effects of publically identifying families or children as "AIDS-affected" or "AIDS orphans."

Targeting Transfers: Are AIDS-affected Households and Orphans the Most in Need?

Answering the first and second questions requires an examination of the relationships between poverty and AIDS, and poverty and orphans. With respect to AIDS, a recent review of the literature found that because HIV has different drivers across socioeconomic groups, poorer groups are not necessarily more at risk to HIV exposure than are wealthier groups. What is clear, however, is that poor families are likely to be hit harder by the downstream impacts of AIDS. They are less able to cope, and AIDS will almost certainly make them poorer. There are many reasons for this. Downward spirals involve reduction and fluctuations in income due to labor constraints from ill or deceased breadwinners; reductions in purchase and application of agricultural inputs and access to extension; increased expenditure on health care, transportation, funerals, expenses for fostered children, and food to replace that formerly accessed through subsistence agriculture; reduction in savings and selling of assets; and reduced access to credit and/or increases in debt at unfavorable terms.[6]

The evidence is thus strong that targeting AIDS-affected families is likely to reach families that are poor and in need of social protection. Two problems remain, however: First, many affected by AIDS are not poor, and second, many people are extremely poor due to other causes. For example, recent work has highlighted the importance of assets in explaining persistent, structural poverty.[7] In a study based on data from six southern African countries, Caldwell found household asset ownership to be a better predictor of food security than chronic illness, presence of orphans, and gender of the household head.[8] Thus, targeting on multiple criteria capturing poverty and vulnerability, including but not limited to indicators associated with AIDS, can capture AIDS-affected families but not exclude others in need.

Another case for targeting poverty is based on evidence that poverty also is a driver of HIV infection. Targeting families or individuals who are poor but not yet AIDS-affected can thus reduce HIV risk. Poverty and food insecurity can lead women and children into transactional sex, or prevent economically dependent women from refusing unsafe sex. A recent review of the evidence finds a number of studies that support this relationship between poverty and risky behavior,[9] although there are also contextual caveats and specificities.[10] In South Africa, Hallman shows that, controlling for wealth and other factors, orphanhood confers added risk for unsafe sexual behaviors.[11] Also in South Africa, Operario et al. found a positive association between young adults (15–24 years of age) who had experienced parental death and HIV status, controlling for socioeconomic status and age.[12] Furthermore, they had a higher likelihood of behaviors linked with HIV transmission, including multiple sex partners among females and unprotected sex among males (this was a nationally representative but cross-sectional sample). Additional evidence from South Africa found that orphaned youth aged 14–18 were more likely to have had sex, and at a younger age, than were nonorphans.[13] Associations were found between orphan status and risk of HIV and herpes simplex virus (HSV)-2 infection among female adolescents in Zimbabwe.[14] Another hypothesized although less researched causal pathway is one in which malnourished people are more likely to suffer weakened immune systems, which may increase risk of HIV transmission in an unprotected sexual encounter. Gillespie, Kadiyala, and Greener's review of the evidence concludes that this directional relationship between poverty and AIDS is not straightforward, in part because research on the association between socioeconomic status and the spread of HIV is still in a rudimentary stage, and because of the complexity and context-specificity of pathways.[15] Although the conclusion is that poor people are not necessarily more likely than wealthier people to be exposed to HIV, poverty has powerful risk drivers, and the poor are less able to cope with the impacts of HIV and AIDS, as they have less access to treatment and fewer assets to draw on. Interventions that target poverty can both reduce vulnerability to HIV and its devastating economic impacts on families.

Turning now to the question of whether to target orphans, several thorny issues emerge. The first is the definitions of orphans, which vary greatly across contexts and do not necessarily resonate among local populations.[16] The second issue is whether orphans, however defined, are more disadvantaged than nonorphans. This is the subject of a large body of research that provides highly disparate answers: Some research shows that orphans are more vulnerable and disadvantaged, and other research shows that they are not. The evidence is less contradictory when contingent on variables such as the relationship between child and caregivers, poverty status, and household demographics and structure. Ainsworth and Filmer's review of 102 datasets from 51 countries found mixed results on whether fostering households were poorer or better-off than households without orphans. In about two-thirds of the studies, paternal orphans were more likely to be in relatively poorer households, whereas maternal orphans were in poorer households in only about one-third of the countries.[17] Results varied even more for double orphans (those who had lost both mother and father)—in ten studies they were in poorer households, whereas in 22 studies they were in relatively richer households. This latter result probably reflects the fact that some deceased parents were from better-off families, and richer households may be better able to care for orphans and thus take more in.

With respect to food security and nutrition, the evidence also points in two directions. Orphans might be expected to be worse off than nonorphans because they came from or are in households where at least one parent has died and another may be ill, with the resultant economic impacts, or because, when both parents die, their fostering households may be poor or discriminate against them. A number of studies have found orphans to be more food-insecure and malnourished, and less healthy than nonorphans.[18]

However, other studies have found small or no differences in health and nutrition between orphans and nonorphans. For example, Lindblade et al. found no difference in most indicators, particularly among paternal orphans and those orphaned more than 1 year.[19] A review by Rivers, Silvestre, and Mason found evidence that households caring for one orphan were less food-insecure than were households without orphans, but that 40% of households with more than one orphan were food-insecure.[20] Analysis of Demographic and Health Survey (DHS) data from five countries found that orphans did not necessarily have poorer nutritional outcomes than nonorphans, when controlling for age, sex, household wealth, and household demographics.[21] The main factor consistently and significantly affecting nutrition was wealth, and in some cases, relationship of orphans to household heads. Within the poorest two quintiles, there is evidence of orphan disadvantage in Zambia and Tanzania, where orphans in blended households (those with orphans and nonorphans, where discrimination might be expected) had greater evidence of stunting than did nonorphans. In Kenya, those in blended households had lower weight-for-age scores when they lived in grandparent-headed households, consistent with findings elsewhere that discrimination is affected by distance in kinship ties. Other findings further complicate the picture: Nonorphans in blended households were better off than nonorphans in nonblended households, providing further evidence that fostering households may have greater capacity to care for children than households that do not take in children. These results are all for younger children, who may be more easily assimilated than older children.

With respect to education, even more evidence points in two directions. If children are more easily assimilated at earlier ages, then one might expect more evidence of discrimination with respect to education if orphans are older (i.e., of school age) when they enter the household. This risk could be exacerbated by high school expenses, the need for and ability of older children to work or care for the ill, and the perception that education is more expendable than food. The question of whether orphans are disadvantaged with regard to schooling has received considerable research attention, but again, the answer is not straightforward. Ainsworth and Filmer's review of 102 nationally representative datasets from 51 countries found statistically significant deficits in enrollment (controlling for enrollment differentials associated with economic status) in 38% and 46% of the surveys for paternal and maternal orphans respectively, climbing to 58% for double orphans.[22] There was a strong systematic association, however, between enrollment and economic status, with the latter a much stronger predictor of enrollment than paternal, maternal, and double orphan status in most countries. Girls tend to be disadvantaged compared to boys, but not significantly more so than nonorphan girls. The overall picture is one of considerable difference across countries. A UNICEF analysis of DHS and Multiple

Indicator Cluster Survey data for 24 countries compared school attendance of orphans and nonorphans and also found wide variation across countries.[23] The implication is that it makes more sense to work harder at targeting orphans in some contexts than in others. Countries with overall low enrollment rates among the poor can focus on the overall group and catch orphans in the process. In countries with overall high enrollment rates but large gaps among orphans, orphan-focused policies are more defendable.

Case, Paxson, and Ableidinger found a different outcome than Ainsworth and Filmer. Using 19 DHS surveys from ten countries between 1992 and 2000, they found that paternal, maternal, and double orphans have significantly lower enrollment rates, in eight, eight, and 13 of the surveys, respectively. They also compare enrollment rates for orphans with that of nonorphans living in the same households, finding significantly lower enrollment rates for paternal, maternal, and double orphans in nine, seven, and 17 of the 19 surveys, respectively. Orphans tended to be poorer on average than nonorphans, but schooling outcomes were explained by neither poverty nor gender, but rather by the "closeness of biological ties"—the degree of relatedness of the orphan to the household head. Children living in households headed by nonparental relatives were systematically worse off than those in households headed by parental relatives, and those living with nonrelatives fared even worse. Where intrahousehold discrimination exists, Case et al. recommended targeting orphans, as income support to families may not benefit them.[24]

Country-level studies present more insights, with gender implications: Using longitudinal data from the KwaZulu-Natal (South Africa) DSA, Case and Ardington found that maternal orphans were significantly less likely to be enrolled and to have completed fewer years of school, and that those enrolled had less money spent on their education, compared to children whose mothers were alive. These results held regardless of the age or sex of the children. These disadvantages were not found for paternal orphans, however.[25] Using a 5-year panel study of 20,000 children in Kenya, Evans and Miguel found a substantial and highly significant drop in primary school participation following the death of a parent, and a smaller drop just before death. Impacts are over twice as large following maternal deaths compared to paternal deaths.[26] Results from a panel survey conducted in Malawi in 2000 and 2004 found that maternal and double orphans tend to face higher mortality risks and worse schooling outcomes than paternal orphans and nonorphans, especially in the case of boys.[27] This study and panel data from Uganda suggest that introduction of universal primary education reduces orphan disadvantage.[28]

Although many studies focus on orphans, these do not capture the experiences of children before they become orphans, which may have an even greater impact on education and other areas. In a study in Uganda, Gilborn et al. found that older children (aged 13–17) living with an ill parent had lower school attendance rates than double orphans, and that the former had declines in school attendance due to parental illness, whereas the latter reported increased attendance following parental death.[29] Orphaning in the context of HIV/AIDS is a process that begins long before the death of a parent.[30] Bicego, Rutstein, and Johnson describe HIV/AIDS as a family crisis involving deterioration of the family unit and trauma in the emotional, psychological, and material life of the child.[31] This process can involve new workloads and responsibilities, withdrawal from school, abandonment, migration, fear, family dissolution, and stigma, all of which may prevent parents and children from accessing resources that can strengthen the capacities of children to deal with these challenges.[32] Targeting orphans would exclude these children whose parents are still alive, but whose needs for support are just as great.

The overall conclusion of this section then, is that it is not possible to claim that orphans are categorically worse off than their nonorphan counterparts, nor that they never are. If the capacity is available, it is possible to use data collection and economic analysis at the country level to determine the relative disadvantage of orphans versus other types of vulnerable children. This can draw important attention to the extent to which policy is needed to address a problem, which may be better addressed through interventions other than transfers (e.g., school uniforms or fee waivers). However, it is difficult to draw a single conclusion about orphan status within one country. The evidence suggests that, with respect to poverty, health, nutrition, and education, the condition of orphans will depend on poverty levels, demographic characteristics, household structure, and orphan–caretaker relations, as well as country-level poverty characteristics. Targeting economic support to respond to these various permutations—for example, targeting orphans who have lost mothers but not those who have lost fathers—would likely be difficult for communities to understand and accept, and some criteria would be too administratively complicated. Furthermore, if the outcome of concern is poverty, health, nutrition, or education, then targeting transfers based on who is more disadvantaged in these indicators—rather than based on orphan status—is more logical and easier to operationalize. If orphans are targeted for resource transfers when their conditions are no worse than those of nonorphaned children affected by chronic poverty, family illness, or other forms of shock or discrimination, then a fundamental problem of equity arises; this point is made persuasively in the South African context by Meintjes et al. who argue that targeting resources to orphans that are significantly larger than those available to other poor children "is *inequitable*. Due to the pervasiveness of poverty across South Africa's child population, directing interventions on the basis of children's orphanhood substantially mistargets resources aimed at reducing vulnerability."[33]

Stigma

Targeting based on AIDS-related criteria or orphan status also raises a separate problem of stigma—the negative effects that can come from the government or other organization publicly labeling children by targeting them based on their status of "orphan." Targeting families and children based on poverty status, rather than the presence of orphans, avoids this type of labeling. Meintjes and Giese found that, in South Africa, local notions of vulnerability and orphanhood correspond poorly with international definitions. Local notions have negative connotations, derived in part from local translations of the terms, which are associated with abandonment and destitution. These local terms are "steeped in stigma," and the authors argue that labeling a child as an orphan is stigmatizing for the child and an insult to those providing care and support to the child.[34] Although the reality of illness, poverty, and the death of breadwinners and loved ones is arguably disempowering enough, public stigma, social exclusion, and self-identification as a victim of AIDS or as an orphan compound the problem. In urban areas of South Africa, Cluver, Gardner, and

Operario found that AIDS-orphaned adolescents reported higher levels of stigma and fewer positive activities than did other groups, although there were no reported differences in bullying or community violence, and they found that stigma signifi-cantly mediated associations between AIDS orphanhood and poor psychological outcomes.[35] Stigma resulting from targeting on AIDS-identified criteria in the con-text of a food distribution program for adults on antiretrovirals (ARVs) was found in a study in Kenya. Many beneficiaries were keeping the food collection a secret from family and friends because of fear of revealing their HIV-positive status and facing discrimination. Problems included the visibility of the food distribution points and the fact that some food packets were labeled with AIDS awareness messages.[36] This visibility can be greatly reduced, but not eliminated in this type of program. In their analysis of the conditions of orphans in sub-Saharan Africa, Subbarao and Coury argue that even when targeting orphans may be appropriate, it can create stigma within families and communities. They suggest minimizing this by targeting a greater number of children within a family, or targeting all children who are at high risk of dropping out of school. They further suggest the following: assess the country situation; delimit the geographic zone of the intervention to areas with high HIV prevalence and orphan and vulnerable children (OVC) vulnerabilities (unless they are widely distributed); map existing forms of support to fill the gaps; assess community strength, resources, and cohesion for providing support for OVCs; and select the children most in need with close collaboration with communities and governments.[37]

In light of these concerns around accuracy, equity, and stigma, many researchers and program implementers have called for targeting transfers based on poverty and multiple vulnerability criteria, with attention to the *context* of AIDS, rather than on AIDS-affected or orphan status alone.[38] This is not a complete consensus,[39] and there is ample need for caveats and context. The research on orphan status can help us contemplate, however, how AIDS-related conditions, articulated with other social and contextual specificities (based on region, gender dynamics, or household struc-ture, for example) can inform the development of proxies for capturing OVCs, as well for as targeting of other types of interventions for which orphans and AIDS-affected families may have unique needs.

TARGETING OTHER FORMS OF ASSISTANCE: FOOD TRANSFERS, LIVELIHOODS PROGRAMS, AND SOCIAL SERVICES FOR AIDS-AFFECTED FAMILIES

Food Assistance and Nutrition Programs

The argument for poverty targeting does not extend to all forms of social protection. For example, some organizations implementing food- and nutrition-based interven-tions argue that school feeding and take-home rations should be universal for all children in poor communities, but that interventions such as prevention of mother-to-child transmission (PMTCT), home-based care, growth monitoring, and nutri-tional rehabilitation services, as well as pediatric hospices and foster care programs, can be a means to target children with specific AIDS-related vulnerabilities and needs.[40] These children can be identified through hospitals and clinics providing antiretroviral therapy (ART) and care for the ill, school teachers, social workers, and government departments, nongovernmental organizations (NGOs), and community-based organizations (CBOs) engaged in AIDS outreach, home-based health care, and other community services. Many food- and nutrition-based interventions have different objectives than cash transfers, with different implications for targeting. A clear example is targeting of benefits for people on ART. Responding to evidence on interactions between HIV/AIDS, food security, and nutrition—including findings that ART is more effective for people who are well-nourished due to an increase in caloric intake and decrease in side effects that reduce adherence[41]—clinical care and treatment programs are teaming up with food aid programs.[42] A study in Kenya comparing 2,200 people receiving food aid and ARVs with people on ARVs alone found that the benefits of the food were substantial with respect to improved health, strength, and other measures of well-being,[43] although, as noted earlier, stigma was a problem.

These findings have two potentially contradictory implications for targeting. On the one hand, they demonstrate the importance of these food transfers for ART patients. On the other hand, they illustrate the stigma problem and raise the equity question—is it right for this group alone to receive social assistance if their HIV-negative neighbors are also hungry? The answer is that the lives of symptomatic people may depend on these transfers. Given the importance of adequate nutrition for people on ART, it is difficult to argue against programs providing them with food assistance. Although cash assistance for those on ART should also be explored, since it can help to fund other necessary expenses such as transportation to the clinic, food and nutrition assistance ensures that people get the calories and micronutrients that they need, a "prescription food." This is more akin to an emergency response than the long-term social protection system that a poverty-targeted cash transfer program represents.

Targeting cash only to those on ART would be more difficult to sustain in the long run. Furthermore, a poverty-targeted program could improve the nutrition of HIV-positive people who are asymptomatic, possibly delaying their need for medication.[44] If well implemented, poverty targeting would reach those who are ill and need the financial assistance, since not everyone on treatment is poor. The ideal combination might be a food transfer for the patient, and a cash transfer for the family, in which the family is selected based on the poverty-targeting criteria, although no research has yet systematically tested and compared these combinations.

Livelihoods Programs and Productive Activities

A remaining issue is how to target social assistance approaches that use livelihoods programs, such as microenterprise support and microcredit, as well as public works. The two key issues discussed above, equity and stigma, are relevant to these types of programs as well. Programs such as those run by The AIDS Support Organization (TASO) in Uganda provide support for small enterprise activities for their HIV-positive clients. Although this has been an important source of support, program staff discuss the difficulties inherent in targeting only their clients, as opposed to the wider community.[45] Furthermore, given labor constraints, dependency ratios, and extreme poverty among the families hardest hit by HIV and AIDS, there are reasons why microenterprise, credit, and public works programs are not the best for reaching large numbers of these families quickly, reliably, and sustainably. Livelihoods programs require higher capacities of families—labor, time, investments, and repayments—as well as higher capacities of implementers in terms of the complexities of administration and delivering client training. They are thus slower to scale up, and they reach fewer people than do cash- and food-based interventions. Adato and Bassett provide a longer discussion of these issues, along with examples of ways in which such programs have been tailored to be more appropriate for AIDS-affected families.[46]

Nevertheless, AIDS-affected families are diverse with respect to their degree of "affectedness"—some are not labor-constrained, or are less so, and are otherwise better positioned to take advantage of interventions that provide more than a cash transfer. For these households, public works and livelihoods approaches can be particularly helpful. The government of Malawi, with support from UNICEF and others, has designed a social support program schema that provides useful guidance for targeting different population groups with the appropriate forms of social protection. Here, the 22% of Malawi's population that can be considered "ultra poor" is divided up into those with and without labor capacity, and appropriate interventions are noted for each: cash transfers and feeding schemes can be targeted to the ultra poor and labor-constrained, whereas public works, cash and food assets, and skills-building programs are targeted toward those with labor capacity, although school feeding for children and supplementary cash support for working adults is appropriate here as well. The moderately poor, between 22% and 52% of Malawi's poverty line, can be reached through agricultural inputs subsidies, public works, insurance programs, and microfinance. More of these types of targeting exercises need to be brought into social protection discussions and planning.[47]

Psychosocial Support and Social Services

Another area where the conditions of orphans are different from those of other poor children relates to psychosocial vulnerability. Living with ill parents and the experience of parental death are traumatizing, and AIDS compounds this experience through stigma and multiple and serial deaths within a family. As noted above, stigma has adverse psychological outcomes among AIDS-orphaned adolescents in South Africa.[48] In South Africa, children orphaned by AIDS are more likely to report symptoms of depression, peer relationship problems, post-traumatic stress, delinquency, and conduct problems than are children orphaned by other causes and non-orphaned children.[49] In Uganda, AIDS orphans had greater risk of anxiety, depression, and anger than did nonorphans.[50] A study in Zimbabwe found that children's AIDS-related bereavement tends to be particularly complicated and difficult to manage, and that adults in their households are ill-equipped to identify and respond well to teenage distress.[51] A global literature review found a consistent picture of negative effects of parental death on a wide range of physical, socioeconomic, and psychological outcomes.[52] Other implications for children experiencing parental illness and death are loss of intergenerational transfer of knowledge; lack of communication with adults; physical, verbal, or sexual abuse; and loss of property.

Programs that respond to the needs of these children may involve home-based health care for ill relatives, psychological counselling and group support, spiritual support, creative activities to maintain family memories, recreational activities, support for communications between adults and children around parental illness and death, sex education, community education around stigma and children's rights, succession planning, care arrangements, wills, legal literacy and protection, and assuring children's continued access to education and health care.[53] This suggests that material support—although critical to any holistic and adequate support strategy—is insufficient for children affected by AIDS. But these other forms of support need to be targeted differently than the forms of material support discussed earlier in this chapter. First, the needs identified here are specific to children affected by AIDS, not necessarily to the wider community of poor children (although neither are they exclusive to AIDS—many will also apply to other epidemics, war, or natural disasters). Targeting cannot be done based on poverty indicators at a geographical or household level, as is the case in targeting transfers to poor communities. Data on HIV prevalence, adult deaths, and dependency ratios can be used to determine geographical priorities for targeting these types of services. Within communities, however, targeting of OVC needs to occur through CBOs, NGOs, youth groups, teachers, school psychologists, school-based committees, social workers, health care workers, traditional healers, and religious leaders. These can be aided by data collection exercises, and support from government departments. Foster argues strongly for the role of CBOs in targeting support for children because of their understanding of the situation on the ground and knowledge of which children are in need, although these organizations may need assistance.[54] In the context of AIDS-related household dissolution and mobility of children, community members are also likely to know where children have moved before or following the death of parents. Foster writes that a community-based approach encourages self-help and builds on local resources, culture, realities, and perceptions of child development.[55] While many resources have been devoted to orphan welfare, they have been highly fragmented, with low coverage.[56] Although this criticism tends to be aimed at international and national programs, with calls for more support for community-based approaches, communities on their own cannot solve the fragmentation and undercoverage problems. One of the main tasks for targeting these services is to establish coordination within geographical areas, mapping out service coverage and gaps. Phiri and Webb call for the strengthening of local/district government departments to coordinate the activities of local organizations by monitoring and evaluating responses to support orphans, and for providing technical assistance for partnerships between government, NGOs, and CBOs at different levels. Similar partnerships will need to be used for coordinated targeting of services.[57]

METHODS FOR TARGETING TRANSFERS

Five main targeting systems are found across social transfer programs. The system selected reflects policy objectives and priorities, budgets, and ideology: categorical targeting, self-targeting, geographic targeting, household targeting, and community-based targeting. This section provides an overview of these methods, followed by examples of uses of some of these methods for reaching children in AIDS-affected contexts. Table 10.1 summarizes these methods, how they can be used to reach children affected by AIDS, and their advantages and disadvantages.

Categorical targeting directs benefits toward a group that is relatively easy to identify (e.g., the elderly or families with children). Characteristics such as gender, age, land ownership, or employment status can be used, usually when these are correlated with poverty,[58] although not always, as in the case of a non–means tested old age pension. Targeting resources toward people affected by HIV and AIDS or to orphans, would be a form of categorical targeting, although this is a more difficult group to identify and involves the equity and stigma problems discussed above. Identifying beneficiaries through a categorical method is more straightforward and likely to be less administratively costly and complicated than methods using means tests, but may do less well in reaching those most in need and can increase costs by covering a larger population.

Self-targeting refers to a method whereby anyone is free to participate, but the program is designed to discourage the participation of people with less need. The most common example is a public works program that sets wages at or below market wages, so that, in theory, the poorest people without better labor market alternatives self-select into the program. Another form of self-targeting is employed through price subsidies, where, for example, subsidies are put on foods disproportionately consumed by the poor. Self-targeted public works programs can be used in contexts of high HIV-prevalence but may be less likely to attract AIDS-affected families when physically demanding work is required. However, programs have been designed to be appropriate to these families through lighter work activities and flexible contracts in which different family members can contribute labor.[59] Harvey argues that participation of asymptomatic HIV-positive individuals who may be "vulnerable but viable" is an important way to minimize stigma.[60]

In geographic targeting, a region is selected because of the profile of its population, based most often on poverty indicators. Geographic targeting often means that everyone in the region is included, but it can also be the first stage of a process that is followed by the targeting of a specific subset of households within that geographic area. In Mexico, for example, a "marginality index" was used to target its CCT program at the locality level, followed by household targeting. In contrast, El Salvador's CCT program covers all households with children under 15 in geographically targeted areas. Geographic targeting of a social assistance intervention in an area with high HIV prevalence is an effective way to target AIDS-affected families, and reduces stigma if all of the population is eligible. Such universal eligibility is more expensive, involving higher "leakage" (a term economists use to refer to where the "non-poor" receive benefits), although it avoids the administrative costs and complexities associated with household targeting.

There are several methods of household targeting. Many Latin American CCT programs involve a proxy means test through a census. Data collected include indicators such as housing, durable goods, demographic structure of the household, education, types of work, expenditures, or reported income. Complicated formulas are sometimes used to weigh variables and calculate a score, as in Mexico's CCT program.[61] In Mexico and Nicaragua, a community assembly was then supposed to review and recommend revisions to the list, although in practice this seldom happened.[62] Another method of household targeting is an application-based process, in

Table 10.1 OVERVIEW OF METHODS FOR TARGETING SOCIAL TRANSFERS

Targeting Method	Description	Examples of How Method Can Be Used to Reach OVCs	Advantages	Disadvantages
Categorical targeting	Resources targeted to a class of people based on an identifiable characteristic (e.g., age; caring for children)	A pension system for the elderly, used to reach grandchildren living with them; a cash transfer given to families caring for OVC; food packages for adults on ART	Easily identifiable target group; no expensive or complicated identification process	Category not necessarily correlated with poverty, so resources may go to those with less need; may miss households with children; stigma associated with identification as member of a category
Self-targeting	People self-select based on program conditions (e.g., poor willing to work for low wage rate when better alternatives are absent; low-intensity labor requirements)	Public works program for poor households; low-intensity labor and flexible family contracts for AIDS-affected families	No exclusionary criteria; no need for expensive/complicated identification process; low stigma	Often used with work-based programs that may be infeasible for households with ill adults or elderly; availability to all may result in greater "leakage" to those who need it less
Geographic targeting	All households receive support in a given locality or region	Transfers available to all families in locality or region	Well targeted to poor with good data and analysis; no OVC HHs will be missed; no expensive/complicated identification process; low stigma	May be more costly to cover all households; will include some with less need

Table 10.1 (Continued)

Targeting Method	Description	Examples of How Method Can Be Used to Reach OVCs	Advantages	Disadvantages
Household targeting through proxy means surveys/ census or applications	Households selected by needs-based criteria and data collection methods; households selected by program officials; List can be reviewed by community	Transfers to poor households, and/or those with OVC; data collection to identify the eligible	Tends to be well targeted to the poor; selection criteria can be designed to include OVC in HH; sophisticated data collection increases accuracy	Data collection can be expensive, require high administrative and technical capacity, or be geographically challenging; eligible households can be missed through enumerator error or poorly designed surveys; poverty line for eligibility may not be transparent or can appear arbitrary or unfair to communities
Household targeting through community-based methods	Households selected by relatively simple needs-based criteria, followed by assessment and decisions by community committees	Transfers to households who are poor and/or contain OVC; data collection and local knowledge to identify eligible	Can be well targeted to the poor; selection criteria can be designed to include OVC in HH; community members may be best informed about household characteristics and needs	Selection process can be complicated and require strong organizational capacity, training, and support; community members on selection committees may hold biases; checks and balances needed to assure quality and fairness

ART, antiretroviral therapy; OVC, orphans and vulnerable children; HH, household.

which people go to government offices and fill out an application form that includes a means test. Program staff may then do a random or systematic verification of information at the household. Application methods are sometimes used in urban areas where both household census visits and community-based processes are not easy to implement, although in South Africa this system is used in urban and rural areas.

The trend toward more data-intensive systems for targeting has been motivated by efforts to make the distribution of benefits fairer and less subject to political manipulation, and in light of evidence that antipoverty programs have often not done well in reaching the poorest people. According to a review of 122 targeted social assistance programs by Coady, Grosh, and Hoddinott, over 25% of the programs had regressive outcomes, meaning that the poor get a share of program resources that is less than their share of the population.[63] Proxy means test methods have been evaluated as largely successful for poverty targeting in many of the Latin American CCT programs in which they have been used, having the advantage of measuring many poverty-related variables with precision. However, they are costly,[64] complex to administer and analyze, and often require travelling large distances to reach remote locations—all characteristics that make them less practical for many countries in sub-Saharan Africa. Even in Latin America, several cautions have been raised. Skoufias, Davis, and De la Vega advise that the additional cost of household targeting over geographic targeting should not exceed the benefits, finding that for Mexico's CCT program household targeting was worthwhile only for the extremely poor.[65] Furthermore, qualitative research found social costs arising from people not understanding or resenting the household selection process.[66] Data-based household targeting has advantages for reaching OVCs, providing the possibility of selecting specific characteristics such as high dependency ratios, presence/absence of able-bodied working age adults, and deaths.

A final method is community-based targeting. This usually involves a community-based committee or a general assembly that applies a set of criteria (determined by another community process or by program officials) for the selection of households within their communities. The process usually involves organization or oversight by local or regional government officials, traditional leaders, or other elites, local organizations, and international NGOs. As seen later in this chapter, this method is used for targeting cash transfer programs in Malawi and Zambia, with selection criteria designed to capture OVC and AIDS-affected households, as well as the poorest of the poor. Community-based methods often require some data collection at the household level, but involve a simpler set of variables than those used in a large-scale census. Although this approach sacrifices some degree of precision, simpler surveys are easier for people to understand, and, especially when criteria are locally developed, they are likely to be more easily accepted in communities. In a study of community-based targeting in public works programs in South Africa, Adato and Haddad found that the criteria applied reflected local perceptions of fairness, need, and entitlement, even if they looked quite different from international norms for proxy means tests.[67] Community-based targeting processes draw on local people's knowledge of local norms and household circumstances. They are not, however, a panacea for reaching those most in need, and can be subject to error and the elite influence that the survey-based approaches have been successful at avoiding. Where strong systems of patronage exist, or the target group has little representation, a categorical approach might be better.[68] Community-based systems can, however, be designed with reviews built-in that strengthen transparency and accountability, as will be seen in examples below.

The targeting system selected will depend in part on the resources available, a country's wealth, economy, development assistance, politics, history, and legal framework, as well as on the geographic distribution of poverty and vulnerability. Selection of a targeting system, and the complexity of its data collection, will further depend on administrative and technical capacities. Whether targeting is done in a centralized manner or by community organizations depends again on the feasibility of data-intensive methods, as well as norms associated with community participation and transparency in the distribution of resources. Examples of these different targeting approaches used in these different contexts, as well as the context of HIV and AIDS, are provided in the next section.

Finally, in all of these methods there are risks of missing certain kinds of households and individuals, for example, households living in remote areas, migrants, child-headed households,[69] and street-children. Although community-based methods tend to be better at identifying some of these groups, they may still exclude others, such as people who self-exclude or face discrimination by other community members due to race, ethnicity, caste, mental or physical disability, stigma, or other factors. Reaching these groups requires that they are explicitly considered in community-based processes, captured in a census, or reached through programs designed specifically for their circumstances.

TARGETING APPROACHES IN AIDS-AFFECTED CONTEXTS: EXPERIENCE WITH COMMUNITY-BASED, CATEGORICAL, AND APPLICATION-BASED METHODS

Community-based Targeting in Eastern and Southern Africa

The major new cash transfer schemes of the governments of Zambia, Malawi, and Kenya use community-based targeting, as have several NGO-run programs. Five case studies are reviewed below to illustrate the different forms that community-based targeting can take, the strengths and weaknesses with respect to reaching target communities and AIDS-affected families, and lessons learned. Several key points are of interest: the structure of the community forums; the systems for data generation; the criteria used as proxies for poverty, vulnerability, and "AIDS-affected"; and the nature of checks and balances on community processes.

Zambia's Social Cash Transfer Scheme (SCTS) stated the following rationale for use of a community-based method: geographic areas are too large, remote, and sparsely populated to enable a reliable census; rural poverty levels are not sufficiently different to be detected in a survey; and finally, Zambia already had a public assistance scheme that used voluntary, community-based processes for beneficiary identification. The targeting process works as follows:[70] The community is briefed about the program at the outset, including the targeting system and criteria, so that people understand the basis of the selection. A volunteer Community Welfare Assistance Committee (CWAC) makes a list of all eligible households based on the following criteria: (1) extremely needy (hunger, malnourishment, begging); (2) incapacitated: bread winners are sick or have died; no able-bodied person of working age; a dependency ratio of 3 or higher; (3) no valuable assets (e.g., no cattle or functioning TV); (4) no regular and substantial source of income (business in town, renting out houses, regular support from relatives).[71] All four criteria capture extreme poverty. Criteria (2) also capture AIDS-affected families and OVC, but do not state that they target these groups; rather, they have the advantage of doing so indirectly.

The CWAC representatives visit each listed household and fill out an application form with questions about external support, livelihoods, assets, and household problems. This information is verified by the village headman. The CWAC reviews the information and selects the neediest 10%, a cap derived from a study indicating that about 10% of Zambians are destitute and incapacitated. Those ranked just outside of the 10% can enter if others leave the program. The ranking is presented to the community, which can propose additions or subtractions, and a consensus is reached. To avoid the nepotism to which this system could be prone, and to otherwise check for errors, a system of checks and balances has been instituted: the final list is reviewed by an Area Welfare Committee, a District Social Welfare Officer, and a District Welfare Assistance Committee official for final approval. Questionable cases are investigated. A reassessment process takes place every 2 years, graduating households with new productive members and allowing others to be included in their place.[72] Although the process was seen to work fairly well, the Technical Working Group on Social Assistance, which developed the implementation framework for the expanded program in Zambia, proposed several formal improvements to the assessment process (e.g., improved training, standardized forms), the eligibility criteria, and the data collected on income, assets, and other variables.[73] A study of the expanded SCTS in Zambia compared different targeting approaches and found that categorical targeting is cheaper than a proxy means test, but that additional criteria must be applied to capture the poor. The study found that, in two out of three districts, community-based methods were effective at identifying the poorest households (compared with poverty deciles). The poorly performing district had less easily identifiable ultra-poor and more clustering around the mean. The study authors thus recommended that targeting methods be selected based on local conditions, suggesting these guidelines: for wards with very high poverty prevalence and severity, geographical targeting only; for medium to medium high poverty, community-based if community structures are adequate (otherwise use proxy means test); for low prevalence and hard to identify poor in urban contexts, means-testing with household verification, if means-testing is found to be over 85% accurate.[74]

Malawi's SCTS uses a similar process to that of Zambia's: Targeting criteria also include variables to capture extreme poverty and, indirectly, AIDS-affected households: (1) being "ultra poor"—that is, the lowest expenditure quintile, and under the ultra poverty line, measured in terms of consuming one meal per day, unable to purchase essential nonfood items, begging, and no valuable assets. This assessment is based to some extent on community perceptions of poverty and on the knowledge of community members, committees, and extension workers. (2) Being "labor constrained"—that is, with no able-bodied household member aged 19–64 years who is fit for work, or with a dependency ratio of over 3. The Community Social Protection Committee (CSPC) at village level lists, visits, and interviews all households that are believed to meet the criteria and ranks them according to perceived need. The ranking is presented to a community meeting for comment, revision, and consensus. A Social Protection Committee at the district level, assisted by extension workers, monitors the fairness, transparency, and results of the process. Among eligible households, those in the neediest 10% are approved to receive the grant.[75]

An evaluation of the targeting system in Malawi identified several problems, not with community participation per se, but with aspects of its implementation. The concepts of ultra poverty and labor-constraint were not well enough understood at the village level, and more guidance is needed for their application. The main problem appears to be the fact that the generic 10% cutoff for inclusion is too narrow and inevitably led to exclusion errors: Given that the rate of ultra poor and labor constrained in Mchinji is higher than the national average, the SCTS must cover 16%–20% of all households to reach all those that meet the eligibility criteria. The coverage rate was approximately 62% of those who should be eligible. Those excluded were found to be eating one to two meals per day, wearing rags, and lacking blankets and adequate housing. Thirty-two percent of community members believed that the SCTS was unfair, creating jealousy and conflict within communities. The study recommends that, rather than applying 10% generically, the cutoff be set using district-specific national data, poverty maps, and household listing data. In addition, better training is suggested on use of the eligibility criteria, a scoring system is recommended to reduce some of the subjectivity in the ranking, and greater involvement is called for among all stakeholders to improve the quality of implementation and increase transparency and the perception of fairness.[76]

A question that emerges is how effective are these systems at reaching AIDS-affected families? Assessing this is difficult because data will normally not indicate whether a household is affected by AIDS. Schubert et al. devised a way to assess this through proxies, in the context of the pilot Zambia and Malawi schemes. In Malawi, after comparing households in the scheme with those in the Integrated Household Survey for 2004, and using a number of assumptions (as empirical verifications were not available) as to the extent to which household categories (such as elderly-headed, female-headed, and with orphans) are related to AIDS, the analysis estimates that 53% of the households receiving transfers had someone who died due to AIDS, and of those 47% remaining, 34% had absorbed children orphaned by AIDS.[77] This adds another 16% to the total of AIDS-affected households, meaning that about 70% of the households were AIDS-affected, plus some additional number that were likely to be living with AIDS.

The same method was used to assess the targeting performance of the pilot program in Zambia. Data from the program baseline were again compared to a national 2004 Living Conditions Monitoring Survey (LCMS). The proportion of program households headed by someone 55 or older was 79% versus 19% in the LCMS. Among these, two-thirds were female-headed. Of those under 55, over half were female-headed and 63% widowed. From there, an estimation of AIDS deaths and AIDS orphans led to the estimation that 68% of participants were AIDS-affected. Based on the Zambia and Malawi experiences, Schubert et al. concluded that cash transfer programs can have a high mitigation impact on HIV/AIDS-affected children if they target households that are ultra-poor and labor constrained, use targeting criteria with exclusion errors under 20%, and link beneficiaries to services such as ART, home-based care, and psychosocial counseling.[78]

Kenya's Cash Transfer Scheme for Orphans and Vulnerable Children made the most explicit effort to target using criteria that resemble proxies for orphans and

AIDS-affected households. The pilot in three districts started with a community-based household listing process, using community-developed criteria based on broad guidelines from UNICEF. These included poverty, vulnerable children, chronically ill caretakers, lack of able-bodied adults, and others. A community discussion followed to finalize the selection.[79] Kenya's subsequent scaled-up cash transfer program adopted similar criteria. Location OVC Committees (LOCs) meet with village elders and community leaders to collect information on potentially eligible households. A preliminary form is filled out on the household. Enumerators visit the households and fill out a detailed questionnaire, and this information is entered into a management information system (MIS), which ranks the households. Households are classified into high, medium, and low vulnerability depending on whether they have 1–3 of the following characteristics: (1) at least one orphan younger than 18; (2) a household head younger than 18; and (3) at least one child, parent, or guardian is chronically ill (easily identifiable illness, e.g., AIDS). The ranking is reviewed in a public meeting and questionable cases sent for review by the LOC, supported by the District OVC Subcommittee.[80]

Findings from the 2007–2009 evaluation of this program illustrate the equity issues inherent in OVC-focused programs that do not also have poverty as a central criterion. As noted in this report, "the Program was not intended, primarily, to address poverty, but decided to support poor OVC households in the face of limited resources."[81] The evaluation found that the program was successful in reaching its target group: about 96% of enrolled households met the criteria. However, a poor OVC household had only an approximate 13% higher chance of inclusion than an "average" OVC household. The result was that an estimated 43% of the poorest OVC households in program areas did not receive benefits, whereas about 13% of program recipients were in the top (best-off) consumption quintile. Qualitative research supported this finding and further found that omissions could not be rectified by the community review process before the list of recipients was finalized. The evaluation report recommends better calibrating the proxy means test, revising the eligibility criteria, and setting quotas that reflect the geographic distribution of poverty. Another important finding of the qualitative research was that households in which caregivers became ill or died following the targeting process were not eligible, pointing to the need to review and update enrollment.[82]

Two NGO-led cash transfer programs in Malawi also provide useful guidance on the design and effectiveness of different community-based targeting methods in reaching AIDS-affected families. Concern Worldwide's short-term Food and Cash Transfer program (FACT) used a "community triangulation" method that divided communities into three groups and asked each to make a list of the neediest households. The three groups' lists were compared in a public forum, and those households appearing on all three lists were included, while those appearing on one or two lists were discussed and a consensus reached. Criteria were defined by each community, although Concern field staff and committees gave guidance. Although FACT was supposed to respond mainly to a food crisis, this guidance included criteria related to illness and disabilities, orphans, and food insecurity.[83] An evaluation of FACT found that the community triangulation method was a good system when it was used as planned, but there were several problems in implementation. First, the methodology was not strictly applied in some areas; for example, in one area, 75% of households were selected because they were caring for orphans or the elderly, or because they had a disability or poor health. Although these are indicators of chronic poverty and vulnerability, they were not necessarily related to the harvest failure that the program was designed to mitigate. Only 3 out of 900 households were selected because they were "food insecure" or suffering from "poor nutrition." Second, the most vulnerable households may not have participated in the selection process because they did not have the time, or might have been out of the village, looking for work or in the hospital. Third, influential elites, such as village headmen or their wives, managed to find their way into the program. Fourth, poor coordination meant that some families got double benefits, while some got none. The study authors emphasize the importance of using the community's own criteria of vulnerability and need. They also recommend that errors of exclusion (where those in need are left out) are taken as a bigger problem than errors of inclusion (where those less in need are included), arguing that the inclusion of some non-needy or politically influential people is a small price to pay to ensure that desperate people are not left out. They further suggest giving the cash to women rather than men (women sometimes asked for this change) to improve spending and avoid disadvantaging women in polygamous households, and to use female-headed households as a proxy for vulnerability.[84] Studies in Latin America and South Africa found that giving cash transfers to women is widely accepted by women and men, because cash transfers are seen as intended for food and children's needs, and because both perceive that women are more likely to use such cash for these expenses.[85]

Oxfam's cash transfer program in Zambia also used a community-based process in which community committees were responsible for targeting decisions, but without formal checks and balances, and a number of additional risks were discovered as a result. First, it appears that some committees were cementing inequalities, leading to elite capture and inclusion errors. Second, there was confusion over concepts of vulnerability, and some relatively wealthy households who had taken in orphans or had ill members were using these criteria to justify their inclusion. Some areas were excluding people who did not have National Registration Cards, which the elderly, migrants, or people designated to pick up benefits on behalf of someone else might not have.[86]

Several main lessons on community-based targeting can be drawn from the evidence from these case studies. These include the need for, first, data collection and good indicators; second, the use of geographical targeting in areas with high poverty rates and more selective household targeting where there is less; third, the use of criteria that simultaneously captures the extremely poor and AIDS-affected families, without explicit reference to the latter category, thus avoiding stigmatization; fourth, setting caps that accurately reflect need within communities (i.e., not setting them too low, resulting in large exclusion errors); fifth, capacity building for committee members, transparency, and guidance and oversight provided by higher (e.g., district) level committees or representatives; and sixth, vigilance and oversight to ensure that the most vulnerable are not left out and to avoid elite capture.

Means Tests and Categorical Targeting in South Africa

South Africa's targeting system for cash transfers, including the Old Age Pension (OAP), Child Support Grant (CSG), Foster Care Grant (FCG), and others, use application-based means tests. The OAP has been found to be well-targeted to poor households and to households caring for children, with three-generation and skip-generation households (in which grandparents are caring for children with no parent present) accounting for almost three-quarters of pension-receiving households.[87] Although the OAP is means tested, it is closer in effect to a categorical approach, nearly universal with respect to poor black South Africans.[88] Old age pensions tend to be well targeted toward AIDS-affected children, as the AIDS epidemic shifts the responsibility of caring for orphaned children onto elderly-headed households. Over 60% of orphaned children in Namibia, South Africa, and Zimbabwe, and over 50% in Botswana, Malawi, and Tanzania are living with their grandparents. In Namibia, the overall percentage of orphans living with their grandparents increased from 44% in 1992 to 61% in 2000.[89] The Lesotho old age pension also seems to be benefitting children: there are data indicating that 60% of pensioners in Lesotho have household members in school, most of whom receive support for education and associated cost, and that 20% of the pension is spent on caring for dependent orphans.[90]

The South African CSG is found to be well targeted in terms of those who have it (i.e., there are low inclusion errors). With respect to exclusion errors, the CSG did poorly in early years but has improved sharply. One study finds that exclusion errors dropped from 91% in 2000 (2 years after its introduction) down to 45% in 2004.[91] A national study from 2008 that sampled lower-income areas found inclusion errors of 13% and exclusion errors of 21% (although this figure may have fallen since then due to ongoing outreach and improvements of the application process).[92]

Why has this last 20% been difficult to reach, and how can these obstacles be overcome? Two studies have found that the poorest families are those who are the least likely to access the CSG,[93] although larger studies are needed that are representative at the provincial level. The criticisms of the eligibility criteria have been that the poverty thresholds for the means test have not kept pace with inflation,[94] the poverty line has not taken into account household size, and families with many dependents—including families fostering orphans—have been disadvantaged. For those who apply, however, only about 0.5% of applications are rejected, suggesting that the means test criteria are not very restrictive.[95] The CSG is not rationed in the sense that there are no caps (such as the 10% limit in Zambia and Malawi), although the overall budget restrictions have created a cap in practice, affecting primarily the age of children covered. In 1998, the CSG started targeting children under 7, gradually extended through age 15 by 2010, and has been projected through age 17 by 2012.

Errors of exclusion have had more to do with gaps in uptake among eligible households, based on lack of knowledge about the grant and its documentation and procedural requirements. The earlier problem has been greatly reduced—people generally know about the grant—although outreach remains important. The KwaZulu-Natal Income Dynamics Study found that the main reason why people do not apply for the grant is the difficulty of obtaining documents, including cost, time, complications, and difficulties accessing documents needed to obtain other documents.[96] For example, birth certificates were required to access the CSG (affidavits are now accepted), but there are many reasons why births are not registered. A review of studies of birth registration in South Africa found considerable provincial and local variability, with an inverse correlation between poverty and birth registration.[97] Another problem with the South African application method has been that the administration is too burdensome on the welfare offices.[98] In fact, some in South Africa argue that the means test should be eliminated because of the high monetary costs and other burdens it places on administrators and beneficiaries, and the fact that these burdens are at least in substantial part responsible for undercoverage of the poor.[99] These problems remain, although increased uptake figures and qualitative data[100] suggest that administration, information, and the application process have improved substantially over the years.

Evidence is limited on how well the CSG has reached AIDS-affected households. Most studies that attempt to assess the effectiveness of social grants in reaching AIDS-affected households use evidence on the impact of grants on children in high-prevalence regions, or on the impact of pensions on children, with assumptions made as to the covariance of AIDS and poverty, and of AIDS-affected and fostering households. Case, Hosegood, and Lund's study in a region in KwaZulu-Natal found mixed results, based largely on low uptake: only one-third of all age-eligible resident children had the grant accessed on their behalf; among the poorest households, only 50% were receiving the grant. Among those with the grant, however, it appeared to be well-targeted: Recipient households were likely to have less educated and less employed parents and fewer assets and luxury items. This may be a self-targeting process, in which better-off households for whom the grant would make up a smaller proportion of their household income find the time costs of applying and picking up the grant not worth the benefits. Children with deceased fathers were more likely to receive the grant, but children living with deceased mothers were particularly at risk of not receiving the grant.[101] This points to the importance of reaching out to children living in households without mothers.

Additional information on how well the CSG is reaching AIDS-affected households is provided by data from the 2004 KwaZulu-Natal Income Dynamics Survey (KIDS). This analysis uses prime-age adult mortality between 1998 and 2004 as a proxy for AIDS-affected households.[102] Figure 10.1 shows CSG receipt by number of household prime age deaths. As the number of prime age deaths per household increases, the percentage of households receiving the CSG increases. However, Figure 10.1 also shows that many households, even those with two or more prime age deaths, do not receive the CSG—more than half in most cases. This subset of data on prime age adult mortality is relatively small, however, particularly for those with two or more cases, and the analysis does not enable conclusions about causality. Only 30% of households fostering orphans (another proxy for AIDS-affected households) were receiving the CSG. The small overall sample size of 207 fostering households limits the conclusions one can draw from this, but the data suggest that the CSG might be missing a significant proportion of this category, and/or that the data include better-off households (those not eligible for or choosing not to access the CSG) fostering orphans.

Booysen's study in Free State Province in South Africa is able to directly assess targeting of AIDS-affected households because his sample uses households identified as experiencing morbidity or mortality due to AIDS. Over 80% of these households received the OAP (in two periods by as much as 90%), but these numbers fell to 15%–35% over a 19-month period in the case of CSG. The Foster Care and Disability Grants reached fewer households. This dataset is small, representing under 300 households in two communities, but it suggests that the OAP was reaching AIDS-affected households, whereas the CSG appeared to suffer from uptake problems.[103] This, at least in part, reflects the lower uptake levels nationally at that time, which would have improved by now.

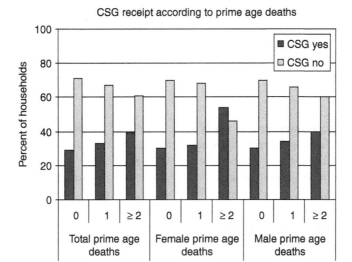

Figure 10.1 Child Support Grant (CSG) targeting of AIDS-affected households.[104]

The South African grants that could arguably be most directly targeted to AIDS-affected families are the Disability Grant and the FCG, although they were not intended for this. The Disability Grant can be obtained by adults who are HIV positive when their CD4 count falls below 200. The uptake rate was about 36% in 2000, but its potential reach for AIDS-affected families is very limited. The FCG is a means-tested grant for children determined to be "in need of care" regardless of whether their biological parents are alive. It is a much higher payment (about three times) than the CSG but much more complicated to obtain and monitor, involving court orders and referrals to social workers. It has increasingly been used to support families fostering children orphaned through AIDS, although take-up by potentially eligible households is very low. Among households that have accessed the grant, however, it appears to be well-targeted toward AIDS-affected families. Schubert et al. estimate that, among FCG recipients, about 50% are AIDS-affected.[105] The FCG has been given considerable attention in social assistance policy for children affected by AIDS: The national Minister of Social Development said in a 2002 address that, "The Department of Social Development [DSD] is encouraging relatives to take care of orphaned children under the foster care package," and reaffirmed this in October 2004 in a DSD document stating that one of the department's priorities was the "intensification of . . . registration of orphans for the Foster Care Grant."[106]

Although the higher FCG provides much better support for households than does the CSG, a strong case has been made for why it is an inappropriate response.[107] Aside from issues of prohibitive application burdens on beneficiaries, administrators, and social workers (much greater than the CSG), it is argued that the FCG is fundamentally inequitable. As discussed earlier in this chapter, the concern is that many children living with biological parents are just as impoverished and at risk (especially since many are living with ill parents) as children living with other relatives. The vast difference in the size of the payment between the FCG and the CSG makes the equity argument even starker. The funds for the FCG could instead go to raising the level of the CSG. The FCG perhaps best illustrates the equity dilemma and the constraints of political economy: While it is one of the few grants large enough to provide adequately for the needs of orphans and their fostering families, many advocates for child welfare do not see it as a viable option.

CONCLUSION

Targeting social protection to reach children affected by HIV and AIDS involves several key challenges. The first is whether to target individuals or households based on some direct measure of their being "AIDS-affected" or to target the poor or "extreme poor" in geographic areas heavily affected by HIV and AIDS. For targeting transfers, a strong case can be made for targeting on poverty criteria, thereby capturing AIDS-affected families and children who need the economic support and leaving out those who do not. This is more equitable—including people whose livelihoods have been undermined by something other than HIV (e.g., tuberculosis or malaria, drought, or structural disadvantages resulting in chronic poverty)—and avoids the stigma that would negatively affect grant recipients based on an association with HIV. Furthermore, targeting poverty can also reduce the number of families affected by HIV through economic assistance that reduces risk factors such as transactional sex and migration, or that slows down disease progression through improved nutrition and ART effectiveness. Ideally, a social protection system like South Africa's covers all poor households with children, so that all AIDS-affected households and children are reached. Where this is not on the table either for financial or political reasons, a targeting system that covers the poorest quintile or decile (as used in Malawi and Zambia) and further overlays the criteria of labor constraints and high-dependency ratios can target HIV without being explicit or inequitable. That does not mean, however, that an AIDS support organization should not take measures to promote the participation of its client base in poverty-targeted programs.

The question of whether to target orphans is addressed by a large literature on whether orphans are worse off than other children who are living with one or both parents. There is no simple answer to this question. Differences in poverty, food security, nutrition, and education depend on several, sometimes interrelated factors: the wealth status of fostering households, household structure, relatedness of children to caregivers, and gender, as well as other country-specific differences. Poverty targeting thus emerges as the most equitable and least stigmatizing solution—the most disadvantaged children will be reached regardless of whether any of their biological parents are living.

There are, however, conditions under which certain forms of social protection are appropriately targeted to orphans or to people living with HIV or AIDS. Targeting food and nutrition assistance to people who are HIV positive or living with AIDS addresses their unique caloric and micronutrient requirements, including those necessary for the effectiveness of ART. Orphans or children whose parents will die of AIDS are dealing with unique problems for which certain forms of social protection need to be targeted to them. These include psychological support, home-based care, legal literacy, and other services designed to help children and families deal with illness, death, and stigma. These services cannot be targeted with standardized indicators nor capped at a percentage of the population. Instead, they must be targeted through individuals, organizations, and agencies with local knowledge of communities and households, which can monitor, identify, and communicate needs.

The choice of system for targeting transfers, and the complexity of the data used to make targeting decisions, depends on a number of factors (see Table 10.1). If poverty, HIV, and OVC are highly concentrated in specific areas, inequality is low, and budgets are sufficient to cover these areas, then geographic targeting that provides benefits to all households may be more efficient, effective, and acceptable to communities than household targeting. If one or more of the reverse conditions are present, then a system for identifying the households most in need is necessary. The approach to means testing chosen (i.e., the level of complexity, and location and means of data collection) depends on administrative, technical, and financial capabilities; geographic distribution of households; and norms associated with centralization versus democratization of resource distribution decision-making. Categorical targeting can be used when an easily identifiable group is seen to be most in need or when it is most effective for meeting a policy objective (e.g., when old age pensions are used to protect the elderly as well as reach children) and when coverage is affordable.

Ultimately, the choice of targeting system reflects choices around levels of coverage in a society—how many categories of people and what percentage of the population will be covered by a system of social protection. This will reflect the political economy of social welfare in a given country as well as globally, involving financial realities, politics, ideology, and societal views on rights and entitlements, and beliefs about the role of different types of investments for poverty reduction, as well as beliefs about the role of economic support, as opposed to a narrower medical focus, in HIV responses and expenditures.

ACKNOWLEDGMENTS

Support for this research was provided by the Regional Network on AIDS, Livelihoods, and Food Security (RENEWAL) of the International Food Policy Research Institute (IFPRI), and by the Joint Learning Initiative on Children and AIDS (JLICA). Thanks to Lucy Bassett and Elisabeth Becker for their research assistance. This chapter was written when the author was an employee of IFPRI. The views expressed are her own and not those of IFPRI nor of her current employer, the Millennium Challenge Corporation.

NOTES

1. In this chapter, the terms social protection and social assistance are used largely interchangeably, although social protection is a broader concept and tends to refer to a broader set of programs. Social assistance refers primarily to material support.
2. Richter, L., et al. (2009). Strengthening families to support children affected by HIV and AIDS. *AIDS Care, 21*(S1), 3–12.
3. A "categorical" targeting approach is sometimes confused with a "universal" program. For example, a pension program is sometimes called a "universal" program, but actually uses categorical targeting of the elderly.
4. Yaschine, I. (1999). The changing anti-poverty agenda: What can the Mexican case tell us? *IDS Bulletin, 30*(2), 47-60.

5. Besley, T. & Kanbur, R. (1993). The principle of targeting. In M. Lipton, & J. van der Gaag (Eds.), *Including the poor* (pp. 67–90). Washington, DC: World Bank.

6. Gillespie, S., Haddad, L., & Jackson, R. (2001). *HIV/AIDS, food and nutrition security: Impacts and actions* (Nutrition policy paper no. 20). Geneva, Switzerland: United Nations SCN; Harvey, P. (2004). *HIV/AIDS and humanitarian action* (HPG research report no. 16). London: Overseas Development Institute; Stokes, C. S. (2002). *Measuring impacts of HIV/AIDS on rural livelihoods and food security.* Rome: FAO. Also, see Gillespie, S. & Kadiyala. (2005). HIV/AIDS and food and nutrition security: From evidence to action (Food Policy Review 7). Washington, DC: International Food Policy Research Institute, for a review over 150 studies examining these and other linkages between HIV/AIDS and food and nutrition security. Impacts vary based on economic and social variables at individual, household, community and country levels.

7. Carter, M., & Barrett, C. (2006). The economics of poverty traps and persistent poverty: An asset-based approach. *Journal of Development Studies, 42*(2), 178–199.

8. Caldwell, R. (2005, April). *Food aid and chronic illness: Insights from the Community Household Surveillance surveys.* Paper presented at IFPRI's International Conference on HIV/AIDS and Food and Nutrition Security. Durban, South Africa.

9. Gillespie, S., Kadiyala, S., & Greener, R. (2007). Is poverty or wealth driving HIV transmission? *AIDS, 21*(7), S5-S16; Bryceson, D., & Fonseca, J. (2006). An enduring or dying peasantry: Interactive impact of famine and HIV/AIDS in rural Malawi. In S. R. Gillespie (Ed.), *AIDS, poverty, and hunger: Challenges and responses* (pp. 97–108). Washington, DC: International Food Policy Research Institute; Tladi, L. S. (2006). Poverty and HIV/AIDS in South Africa: An empirical contribution. *Journal of Social Aspects of HIV/AIDS Research Alliance, 3*(1), 369-381; Brook, D. W., et al. (2006). South African adolescents: Pathways to risky sexual behavior. *AIDS Education and Prevention, 18*(6), 259–272; Kaufman, C., et al. (2004). Communities, opportunities, and adolescents' sexual behavior in KwaZulu-Natal, South Africa. *Studies in Family Planning, 35*(4), 261–274.

10. Kimuna, S., & Djamba, Y. (2005). Wealth and extramarital sex among men in Zambia. *International Family Planning Perspectives, 31*(2), 83-89; Weiser, S. D., et al. (2007). Food insufficiency is associated with high-risk sexual behavior among women in Botswana and Swaziland. *PLoS Medicine, 4*(10) e260; Nii-Amoo Dodoo, F., Zulu, E. M., & Ezeh, A. C. (2007). Urban—Rural differences in the socioeconomic deprivation—Sexual behavior link in Kenya. *Social Science and Medicine, 64*, 1019–1031.

11. Hallman, K. (2004). *Socioeconomic disadvantage and unsafe sexual behaviors among young women and men in South Africa.* Policy Research Division Working Paper 190. New York: Population Council.

12. Operario, D., et al. (2007). Prevalence of parental death among young people in South Africa and risk for HIV Infection: Results from a national representative sample. *Journal of Acquired Immune Deficiency Syndromes, 44*, 93–98.

13. Thurman, T. R., et al. (2006). Sexual risk behavior among South Africa adolescents: Is orphan status a factor? *AIDS and Behavior, 10*, 627–635.

14. Birdthistle, I. J., et al. (2008). From affected to infected? Orphanhood and HIV risk among female adolescents in urban Zimbabwe. *AIDS, 22*(6), 759–766.

15. Gillespie, Kadiyala, & Greener. (2007). Is poverty or wealth driving HIV transmission?

16. Sherr, L., et al. (2008). A systematic review on the meaning of the concept 'AIDS Orphan': Confusion over definitions and implications for care. *AIDS Care, 20*(5), 527–536.

17. Ainsworth, M., & Filmer, D. (2006). Inequalities in children's schooling: AIDS, orphanhood, poverty, and gender. *World Development, 34*(6), 1099–1128. Paternal, maternal, and double orphans refer to children whose fathers, mothers, or both are deceased, respectively.

18. Lundberg, M., & Over, M. (2000). Sources of financial assistance for households suffering an adult death in Kagera, Tanzania. *South African Journal of Economics, 68*(5), 1–39; Ainsworth, M., & Semali, I. (2000). *The impact of adult deaths on children's health in northwestern Tanzania* (World Bank Policy Research Working Paper Series). Washington, DC: World Bank; Gilborn, L., et al. (2001). *Making a difference for children affected by AIDS: Baseline findings from operations research in Uganda.* New York: Population Council; Deininger, K., Garcia, M., & Subbarao, K. (2003). AIDS-induced orphanhood as a systemic shock: Magnitude, impact, and program interventions in Africa. *World Development, 31*(7), 1201-1220; Rivers, J., Silvestre, E., & Mason, J. (2004). *Nutritional and food security status of orphans and vulnerable children.* New Orleans, LA: Tulane University.

19. Lindblade, K. A., et al. (2003). Health and nutritional status of orphans <6 years old cared for by relatives in western Kenya. *Tropical Medicine and International Health,* 8(1), 67–72.

20. Rivers, Silvestre, & Mason. (2004). *Nutritional and food security status of orphans and vulnerable children.*

21. Stewart, S. (2008). *No worse than their peers? Orphans' nutritional status in 5 Eastern and Southern African countries* Nairobi, Kenya: UNICEF/ESARO.

22. Ainsworth & Filmer. (2006). Inequalities in children's schooling.

23. UNAIDS/UNICEF/WHO. (2007). *Children and AIDS: A stocktaking report.* New York: UNICEF.

24. Case, A., Paxson, C., & Ableidinger, J. (2003). *The education of African orphans.* Princeton, NJ: Princeton University.

25. Case A., & Ardington, C. (2006). The impact of parental death on school outcomes: Longitudinal evidence from South Africa. *Demography, 43*(3), 401–420.

26. Evans D., & Miguel, E. (2007). Orphans and schooling in Africa: A longitudinal analysis. *Demography, 44*(1), 35–57.

27. Ueyama, M. (2007). *Mortality, mobility, and schooling outcomes among orphans: Evidence from Malawi* (Discussion Paper 00710). Washington, DC: International Food Policy Research Institute.

28. Deininger, Garcia, & Subbarao. (2003). AIDS-induced orphanhood as a systemic shock.

29. Gilborn, et al. (2001). *Making a difference for children affected by AIDS.*

30. Norman, A., Kadiyala, S., & Chopra, M. (2005). *Placing HIV-positive mothers at the centre of planning for orphans and vulnerable children: A case study of South Africa.* Washington, D.C.: IFPRI.

31. Bicego, G., Rutstein, S., & Johnson, K. (2003). Dimensions of the emerging orphan crisis in sub-Saharan Africa. *Social Science and Medicine, 56*(6), 1235–1247.

32. Adato, M., et al. (2005). *Children in the shadow of AIDS: Studies of vulnerable children and orphans in three provinces in South Africa* (RENEWAL Discussion Paper). Washington, DC: International Food Policy Research Institute; Norman, Kadiyala, & Chopra. (2005). *Placing HIV-positive mothers at the centre.*

33. Meintjes, H., et al. (2003). *Children "in need of care" or in need of cash? Questioning social security provisions for orphans in the context of the South African AIDS pandemic.* Cape Town, South Africa: Children's Institute, and the Centre for Actuarial Research, University of Cape Town.

34. Meintjes, H. & Giese, S. (2006). Spinning the epidemic: The making of mythologies of orphanhood in the context of AIDS. *Childhood, 13*(3), 407–430.

35. Cluver, L. D., Gardner, F., & Operario, D. (2008). Effects of stigma on the mental health of adolescents orphaned by AIDS. *Journal of Adolescent Health, 42*(4), 410–417.

36. Byron, E., Gillespie, S., & Nangami, M. (2006). *Integrating nutrition security with treatment of people living with HIV: Lessons being learned in Kenya* (RENEWAL Working Paper). Washington, DC: International Food Policy Research Institute.

37. Subbarao K., & Coury, D. (2004). *Reaching out to Africa's orphans: A framework for public action.* Washington, DC: World Bank.

38. See, for example, Subbarao, K., Mattimore, A., & Plangemann, K. (2001). *Social protection of Africa's orphans and vulnerable children—Issues and good practices program options.* Washington, DC: World Bank; Slater, R. (2004). *The implications of HIV/AIDS for social protection.* London: Overseas Development International; Harvey (2004). *HIV/AIDS and humanitarian action*; Schubert, B., et al. (2007). *The impact of social cash transfers on children affected by HIV and AIDS: Evidence from Zambia, Malawi, and South Africa.* Lilongwe, Malawi: UNICEF/ESARO; Devereux, S., et al. (2005). *Making cash count: Lessons from cash transfer schemes in east and southern Africa for supporting the most vulnerable children and households.* London: Save the Children, HelpAge International, Institute of Development Studies, University of Sussex.

39. Evans & Miguel (2007). Orphans and schooling in Africa.

40. Greenblott, K., & Greenaway, K. (2007). *Food security and nutrition: Meeting the needs of orphans and other children affected by HIV and AIDS in Africa* (Report for World Food Programme/UNICEF). Rome: World Food Programme.

41. Paton, N., et al. (2006). The impact of malnutrition on survival and the CD4 Count Response in HIV-infected patients starting antiretroviral therapy. *HIV Medicine, 7*(5), 323–330; Zachariah, R., et al. (2006). Risk factors for high early mortality in patients on antiretroviral treatment in a rural district of Malawi. *AIDS, 20*(18), 2355–2236.

42. A recognition of the importance of integrating food and nutritional support into HIV/AIDS programming is reflected in policy declarations by several organizations, including the World Health Assembly, UNGASS, and the Africa Forum 2006. See Byron, Gillespie, & Nangami. (2006). Integrating nutrition security with treatment.

43. Byron, Gillespie, & Nangami. (2006). Integrating nutrition security with treatment.

44. Current research is also testing whether better nutritional status for asymptomatic HIV-positive individuals may delay the need to start ARVs. See Byron, Gillespie, & Nangami. (2006). Integrating nutrition security with treatment.

45. Personal communication with Rahul Rawat.
46. Adato, M., & Bassett, L. (2008). *What is the potential of cash transfers to strengthen families affected by HIV and AIDS? A review of the evidence on impacts and key policy debates* (Technical report for the Joint Learning Initiative on Children and HIV/AIDS, Learning Group 1: Strengthening Families). Boston: JLICA.
47. These figures were presented by UNICEF at a conference in Johannesburg in February 2009. Its source is Government of Malawi, but it also appears in a paper on targeting in the Malawi SCTS: Schubert, B. (2009). *Targeting social cash transfers: The process of defining target groups and designing the targeting mechanism for the Malawi social cash transfer scheme.* Johannesburg, South Africa: Regional Hunger and Vulnerability Programme.
48. Cluver, Gardner, & Operario. (2008). Effects of stigma on the mental health.
49. Cluver, L., Gardner, F., & Operario, D. (2007). Psychological distress amongst AIDS-orphaned children in urban South Africa. *Journal of Child Psychology and Psychiatry, 48,* 755–763.
50. Atwine, B., Cantor-Graae, E., & Bajunirwe, F. (2005). Psychological distress among AIDS orphans in rural Uganda. *Social Science & Medicine, 61*(3), 555–564.
51. Wood, K., Chase, E., & Aggleton, P. (2006). "Telling the truth is the best thing": Teenage orphans' experiences of parental AIDS-related illness and bereavement in Zimbabwe. *Social Science & Medicine, 63,* 1923–1933.
52. Sherr et al. (2008). A systematic review.
53. Wood, Chase, & Aggleton. (2006). "Telling the truth is the best thing"; Foster, G. (2005). *Bottlenecks and drip-feeds: Channelling resources to communities responding to orphans and vulnerable children in southern Africa.* London: Save the Children; Gilborn et al., *Making a difference for children affected by AIDS,* 2001; Fox, S. (2001). Investing in our future: Psychosocial support for children affected by HIV/AIDS. A case study in Zimbabwe and the United Republic of Tanzania (U.N. AIDS Case Study). Geneva: UNAIDS; Richter, L,. Manegold, J., & Pather, R. (2004). *Family and community interventions for children affected by AIDS.* Cape Town, South Africa: HSRC Publishers.
54. Foster. (2005). *Bottlenecks and Drip-feeds.*
55. Foster, G. (2002). Beyond education and food: Psychosocial well-being of orphans in Africa. *Acta Paediatrica, 91,* 502–504.
56. Richter, Manegold, & Pather. (2004). *Family and community interventions;* Subbarao & Coury. (2004). *Reaching out to Africa's orphans;* Williamson et al., 2001, cited in Phiri, S., & Webb. D. (2007). The impact of HIV/AIDS on orphans and programme and policy responses. In G. A. Cornia (Ed.), *AIDS, Public Policy and Child Well-Being* (pp. 317–342). Florence, Italy: UNICEF.
57. Phiri & Webb. (2007). The impact of HIV/AIDS on orphans.
58. Coady, D., Grosh, M., & Hoddinott, J. (2004). *Targeting of transfers in developing countries: Review of lessons and experience.* Washington, DC: World Bank.
59. McCord, A. (2005). *Public works in the context of HIV/AIDS.* Cape Town, South Africa: Public Works Research Project, Southern Africa Labour and Development Research Unit; Slater. (2004). *The implications of HIV/AIDS for social protection.*
60. Harvey. (2004). *HIV/AIDS and humanitarian action.*
61. Skoufias, E. Davis, B. & de la Vega, S. (2001). Targeting the poor in Mexico: An evaluation of the selection of households into PROGRESA. *World Development, 29*(10), 1769–1784.

62. Adato, M. & Roopnaraine T. (2010). Women's status, gender relations, and conditional cash transfers. In M. Adato, & J. Hoddinott (Eds.), *Conditional Cash Transfers in Latin America* (pp. 284–314). Baltimore: Johns Hopkins University Press.

63. Coady, Grosh, & Hoddinott. (2004). *Targeting of transfers in developing countries.*

64. Caldés, N., Coady, D., & Maluccio, J. (2006). The cost of poverty alleviation transfer programs: A comparative analysis of three programs in Latin America. *World Development, 34*(5), 818–837.

65. Skoufias, Davis, & de la Vega. (2001). Targeting the poor in Mexico.

66. Adato & Roopnaraine. (2010). Women's status, gender relations, and conditional cash transfers.

67. Adato M., & Haddad, L. (2002). Targeting poverty through community-based public works programmes: Experience from South Africa. *Journal of Development Studies, 38*(3), 1–36.

68. Department for International Development (DFID). (2005). *Social transfers and chronic poverty: Emerging evidence and the challenge ahead: A DFID Practice Paper.* London: DFID.

69. DHS data from 2000–2004 in nine countries in sub-Saharan Africa show that under 1% of households were headed by children; still, these households are likely to be among those most in need.

70. This description reflects both the pre-2006 pilot and the expanded program, which were largely similar.

71. Ministry of Community Development and Social Services, Government of Zambia/German Technical Cooperation (MCDSS/GTZ). (2006). *Evaluation report: Kalomo Social Cash Transfer Scheme.* Lusaka, Zambia: MCDSS/GTZ; World Bank. (2007). *Impact evaluation design: Cash transfer pilot in Zambia.* Unpublished concept note. Washington, DC: World Bank.

72. MCDSS/GTZ. (2006). *Evaluation report*; World Bank. (2007). *Impact evaluation design.*

73. Ministry of Community Development and Social Services, Government of Zambia/Technical Working Group on Social Assistance (MCDSS/TWG). (2007). *Kalomo evaluation - Way forward?* Lusaka, Zambia: MCDSS/TWG; World Bank. (2007). *Impact evaluation design.*

74. Watkins, B. (2008). Alternative methods for targeting social assistance to highlyvulnerable groups (Report submitted to the Technical Working Group Social Assistance, Zambia). Washington, DC: Kimetrica International Limited.,

75. Schubert. (2009). *Targeting social cash transfers.*

76. Miller, C., Tsoka, M., & Reichert, K. (2008). *Targeting report. External evaluation of the Mchinji social cash transfer pilot.* Boston: Boston University.

77. Schubert et al. (2007). *The impact of social cash transfers on children.*

78. Ibid.

79. Acacia Consultants Ltd. (2007). *Evaluation of cash transfer programme in Nairobi, Kwale, and Garissa districts: Final report.* Nairobi, Kenya: Acacia Consultants/UNICEF Kenya Country Office.

80. Office of the Vice President & Ministry of Home Affairs, Government of Kenya. (2006). *Cash transfers for orphan and vulnerable children (OVC).* Nairobi, Kenya: Government of Kenya.

81. Ward, P., et al. (2010). *Cash transfer programme for orphans and vulnerable children (CT-OVC), Kenya, Operational and impact evaluation, 2007–2009, Final report.* London: Oxford Policy Management.

82. Ibid.

83. Devereux, S., Mvula, P., & Solomon, C. (2006). *After the FACT: An evaluation of Concern Worldwide's Food and Cash Transfers Project in three districts of Malawi.* Brighton, U.K., and Lilongwe, Malawi: Institute of Development Studies (IDS), University of Sussex, and Concern Worldwide Malawi.

84. Ibid.

85. Adato, M., & Roopnaraine, T. (2010). Conditional cash transfer programs, participation and power. In M. Adato, & J. Hoddinott (Eds.), *Conditional cash transfers in Latin America* (pp. 315–347). Baltimore: Johns Hopkins University Press; Hunter, N., & Adato, M. (2007). The Child Support Grant in KwaZulu-Natal: Perceptions and experience inside the household (Research Report 73). Durban: University of KwaZulu-Natal.

86. Harvey, P., & Marongwe, N. (2006). *Independent evaluation of Oxfam GB Zambia's emergency cash-transfer programme.* London: Overseas Development Institute.

87. Case, A., & Deaton, A. (1998). Large cash transfers to the elderly in South Africa. *Economic Journal, 108,* 1341.

88. Palacios, R., & Sluchynsky, O. (2006). *Social pensions part I: Their role in the overall pension system.* Washington, DC: World Bank.

89. Gorman, M. (2004). *Age and security: How social pensions can deliver effective aid to poor older people and their families.* London: HelpAge International; UNICEF. (2010). *Africa's orphaned generations.* New York: UNICEF.

90. Thulo, D. and Croome, D. (2006, October). *Furthering national action to realise commitments to social transfers in Africa: The case of Lesotho*; Lesotho Pensions Impact Project. Presentation, Lisbon, Portugal.

91. Samson, M., et al. (2004). *Final report: The social and economic impact of South Africa's social security system* (Research Paper #37). Cape Town, South Africa: Economic Policy Research Institute.

92. Delany, A., et al. (2008). *Review of the child support grant: Uses, implementation and obstacles.* New York: United Nations Children's Fund.

93. Rosa, S., Leatt, A., & Hall, K. (2005). *Does the means justify the end?* Cape Town: Children's Institute, University of Cape Town; Goudge, J., et al. (2007). *Costs and other barriers to health care (the SACOCO study).* PowerPoint presentation, Centre for Health Policy.

94. Budlender, D., Rosa, S., & Hall, K. (2005). *At all costs? Applying the means test for the Child Support Grant.* Cape Town, South Africa: Children's Institute & Centre for Actuarial Research, University of Cape Town.

95. Haarman, D. (1998). *From the maintenance grant to a new child support.* Cape Town: University of the Western Cape; Rosa, Leatt, & Hall (2005). *Does the means justify the end?*; Goudge et al. (2007). *Costs and other barriers to health care.*

96. Woolard, I., Carter, M., & Agüero, J. (2005). *Analysis of the child support grant: Evidence from the KwaZulu-Natal income dynamics study, 1993–2004.* Report to the Department of Social Development, Republic of South Africa, unpublished manuscript; Hunter & Adato. (2007). *The Child Support Grant in KwaZulu-Natal.*

97. Giese, S., & Smith, L. (2007). *Rapid appraisal of home affairs policy and practice affecting children in South Africa.* Cape Town, South Africa: Alliance for Children's Entitlement to Social Security.

98. Rosa, Leatt, & Hall. (2005). *Does the means justify the end?*; Goudge et al. (2007). *Costs and other barriers to health care.*

99. Ibid.

100. Devereux, et al. (2010). *Child Support Grant Evaluation 2010: Preparatory Qualitative Research Report.* Cape Town, South Africa: Economic Policy Research Institute.

101. Case, A., Hosegood, V., & Lund, F. (2005). The reach and impact of child support grants: Evidence from KwaZulu-Natal. *Development Southern Africa, 22*(4), 467–482.

102. Thanks to Futoshi Yamauchi for assistance with analyzing the KIDS data.

103. Booysen, F. (2004, March). The role of social grants in mitigating the socio-economic impact of HIV/AIDS. Paper presented at Centre for the Study of African Economies Conference on Growth, Poverty Reduction and Human Development in Africa, St. Catherine's College, Oxford,

104. Source: KIDS data from 2004

105. Schubert et al. (2007). *The impact of social cash transfers on children.*

106. Government of South Africa. (2004). *Minister and MECs to give priority to the removal of children from prison as well as the provision of more protection for other vulnerable children* (Media Release 6) Pretoria, South Africa: Government of South Africa.

107. Meintjes et al. (2003). *Children "in need of care" or in need of cash?*

11

Whose Responsibility Is It Anyway? Four Perspectives

View 1: Moving from Abrogation to Shared Responsibility

DOUGLAS WEBB ∎

The question of responsibility for children affected by AIDS is a narrative of denial and abrogation. Although in principle the roles and responsibilities for caring for this new "target group" have been defined in policy discourses, the reality of the response has its own geography and rationale that defies any simple categorization. The tension between "reacting" to assist a newly identified group of children rather than situating this group within and among a preexisting group of children who are *already* in need of support is real, continuous, and unresolved. Ascribing responsibility for care implies that actors are aware, able and willing to take up a caring role. The necessary dialogue that this implies has itself taken some time to mature, as manifested at a macro level through the emergence of interagency task teams and global partners fora and, at the opposite end of the spectrum, through supporting community-based structures, with a host of mediating institutions in between.

Before any structured and substantive policy dialogue on responsibility had taken place, responses were organic and reactionary. Initial reactions to the epidemic consisted of denial and processes of "otherization" by those in proximity to its impacts. Fieldwork conducted by the author in South Africa and Namibia in 1992–1993 indicated that communities faced with children affected by AIDS largely expected the government to take care of orphans, either in institutional care or in special houses on the periphery of the community.[1] Household perceptions varied by economic status, with poor households generally showing a more sympathetic response to the children and indicating a preference for family- and community-based support, as opposed to government-organized institutional care. Parents were more likely than dependents to state a preference for community care. Respondents who knew someone with AIDS also stated the desire to see the community take responsibility for care. Those who felt more distant from the disease, those who were closest as they were themselves dependants, and those who were relatively better off, stated that the government should care for the children. Regardless of care preferences, the vast majority of affected children were supported by immediate and extended family members, most often women. The initial response of the majority of respondents was to see the care of children affected by AIDS as a new and external problem that demanded a state response. AIDS-related stigma also played a large part in the common desire to see children—perceived as carrying the secondary guilt from their parents—"removed" from the community, which needed overall protection from this unfamiliar and insidious threat. Politicization of the epidemic in southern Africa in the early 1990s furthered the position that the epidemic was exogenous, and that it was beyond the mandate and capacity of communities to care for those affected, a position mirrored in national debates on AIDS.

Although communities themselves gradually internalized the reality of an unprecedented caring function, the policy response remained muted. The combination of economic nonviability and generalized resistance to the expansion of institutional child care meant that families and indigenous community safety net mechanisms or reciprocity networks bore the brunt of the care burden. State engagement in child care was nonexistent on the whole until the reconstruction and emergence of child-oriented welfare mechanisms in South Africa in the late 1990s. Until that point, the communities had some support from nongovernmental organizations (NGOs), almost all of them foreign-funded. By the mid 2000s, however, even in contexts with a relatively high degree of NGO activity, no more than around one-quarter of AIDS-affected households in high-burden countries were receiving any form of external assistance.[2] For the majority of affected children and families, what scant help there was came from church groups or small-scale NGOs, and state responses were notable by their continued absence.

This position was increasingly regarded as untenable by the international community, which highlighted the plight of communities and extended families unable to cope. Rights-based models of care and responses were brought to the fore, using concepts of rights holders, duty bearers, and hierarchy of responsible institutions (family, kinship care, nonkinship care, state) that defined the centrality of the family to care for children within a "protective" or "enabling" environment. The Convention on the Rights of the Child (1989) mentions that, where such care is unavailable or the best interests of the child are not being upheld while in family care, the state has an *obligation* to provide alternative care until permanent care is found. Limited capacity in state systems has dictated that families have generally been left to provide care unsupported by state actors, in spite of rhetorical advances. This reality contrasts with alternative political models of responsibility, still prevalent in ex-communist countries and states, where child care by the state deliberately replaces that of families perceived to be unable to provide care. Estimates put the number of children in institutional care globally at around 8 million.[3]

Following the United Nations (UN) Declaration of Commitment on HIV/AIDS (2001), the first global consensus statement on support to children affected by AIDS, "A Framework for the Protection, Care, and Support of Orphans and Vulnerable Children Living in a World with HIV and AIDS" (2004), outlined five strategies, namely:

- Strengthen the *capacity of families* to protect and care for orphans and vulnerable children by prolonging the lives of parents and providing economic, psychosocial, and other support.
- Mobilize and support *community-based responses.*
- Ensure access for orphans and vulnerable children to *essential services,* including education, health care, birth registration, and others.

- Ensure that *governments protect* the most vulnerable children through improved policy and legislation and by channeling resources to families and communities.
- Raise awareness at all levels through advocacy and social mobilization to create a *supportive environment* for children and families affected by HIV/AIDS.

In 2011, these strategies remain relevant. What has changed is the perceived role of the state in the caring response. Faced with continued inability of poor households to provide adequate care for AIDS-affected children, the expected role of the state has been amplified, not least in international policy discourse. The emergence of social protection in Africa is a recent phenomenon as far as the role of the state is concerned, and the momentum is considerable.[4] The response centers on the expanded role of the state in providing a modicum of a child-focused social welfare response that includes social cash transfers (such as child and foster grants, and pensions), livelihood support strategies for the most vulnerable, and expanded access to social services for the previously excluded. Although the preferred or optimal social protection construct (and its variability) is yet to be defined, the central role of the state is not disputed. Indeed, the role of the state is mandated by its natural place within a social contract with its own citizenry; rationalist notions of social obligation and entitlement underpin the state's purported role. Although familiar and conceptually convincing to international observers and policy-makers, these notions of state-centered social protection are experiencing resistance from states themselves. Their objections hinge on arguments of affordability, fear of dependency, and the danger of compromising communities.

The case of Ethiopia is illustrative of the shifts of perceived and actual responsibility over the last two decades. Following the removal of the Derg and its institutional infrastructure in 1991, the new government (based around the Ethiopian People's Democratic Revolutionary Front) centered the responsibility for children's welfare in the Ministry of Labour and Social Affairs, whose Developmental Social Welfare Policy of 1997 defined the state's role in supporting the destitute. The later emergence of the HIV/AIDS Prevention and Control Office (HAPCO) and its strategic plans implied that the support of AIDS-affected children lay within its own coordination (and possibly service provision) mandate. Despite high HIV rates throughout the 1990s, the issue of orphans and vulnerable children (OVC) failed to achieve any political traction or financial allocation due to sensitivities over concepts of child protection and children lacking adequate support from family and community structures.

The Global Framework-inspired rapid assessment analysis and action planning process in 2004 and the resultant National Plan of Action for Orphans and Vulnerable Children (2004–2006) was an example of an externally-pushed response that failed to find local political support. Plans to revive the process through a national situational analysis on OVC were on the table in 2006 but were never carried through, and in 2011, the process is still pending. In the interim, the mandate for care of children affected by AIDS has been passed to the Ministry of Women, Children and Youth Affairs (MOWCYA), and HAPCO has similarly transferred any leadership over to MOWCYA. Meanwhile, a large-scale public sector reform exercise resulted in reduced institutional memory and arguably reduced capacity in the core ministries.

The net result is that there is no central strategy or institution empowered to take the lead on the response to AIDS-affected children. With the landscape so devoid of institutions or operational frameworks, the Ethiopian response is in a state of flux. New guidelines on child care are being issued but have limited operational effect. Moreover, the Charities and Societies Proclamation (2009) limited the operations of NGOs in the areas of child rights and social mobilization. Policy concerns now revolve around the expansion of family-based alternative child care, coinciding with heightened international concerns around the state of the intercountry legal adoption infrastructure.

The centrality of the state's response is now being engineered in a different guise through social protection mechanisms, notably the Productive Safety Nets Programme (since 2006), the revision of the Developmental Social Welfare Policy (now called the Social Protection Policy), and the construction of a new National Social Fund. This follows Ethiopia's ratification of the African Union Social Policy Framework (2008), which calls for the development of a national social protection plan. In Ethiopia, as elsewhere, poverty alleviation could be increased through carving out a greater role for the private sector by, for instance, enhancing the role of the microfinance institutions and extending credit outreach to the most vulnerable and those previously excluded, in partnership with an expanded public social welfare sector.

The overall shift in policy has been from families absorbing the costs to families being supported to bear the costs. Yet, while the change in support for AIDS-affected children in the policy arena makes sense on a conceptual level, financially, the outlook is less optimistic. Including children in the national AIDS strategies through the 2000s meant that funding was easier to find, especially from the Global Fund to Fight AIDS, Tuberculosis, and Malaria and the U.S. President's Emergency Plan for AIDS Relief (PEPFAR), which provided hundreds of million dollars for AIDS affected children in the last decade. The gradual engagement of the Global Fund in financing responses for AIDS-affected children was an important shift, although it could be argued that proposals that focus on impact mitigation are generally of a lower quality in what is still a medically-dominated response. In addition, future Global Fund financing is likely to be tied specifically to national AIDS strategies, whether child-inclusive impact mitigation is highlighted or not. Sector-wide financing in the form of sector-wide approaches (SWAPs) has not, to date, been a viable option as no SWAPs cover children affected by AIDS effectively. Social welfare sector SWAPs do not exist, and national development plans also rely on sector-specific inputs. This means that financing has been effectively pushed out of the public sector by the fact that sector-wide plans do not exist, AIDS-specific financing for children affected by AIDS is not part of the budget, and among the high-burden countries, there are no child focused social welfare systems to speak of beyond, arguably, South Africa. State-financed responses are essential if coverage is to be increased to an acceptable standard. In summary, there is no equivalent financing mechanism in existence for the otherwise-popular child-focused social protection movement. There is a real danger, in the Ethiopian context at least, that conceptual advances and resultant mandate shifts may leave the children themselves without a caring environment that has any semblance of secure financing.

This case raises the larger question of financing and the simple fact that AIDS-specific responses have been historically easier to finance than AIDS-sensitive or -inclusive ones. High levels of AIDS funding removed the onus from state structures to finance the social support system—PEPFAR financing reiterated this position—so state roles were limited to normative standards and plan development, but not financing more generally. PEPFAR's history of supporting non–state actors combined with an absence of funding and support to formal (professional and paraprofessional) social work systems has not helped build the sustainable child care systems that are most desperately needed. Large investments have gone into health systems definition and strengthening, but the social sector has been largely ignored in public policy discourse. Donors other than PEPFAR have steered away from support to AIDS impact mitigation due to a perceived saturation, but the reality is that medium- to long-term financing of civil society at the expense of a public-sector financing mechanism is a strategy borne out of an emergency, not developmental outlook.

Even if AIDS exceptionalist responses have a limited lifespan in the coming years, the financing processes will naturally lag and the problem of financing child- (and AIDS-) sensitive social protection will fast become a pressing one. Indeed, the nervousness of governments around financing social protection, given its lack of operational maturity and questionable support across the sociopolitical spectrum, may mean that the community–family nexus, rather than the state–family nexus, will be preferred by policy-makers in the meantime. Constructs of AIDS-sensitive social protection point to strong state–family connections, mediated by community and nongovernmental institutions, as the preferred structure. Political preferences for formalizing or strengthening community-based structures may predominate, and this may well be the case in Ethiopia, which has a robust and revered community-based institution network. Other nation states may be more able to operationalize a strengthened state–family connection, and this is emerging as the dominant policy trend in South Africa, Namibia, and Lesotho. In these contexts, over time and as stigma is reduced, the state accepts more obligation, perhaps as a mirror of social intentions and accepted norms. Cash transfers to AIDS-affected households, for example, have grown in popularity as states recognize their own responsibility to intervene directly.[5] Political capital must be used on behalf of children affected by AIDS as a group of children who have the right to social protection. Lessons must be identified in how this is being done in the African context (as it has been done in Latin America), with the desired trajectory of exogenous funding being replaced by indigenous (tax-based) funding.

As the overall response matures, a balance of responsibility must be attained among actors and layers of agency. The state role should focus on normative standards of care, guidelines of operational support, targeting guidance, macrofinancing management, cost estimations, strategic planning, and multisectoral coordination. Civil society's natural roles are related to supplementary and specialized service delivery, witnessing, case identification and referral, monitoring, follow-up, and program innovation. Community-based organizations will remain vital, and state-led responses will need to support and supplement preexisting community support structures and not replace them—this will remain a challenge for policy-makers and program designers. Households provide immediate familial care and nurturing. The roles of the international community are perhaps the most fickle and uncertain. Inevitable roles for the international community will be encouraging normative standards around state support, technical assistance coordination and provision, operationalization of rights-based responses, and gap financing while advocating for core (tax-based) financing. Between the international community and the states are the regional economic communities in Africa, which will continue to support the evolution of the policy environment, and convene and facilitate policy consistency, learning, and resource mobilization. The UN, as a component of the multilateral response, can focus on normative support and technical assistance, learning, adherence to, and monitoring of rights-based responses.

Supporting children affected by AIDS is complex. Families are the essential and principal sources of care. States in sub-Saharan Africa are finally acknowledging an expanded role in their care, but how this will be manifested—and, more importantly, paid for—is still a subject for debate, research, and incessant advocacy.

ACKNOWLEDGMENTS

Douglas Webb serves as chief of section for adolescent development, protection and HIV/AIDS in UNICEF Ethiopia. The views expressed in this chapter are his own and do not necessarily represent the views of UNICEF.

NOTES

1. Webb, D. (1997). *HIV and AIDS in Africa*. London: Pluto Press.
2. UNICEF. (2008). *Children and AIDS Stocktaking report*. New York: UNICEF.
3. Save the Children Alliance. (2003). *A last resort: the growing concern of children in institutional care*. London: Author.
4. Joint Learning Initiative on Children and AIDS. (2009). *Home truths: Facing the facts on children, AIDS, and poverty*; Handa, S., Devereux, S., & Webb, D. (Eds.). (2010). *Social protection for Africa's children*. New York: Routledge, Oxford.
5. Schubert, B., Webb, D., Temin, M., & Masabane, P. (2007). *The impact of social cash transfers on children affected by HIV and AIDS–Evidence from Zambia, Malawi and South Africa*. Nairobi: UNICEF ESARO.

View 2: Responsibility, Accountability, and Government (In)Action

AGNES BINAGWAHO ■

Previous chapters revealed promising opportunities to strengthen children's well-being in the context of HIV and AIDS. Those discussions also raised urgent questions of responsibility. Although evidence-based strategies have been identified in many areas connected with children's well-being, delivery of these interventions lags. To accelerate progress for children, we must be clear about who stands accountable for executing the actions this book has described.

The question of responsibility does not have a one-line answer. Improving children's well-being requires collaboration among multiple stakeholders. Moreover, the most effective division of tasks will vary across national and local contexts, depending on history, local capacities, the type of intervention, and other factors. Accordingly, my aim here is not to analyze in detail the breakdown of responsibilities in delivering particular programs or interventions, but rather to make a broad argument about the critical role of government in guiding and coordinating the overall agenda of action for children affected by AIDS. I will argue that the governments of affected countries hold primary responsibility for leading the response to children's needs. Today, however, inadequate governmental responses often leave the fight to protect children fragmented and without coordination, effectiveness, and sustainability. My claim is thus twofold. We need to (1) assert the primacy of government responsibility for children affected by AIDS, while understanding previous failures; and (2) identify concrete steps to overcome current bottlenecks and accelerate action.

To stress the central responsibility of governments is not to neglect the contributions of other stakeholders: children and young people themselves; families; communities; national and international nongovernmental organizations (NGOs), including faith-based organizations (FBOs); bilateral and multilateral development agencies; and donors. All these actors exhibit distinctive strengths and perform roles that governments cannot. However, without the coordination, sustainability, and political legitimacy provided by government authorities, the contributions of these other stakeholders will fall short of what they could achieve for children.

Framing the Argument: Human Rights Instruments and Norms

The international human rights framework provides the appropriate conceptual and legal structure within which to discuss responsibility for action on children's well-being. This framework is not universally embraced, nor is it uniformly interpreted by those who do accept it. However, the foundational documents of the international human rights framework, such as the Universal Declaration of Human Rights (UDHR), articulate principles to which the large majority of states and other relevant actors broadly subscribe, even if important divergences in interpretation exist. Moreover, the stipulations of international human rights declarations, treaties and conventions, including the UDHR, are not merely aspirational. They constitute legally binding obligations for the states that have signed and ratified these instruments. Thus, as international jurists such as Alicia Ely Yamin have argued, the most distinctive contribution of the rights framework in health is to recast "misfortunes" as violations that are legally actionable, thus fueling demands for accountability.[1]

Of course, enforcing such accountability in practice, when states may have violated their obligations under the rights framework, is notoriously difficult. International human rights norms nonetheless provide us with a widely recognized set of legal standards for analyzing responsibility and seeking redress in cases of violation. Central to international human rights doctrine is the principle that national governments bear ultimate accountability for the security and welfare of all their people, including children.

Pragmatically speaking, this does not mean that rights language is the only language we should ever be prepared to use in seeking to influence governments or other institutions whose behavior affects children's well-being. Arguments based on economic interests will often carry greater immediate weight with decision-makers. However, I believe that, as we press for implementation of the actions described in this volume, human rights obligations toward children and the national economic interest of countries burdened by HIV will often prove to be convergent, rather than opposed.

Even among countries at similar income levels, governments differ widely in their structures, procedures, and priorities. Thus, effective solutions must always be tailored to national contexts. Analyzing options for any specific state lies beyond the scope of this discussion. My aim is to argue foundational points about political responsibility for children's well-being, while recognizing that the operationalization of these ideas will look very different in different settings. Meanwhile, arguments about government responsibility have little immediate relevance in contexts in which state structures have effectively ceased to operate due to conflict or natural disaster. In such settings, international agencies and nongovernmental partners must temporarily assume the accountability for children's well-being that ordinarily belongs to the state, and work to restore the national government's capacity to manage this critical facet of governance.

The core of my discussion in this chapter will adopt the following structure. As an entry point to my argument about government responsibility, I look at the example of HIV-specific services. Not because these are the only services children and families affected by AIDS require, but because these well-known interventions illustrate a pattern in the division of responsibilities that applies more broadly. I then take up the pivotal issue of resource flows. I argue that the primary obstacle depriving children of their right to needed services is not the amount of money available to the fight against HIV/AIDS, but instead the chronic financial waste resulting from how donors choose to channel funds, and how beneficiaries use and allocate them. Developing this point, I argue that improving efficiency requires integrating action for children into a comprehensive national development plan—something only government can do—and fighting corruption. Finally, I step back to propose a broad response to the question of what it will take to accelerate progress for children now.

GOVERNMENT LEADERSHIP IN ACTION FOR CHILDREN

In many instances, the public sector will not function as the direct provider of the services that children, families, and communities affected by AIDS need. But government is accountable for directing and coordinating service provision and making sure that interventions reach all those who require them. Selected HIV-specific services illustrate this point.

Availability and Accessibility of HIV Services

In each country, HIV-affected children should receive the best care and treatment that is affordable locally. Specific characteristics of HIV highlight responsibilities that only government can legitimately assume. As HIV is a chronic disease with opportunistic infection and requires lifelong treatment, it needs national policies, protocols, and guidelines. Additionally, it requires the integration of pediatric HIV services into basic pediatric care and the commitment to a family-centered, holistic approach.[2] The creation of such a framework and the guarantee of an adequate system of coordination, monitoring, and evaluation can only be assumed by governments.

In addition to establishing technical norms, government plays a critical and unique role in advancing health equity. Only governments can guarantee equitable access for all orphans and vulnerable children (OVC) to HIV services based on finances, geography, age, and gender. The government has a responsibility to create an enabling environment for the fight against discrimination through antidiscriminatory laws and campaigns, and through the promotion of the Greater Involvement of People Living with AIDS (GIPA) concept.

PREVENTION
HIV prevention at all stages of the life cycle points to areas in which government leadership is irreplaceable. Governments should integrate—based on geographic equity—and subsidize prevention of mother-to-child transmission (PMTCT) services in antenatal clinics, supporting, promoting, and, where necessary, providing programs that can identify and draw in pregnant women and expectant fathers. To ensure the broad implementation of a family-centered PMTCT approach requires the formulation of appropriate national norms, as well as changes in the training of health professionals, areas in which government has unique authority.

The distinctive responsibility of government also comes to the fore on prevention during childhood and adolescence. According to the Convention on the Rights of the Child (CRC), governments have the responsibility to provide children with accurate, uncensored, and age-appropriate information on HIV/AIDS as part of educational programs both inside and outside of school.[3] Also, explaining and instructing children on topics regarding HIV/AIDS can help prevent the stigmatization of those who are affected by HIV. In this manner, fulfilling all children's right to HIV education can also help uphold the rights of HIV-infected children to live in a nondiscriminatory environment.

Governments should pay special attention to HIV testing among adolescents, as this is the stage at which individuals tend to first engage in sexual intercourse and other behaviors that increase their risk of HIV infection, such as drug use. Adolescents should have the option of receiving their HIV test results without their parents' knowledge, but children and caregivers must also be properly counseled. In many countries, this implies changes at the central level for laws, policies, and protocols; infrastructure must also be renovated or newly created to allow teenagers free access to HIV care, treatment, testing, and other prevention services without parental approval. As these examples show, government leadership is especially important on issues that challenge traditional social norms, for example sexual activity among adolescents and also homosexuality and sex work.

The actual delivery of prevention messages and services relies on grassroots knowledge and the initiative of affected communities. But grassroots initiatives can only be sustainable if government is on board. For this reason, innovative prevention campaigns, for example among sex workers in India, have emphasized the need for government to ultimately assume coordination and ownership of prevention programs, including those initiated in the nongovernmental sector.[4]

TREATMENT

The expansion of access to antiretroviral therapy (ART) is a critical human rights concern. Governments have committed themselves to achieving universal access to ART for children and adults. The limited progress achieved to date is insufficient. In Africa, the continent with the greatest number of HIV-positive children, when pediatric HIV prevention care and treatment exist, they are still generally not included in basic health services. ART coverage for children is at 35%,[5] and 50% of HIV-positive infants who do not receive treatment die within the first year of life,[6] translating into a high rate of child mortality.[7] Meanwhile, as earlier chapters argued, it is critical to frame treatment and care in a family context, and to recognize that treating HIV-positive parents and caregivers is vital to the well-being of children affected by HIV and AIDS.

Again, in many heavily burdened countries, the public sector will not be the only or even the main direct provider of AIDS treatment. But government alone has the legitimacy to establish norms and to coordinate and integrate the activities of NGOs, FBOs, and private sector providers across the whole national territory.

Allocating Resources

Action to improve the lives of children affected by AIDS requires resources. For too long, the main and in some cases only resources available to help children were those generated at the grassroots level by families and communities.[8] Perhaps more than any other issue, the need for more equitable mobilization and allocation of resources for children highlights the unique responsibility of government.

Governments in many affected countries lack the revenue base to fund all necessary services themselves. However, the role of government in oversight and priority-setting remains crucial to ensure that external funds are used coherently to achieve national goals. For development partnerships to succeed, the use of funds from international donors must be determined by the recipient country's own priorities, not donors' preconceived agendas.

Over the last 9 years, funding for HIV has increased dramatically. Much of this money, however, has not reached children. Although a lack of resources may prevent us from immediately meeting the needs of all HIV-affected people, human rights and the principle of equity dictate that we allocate available resources according to the number of beneficiaries, their needs, and their vulnerability. Still, many donor and beneficiary countries do not apportion enough money for programs that help OVC. The government has a responsibility to advocate for increased and equitable allocation of resources to support HIV-affected children.

As the legitimate primary interlocutor of international funding agencies, government has a natural role to play in ensuring that donor funds are channeled to those actors within the country who will use the resources most efficiently to improve children's lives. The government can broker relationships between international funders and the national and community-level organizations that, today, often remain excluded from the chain of funding for vulnerable children. Local groups and families provide the largest share of support to children. But, instead of flowing to them, money earmarked for children too often remains in donor countries to support organization headquarters, or it is given mainly to international NGOs from the global North. The obstacles that are named to explain why funds are channeled through international NGOs include lack of managerial capacities and the ineffective use of funds within local NGOs and community-based organizations (CBOs). For example, 70% of the U.S. President's Emergency Plan for AIDS Relief (PEPFAR) money goes to international NGOs, and only 30% goes to locally based groups.[9]

Meanwhile, it has been documented that international NGOs spend more money in administrative and overhead costs than do domestic NGOs.[10] The financial loss exists at all levels, with overhead at headquarters compounded by overhead for in-country offices. Along with high transactional costs, high salaries, and multiple business trips, the losses may be up to ten times higher than if funds were channeled directly through families, communities, and local NGOs and CBOs. Despite this, few questions are raised about the enormous loss of money that occurs when funds are channeled in this manner.[11]

Rather than giving the money to these expensive intermediaries, donor organizations should instead consider giving funds directly to local organizations. Such aid should be given in conjunction with capacity building and tools to increase the expertise of local NGOs.[12] In this way, administrative costs could be reduced[13] and local capacity would be improved. Effective government leadership in monitoring and managing resource flows could strengthen nongovernmental actors and enable a more effective overall response. Mechanisms to coordinate and harmonize funding flows under national government leadership have been recognized as critical to sustain local, community-based efforts for children.[14]

Governments as well as development partners have a clear responsibility for the financial losses resulting from transaction and overhead costs.[15] These stakeholders are responsible for improving the monitoring and evaluation of funds raised for HIV-affected children, and for ensuring that HIV money earmarked for children enters the selected countries and goes toward the correct beneficiaries.

This requires that governments better coordinate around HIV funding, which will guarantee that the money is better utilized toward achieving sustainable results, and that they develop national ownership of HIV programs.

Integrating the Fight Against HIV into the National Development Plan

Ultimately, funds for children's well-being can only be used to maximum effect if they are guided by a comprehensive national development plan. Isolated interventions and independent programs can, of course, achieve some good at the local level, reducing the immediate impacts of HIV and AIDS on children, families, and communities. However, this piecemeal mode of response is reaching its limits in many African countries. To reach the next level, we must offer children and families not only short-term protection from the direct effects of HIV, but a future of social stability and economic opportunity. Enabling children's well-being in this broader sense cannot be achieved through fragmented interventions, but only through coordinated policy action across the multiple sectors that contribute to economic and social development. For this reason, action on the specific threats of HIV must be connected to country-appropriate systems of social protection to guarantee the durable well-being of children and families. The whole strategy to address children's needs in the context of HIV and AIDS must also be integrated within a coherent and comprehensive national development strategy that incorporates all aspects of economic activity and social progress.

The African Charter urges states to integrate basic health service programs, including HIV clinical response, into national development plans. Furthermore, the concurrence of the global burden of HIV with the global burden of poverty is so evident that it would not be a stretch to say that HIV can be fought by efficiently battling poverty. Nations should encourage economic growth in general, and promote education and health in particular.[16]

To date, efforts to accelerate economic development in low-income countries have often yielded disappointing results. In part, this is because governments in the global South have failed to use donor aid efficiently and effectively. Hundreds of billions of aid funding dollars have been injected into low-income countries over the last 50 years but far too little progress on development has been made. In general, African citizens are poorer today than in the 1960s,[17] and the majority of the population lives at income levels that are insufficient to meet their basic needs.[18] Moreover, on a continent where more than 60% of children already in live in poverty,[19] the recent global financial crisis will certainly intensify the vulnerability of poor families. This is important, as HIV infection and poverty often overlap and have a cyclical relationship: The virus exacerbates poverty through morbidity and mortality of productive adults, diverting incomes toward treatment, while poverty facilitates the transmission of the infection.[20] Even though, in some specific circumstances, improved socioeconomic status can heighten exposure to HIV,[21] in general, poverty increases one's risk of HIV infection.[22]

Pushing for HIV to be fought within the framework of the overall development agenda does not obviate governments' duty to mobilize funds for OVC-focused HIV response; instead, it provides a link to the development framework of poverty alleviation. There is strong interdependence between them, as addressing HIV in OVC populations also contributes to, and is an asset for, sustainable development and fighting poverty.

The proper use of aid money could have allowed countries to tackle the determinants of HIV infection, such as lack of education and deepening poverty. However, due to corruption, mismanagement, and misuse, aid has failed to prevent the continued impoverishment of Africa and the spread of HIV. If the expenditure of international aid and domestic funds continues in a business-as-usual mode, communities and families will have fewer resources to care for their children, and the next generation will likely remain poor, malnourished, uneducated, and unhealthy.

Not all factors fueling poverty can be controlled at the country level, since external variables like debt burdens and unfair trade regimes also play a role. However, most poverty in sub-Saharan Africa can be attributed to internal factors such as bad governance, lack of opportunities to increase professional capacity, poor public services, and mismanagement.[23] These internal issues enable the external factors to take root, and governments must take leadership in reversing the business-as-usual scenario. Thus, ironically, the frequent failure of government leadership in promoting economic development further underscores government's unique responsibility. When the state fails to exercise its critical role of coordination and stewardship in guiding development, no other actor or institution can durably fill the vacuum.

JUMPSTARTING ACTION: WHAT'S NEEDED NOW

Focusing on the theme of state responsibility raises the question of why, in practice, governments have so often abdicated their responsibilities toward children and have proven unwilling or unable to provide the enabling support that families, communities, and nongovernmental partners seek. There is no uniform answer to this question. The character and causes of states' performance show complex variation. Research using methodologies like the business case study model has begun to generate valuable insights, but much more must be learned.[24]

However, action cannot and need not wait for the results of additional research. Our question is practical and immediate: How should the international community proceed now, based on the best current evidence, to drive implementation of those actions that we know will improve children's lives in the context of AIDS? On this question, my thesis is clear. Although governments have often fallen short of their obligations, we cannot eliminate them from the equation. The ability of other actors and stakeholders to achieve and sustain positive outcomes for children depends, in the long run, on the constructive engagement of state authority. The way to improve states' performance in meeting children's needs is not by giving states less responsibility or attempting to circumvent and marginalize government decision-making structures. On the contrary, the way forward is to engage governments more actively in defining the parameters within which they can lead a coherent national agenda of action for children affected by AIDS.

The issue of coherence and transparency in funding flows is critical. Governments must be in the driver's seat in establishing mechanisms appropriate for their contexts. To stop misuse of funds, governments must create appropriate channels for the in-country flow of aid by establishing proper legal frameworks in the spirit of the Rome and Paris Declarations and the "Three Ones": one coordinating body, one national plan, and one monitoring and evaluation framework. The fight against HIV for OVC must start with a national assessment of OVC needs linked with an assessment of the economic opportunities for families and low-income communities. This assessment, a participatory process involving OVC, families, communities, and partners, will form the basis of a national HIV response plan with which all stakeholders and funding streams will align. Such actions do not require substantial additional funds but do require national ownership, accountability in governance using a participatory approach, and a development process committed to inclusion and equity.

Multisectoral Collaboration Under Government Coordination

The aim of government efforts must be to strengthen families and communities in multiple dimensions, so that they can continue to care for children. This involves reinforcing HIV-related health services, but also fostering expanded economic opportunity and exploring options for national social protection.[25]

In driving a multisectoral approach, government ownership and active engagement by other stakeholders are not in opposition. They reinforce each other. Stakeholder participation and the potential for responsiveness to local needs are enhanced, not undermined, when national government uses its authority to create consistent channels of communication and resource distribution, giving transparency to policy choices and funding flows. Only government authority can create a fair, predictable environment that enables all actors working for children to perform at their best. This realization is critical to get past "business as usual" and create a new model of accountability in action for children affected by AIDS.

What are other stakeholders' most urgent tasks? Governments and donors in the North must critically review their funding channels and stop tolerating the routine loss of large proportions of aid money before it actually reaches children. NGOs and FBOs must provide quality services equitably and align their work fully with the national agenda. Private service providers and clinics must align their areas of coverage with national plans, in order to expand the geographic accessibility, acceptability, and effectiveness of services. Meanwhile, NGOs, communities, families, and children must have a voice in the planning, management, implementation, and evaluation of all child-related services. Participatory processes ensure that children's rights are upheld in practice, not just on paper. Civil society organizations must continue to exercise their watchdog function, using means of democratic participation, information, and critical debate to ensure that governments and all stakeholders are accountable and meet their responsibilities to children and families under human rights law. By aligning their efforts in this way, partners will enhance support to the families and communities who each day provide children with the love and care on which all hopes for a better future depend.

WHAT TO DO WHEN GOVERNMENTS ARE CORRUPT

Corruption is one of the main reasons why development aid does not reach its intended beneficiaries. Corruption occurs at all levels of governance, from local to national, and also within judicial systems. It circumvents legislation, undermines development and democratic processes, and exacerbates inequality and poverty. Corruption concerns not only the public sector, but also the private sector, the military, and civil society. It exists everywhere in the world, in both rich and poor nations. The difference between countries in the North and the South, however, resides in the strength of institutions and legal frameworks in the North, which can be mobilized to fight corruption. Corruption is often difficult to differentiate from other problems such as negligence, mismanagement, and inefficiency, as has been well documented in emergency situations in which the speed needed to save lives conflicts with the time and resources required to minimize corruption risks.[26]

Corruption and human rights are interconnected; corruption exists when incentive meets opportunity, and a government that does not uphold human rights creates an enabling environment for corruption to flourish. The existence of corruption, in turn, hinders governments from guaranteeing numerous fundamental human rights.[27]

Corruption concerns governments at two levels: Governments are either directly involved as the primary perpetrators of corruption, or else they are involved indirectly through failure to protect their citizens from corruption generated by a different sector of society.

One might argue that stopping the flow of aid to Africa will prevent corruption, as aid would no longer provide the incentive and opportunities for corruption. This would be a mistake, however. Cutting aid would negatively impact millions of poor people, especially women and children, more than it would those who are responsible for corruption, as corruption is a system that exists with or without aid (corruption in rich countries is not linked to aid).

The Solution

To control both aid and corruption, we need a multidimensional approach that can provide a comprehensive antidote, all of which must come from within African societies and cultures.

THE CONTROL OF AID

The example of the post-World War II Marshall Plan, which helped improve the devastated European economy with US$13 billion in aid funding (valued at US$100 billion today), shows us that development aid can work. If Africa had strong policies to regulate and monitor aid, we should expect comparable results.[28] Aid should be aligned with proven results through a system of reasonable and accurate evaluation, with progress measured against clear, measurable goals to which government and development partners have agreed. These goals should be relevant to local communities in a sustainable way. The evaluation process should not create operational burdens without bearing any accountability for real results.[29]

Creating an independent monitoring mechanism, guided by international auditing rules, is one step toward combating corruption. There are two sides to corruption, however—the giver and the taker—and the global North continues to knowingly fund corrupt governments in the global South for geopolitical, economic, and strategic reasons.[30] To address this, institutions such as Transparency International, along with international and domestic civil society, must advocate for international laws to prevent the spread of corruption from all angles.

This also concerns aid for humanitarian emergencies, which should systematically apply principles of quality management and good governance. When legal frameworks with enforcement mechanisms are in place, corruption and the mismanagement of aid funding will begin to disappear.[31]

MINIMIZING CORRUPTION

We cannot eliminate corruption overnight, and minimizing it with a zero-tolerance method is a long process. Examples exist, however, showing that over time, this method can work when certain enabling conditions are met.[32] For example, there must be enough direct funding to provide education to citizens. On the other hand, resources must also be used to create appropriate international and national legal frameworks. Such frameworks are essential for spurring institutional reforms to improve public administration and strengthen implementation of the United Nations Convention against Corruption (UNCAC). Education promotes economic literacy and strengthens the minds of citizens to take control of their own destinies. Education also empowers citizens to advocate for needed regulatory changes, to challenge their leaders when required, and to hold their governments accountable. An effective legal framework enables citizens to seek justice through clear, predicable mechanisms, allowing transparency in the operation of local institutions.

Structural measures, such as strengthening education and legal frameworks, are the only way to tackle corruption at the root and thus solve it in the long term. Thus, efforts to get quick results in the anticorruption fight by circumventing government are unlikely to succeed and certain to be unsustainable. The way forward is through mechanisms that reinforce governments' own capacities to monitor and respond to corruption, in dialogue with an informed citizenry empowered to demand accountability.

CONCLUSION

The contributions to this volume show that opportunities exist to improve the lives of children affected by HIV and AIDS through an agenda of evidence-based actions. To date, despite progress in some areas, action for children lags far behind need. Governments in countries affected by HIV, as well as their development partners, bear responsibility for the inefficient use of aid funds. But if governments to date have often fallen short in their support for children affected by AIDS, this only underscores the critical importance of bringing the governments of affected countries on board as drivers of a more adequate response. Without commitment to and ownership of this agenda by states, action for children cannot be sustained.

The response to children's needs must be guided by the international human rights framework. Most of the world's governments have endorsed the World Health Organization (WHO) Constitution and ratified the UDHR, the CRC, and the UNCAC. As signatories to these instruments, governments must respond to HIV/

AIDS with rights-based public health laws and policies.[33] Among the crucial principles derived from the human rights framework is that of a multisectoral response to children's needs. Clearly, this response must encompass the provision of appropriate HIV-specific services, including ensuring full adherence to ART for HIV-infected children. But the human rights framework shows that the delivery of specific health services for affected children and families must be connected to a broader agenda of strengthening social well-being and expanding economic opportunities. This broader agenda engages sectors such as education, labor, infrastructure, and economic development, in addition to health. This again highlights the central role of government, which alone can be held accountable for the well-being of the population in this broad sense.

The national government must lead the national response. But that response can only succeed if it incorporates democratic processes that engage the talents of all stakeholders and gives affected communities a strong voice in decision-making. Broad participation is required to establish a framework for coordination, monitoring, and evaluation of HIV funding and programs, ensuring that all stakeholders are aligned under one national plan. Participatory processes take time, and they can go awry in many ways. The mechanisms of democracy are imperfect—in wealthy countries as in poorer ones. But these mechanisms and the state authority derived from them remain our best hope for accelerating action to improve children's lives.

NOTES

1. Yamin, A.E. (2008). Will we take suffering seriously? Reflections on what applying a human rights framework to health means and why we should care. *Health and Human Rights, 10,* 1, 45–63.

2. Office of the United Nations High Commissioner for Human Rights (OHCHR) and the Joint United Nations Programme on HIV/AIDS (UNAIDS). (2008). *Handbook on HIV and human rights for national human rights institutions.* Geneva: OCHCR and UNAIDS; Rudan, I., et al. (2008). Epidemiology and etiology of childhood pneumonia. *Bulletin of the World Health Organization, 86,* 5, 321–416.

3. Committee on the Rights of the Child. (2003). *General comment no. 3(2003): HIV/AIDS and the rights of the child.* Geneva: Committee on the Rights of the Child 32nd Session.

4. Avahan. (2008). *Avahan—The India AIDS initiative: The business of HIV prevention at scale.* New Delhi: Bill & Melinda Gates Foundation. Retrieved December 14, 2009, http://www.gatesfoundation.org/avahan/Documents/Avahan_HIVPrevention.pdf

5. WHO, UNAIDS, and UNICEF. (2009). *Toward universal access: Scaling up priority HIV/AIDS interventions in the health sector.* Geneva: WHO. Retrieved February 22, 2010, http://www.uniteforchildren.org/files/tuapr_2009_en.pdf

6. Katzenstein, D. et al. (1999). Serum level of maternal human immunodeficiency virus (HIV) RNA, infant mortality, and vertical transmission of HIV in Zimbabwe. *Journal of Infectious Diseases, 179,* 6, 1382–1387.

7. Cohen, D. (1998). Socio-economic causes and consequences of the HIV epidemic in Southern Africa: A case study in Namibia. UNDP HIV and Development Programme Issues Paper No. 31, 1998. Retrieved October 9, 2009, http://www.undp.org/hiv/publications/issues/english/issue31e.htm

8. Joint Learning Initiative on Children and HIV/AIDS (JLICA). (2009). *Home truths: Facing the facts on children, AIDS, and poverty.* Boston: JLICA. Retrieved January 13, 2010, http://www.harvardfxbcenter.org/pdf/JLICA%20Final%20Report.pdf

9. Oomman, N., Bernstein, M., & Rosenzweig, S. (2008). *The numbers behind the stories: PEPFAR funding for fiscal years 2004 to 2006.* Washington, DC: Center for Global Development. Retrieved December 17, 2009, http://www.cgdev.org/files/15799_file_theNumbersBehindTheStories.PDF

10. Phiri, S.N., Foster, G., & Nzima, M. (2001). *Expanding and strengthening community action: a study to explore ways to scale up effective, sustainable community mobilization interventions to mitigate the impact of HIV/AIDS on children and families.* Washington, D.C.: Displaced Children and Orphans Fund of USAID. Retrieved December 17, 2009, http://pdf.usaid.gov/pdf_docs/PNACL778.pdf

11. Oomman, Bernstein, & Rosenzweig. (2008). *The numbers behind the stories*; Phiri, Foster, & Nzima. (2001). *Expanding and strengthening community action.*

12. Oomman, N., Bernstein, M., & Rosenzweig, S. (2007). *Following the funding for HIV/AIDS: A comparative analysis of the funding practices of PEPFAR, the Global Fund and World Bank MAP in Mozambique, Uganda and Zambia.* Washington, D.C.: Center for Global Development; Phiri, S. N., & Webb, D. (2007). The impact of HIV/AIDS on orphans and programme and policy responses. In G. A Cornia (Ed.), *AIDS, public policy and child well-being* (2nd ed., pp. 317–342). Florence, Italy: UNICEF- Innocenti Research Centre. Retrieved December 17, 2009, http://www.aidslex.org/site_documents/CY-0004E.pdf

13. Bhargava, A., & Bigombe, B. (2003). Public policies and the orphans of AIDS in Africa. *British Medical Journal, 326*, 21, 1387–1389.

14. Joint Learning Initiative on Children and HIV/AIDS (JLICA). (2009). *Home truths.*

15. Binagwaho, A. (2008). The missing link in HIV coordination. Paper presented at Implemented Meeting, Kampala, Uganda, August 6, 2008. Retrieved September 3, 2009, http://www.kaisernetwork.org/health_cast/uploaded_files/E10_Binagwaho.pdf

16. WorldMapper. (2010). HIV Prevalence. Retrieved January 29, 2010, http://www.worldmapper.org/images/largepng/227.png; WorldMapper. (2010). Human Poverty. Retrieved January 29, 2010, http://www.worldmapper.org/display.php?selected=174

17. UN Conference on Trade and Development (UNCTAD). (2004). *The least developed countries report, 2004.* Geneva: United Nations. Retrieved January 29, 2010, http://www.unctad.org/en/docs/ldc2004_en.pdf

18. Ibid.

19. Ibid.

20. Ganyaza-Twalo, T., & Seager, J. (2005). Literature review on poverty and HIV/AIDS: Measuring the social and economic impacts on households. Unpublished paper of the Human Sciences Research Council.

21. Gupta, G.R., et al. (2008). Structural approaches to HIV prevention. *The Lancet, 372*, 9640, 764–775.

22. Ibid.

23. Collier, P., & Gunning, J.W. (1999). Explaining African economic performance. *Journal of Economic Literature, 37*, 64–111.
24. Global Health Delivery Project. WHO Maximizing Positive Synergies. Retrieved September 10, 2010, http://globalhealthdelivery.org/research/who-maximizing-positive-synergies/
25. African Union. (2008). *Windhoek declaration on social development.* Addis Ababa: African Union. Retrieved March 14, 2010, http://www.africandecade.org/document-repository/Windhoek%20Declaration%20on%20social%20Development.pdf
26. Bailey, S. (2008). *Humanitarian policy group policy brief 32. Need and greed: Corruption risks, perceptions and prevention in humanitarian assistance* London: Overseas Development Institute. Retrieved August 8, 2010, http://www.odi.org.uk/resources/details.asp?id=2385&title=corruption-risks-perceptions-prevention-humanitarian-assistance
27. Ibid.; International Council on Human Rights Policy (ICHRP)/Transparency International. (2009). *Corruption and human rights: Making the connection.* Geneva: ICHRP. Retrieved March 3, 2010, http://www.ichrp.org/files/reports/40/131_web.pdf
28. Hanlon, J., & Pettifor, A. (2000). *Kicking the habit: Finding a lasting solution to addictive lending and borrowing-and its corrupting side-effects.* London: Jubilee 2000 Coalition. Retrieved August 6, 2010, www.jubilee2000uk.org/reports/habitfull.htm
29. Shah, A. Foreign aid for development assistance. Retrieved September 10, 2010, http://www.globalissues.org/article/35/foreign-aid-development-assistance
30. Hirvonen, P. Stingy Samaritans: Why recent increases in development aid fail to help the poor. Policy paper of the Global Policy Forum. Retrieved August 8, 2010, http://www.globalpolicy.org/home/240-international-aid/45056-stingy-samaritans.html
31. Stockton, N. (2005). Preventing corruption in humanitarian relief operations. Paper presented at conference entitled ADB/OECD Anti-Corruption Initiative for Asia and the Pacific: 5th regional anti-corruption conference, Beijing, PR China, September 28–30 2005). Retrieved August 8, 2010, http://www.oecd.org/dataoecd/63/49/35592702.pdf; Bailey. (2008). *Humanitarian policy group policy brief 32.*
32. Wallis, J. J., Fishback, P. V., & Kantor, S. E. (2006). Politics, relief, and reform: Roosevelt's efforts to control corruption and political manipulation during the New Deal. In E.L. Glaeser & C. Goldin (Eds.), *Corruption and reform: Lessons from America's economic history* (pp. 3–22). Chicago: University of Chicago Press;
33. Patterson, D., & London, L. (2002). International law, human rights and HIV/AIDS. *Bulletin of the World Health Organization, 80*, 12, 964–969.

View 3: Children's Rights and the
Responsibility of All Stakeholders

STEFAN E. GERMANN, STUART KEAN,
AND RACHEL SAMUEL ■

Whose responsibility is it? This is a fundamental question to guide the response to children affected by AIDS. There are many perspectives from which to approach the question of responsibility, each potentially leading to very different answers.

We have chosen to examine this question by drawing on a key framework, namely Bronfenbrenner's ecological model of child development, which maps the relationships of various stakeholders to the child.[1] Within this overarching framework, we consider the use of the human rights approach, as encompassed within the Convention on the Rights of the Child (CRC), which articulates the obligations that state signatories have to the child within the ecology of said child.[2] We also examine state obligations stemming from the conceptualization of citizenship of the child.

The first section of the chapter introduces the framework for analysis and discusses its implications related to the question of responsibility to children in the context of HIV. The next section provides an overview of how responsibilities have evolved over the course of the HIV epidemic, followed by a discussion of the roles and responsibilities of stakeholders, particularly in relation to the theoretical framework that underpins this chapter. Our analysis will also present examples from Mozambique and Switzerland, which illustrate some of the issues discussed.

THE ECOLOGY AND RIGHTS OF THE CHILD
IN THE CONTEXT OF HIV AND AIDS

One of the leading scholars in the field of child developmental psychology, Urie Bronfenbrenner, has been the primary contributor to ecological systems theory.[3] This model (Figure 11.1) looks at a child's development within the context of the system of relationships that form his or her environment. Children do not live in isolation. They live in families and communities, and their lives are influenced by factors from the local to the international environment.

The child ecology model conceptualizes how the child contributes to his or her social environment at all levels, while simultaneously being affected and served by it.

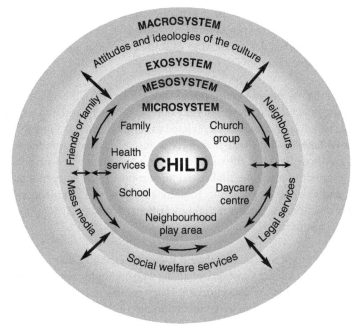

Figure 11.1 View 3: Children in context: Bronnfenbrenner's ecological model.[4]

Thus, this model highlights the interconnectedness between levels leading to child and societal well-being. The interdependence between child and society implies that each adult in the community may influence the growth and development of all children in his or her community; if children are to fare well, all community members will need to contribute to the care of children in the community, especially those most vulnerable.

This model serves as a guiding framework to help identify how responsible stakeholders (such as peers, adults, professionals, and government) can support the holistic development of children *and* embed child rights in their approaches and practices.[5] The child rights approach, embodied by the CRC, to which national governments are signatories, includes the following fundamental principles: (1) to fulfill children's right to survival, well-being, and development; (2) to ensure nondiscrimination; (3) to take into account the best interest of the child; and (4) to encourage their participation in activities aimed at promoting their well-being.[6]

Although only states are bound by the CRC, actions by all stakeholders in support of children in general, and children affected by AIDS in particular, should be guided by the CRC. Child care workers and professionals should ensure that the rights of children affected by AIDS are maintained, and that their voices are heard. States and the international community have obligations to create enabling environments for families and community members to have the means to provide adequate care and support for children affected by AIDS.[7]

In many parts of the world, family and community approaches to child care affirm the notion of "everyone's child." Countries' endorsement of the CRC expands this notion to include "everyone's child, and every child has rights." The conceptualization of the citizenship of the child is intrinsic to our interrogation of rights and responsi-bilities within the ecology of the child.

This combination has the potential to shift the balance of power in communities in favor of children. According to Dominelli:

> [P]ursuing the objective of empowering children [is critical] because these can make caring for children a responsibility that can be discharged by a large group of people which are not necessarily related to children through kinship ties, but who, nonetheless, accept that they have a duty of care towards them. These people are those living in the same community as them and who share with them a number of attributes and social links rooted in interdependence, reci-procity, and citizenship. For adults to share a reciprocated interdependent citi-zenship with children requires the empowerment of children, that is, their being treated as citizens from birth.[8]

As a result, children's upbringing should focus on enabling them to realize their rights as citizens—with the assistance of adults who are supported in that duty by the state—from the day they are conceived until they are able to fend for themselves. The way to do this varies for each child, but should be conducted as a publicly account-able process whereby the child should never lose citizenship rights and entitlements. Treating children as equal citizens does not mean that they are "little" adults, and childhood needs to be given a special status. However, it is critical to accept that children are people in the process of becoming adults from the day that they are born, and that they do not embark on this process only when they reach a certain age.[9]

The implications of this are clear—children do not "belong" to their parents or guardians in a proprietorial sense. They are "citizens" in their own right and there-fore have a right to care and support, and the state has clear obligations towards them. Further, citizenship in this context is not the "status that is acquired as one grows up," which is limited to the boundaries of a nation-state. It is more along the lines of a "portable citizenship right" that starts from birth, regardless of place of abode,[10] underscoring as an issue of justice the responsibility of the international community and its solidarity to children affected by AIDS in all parts of the world.

Thus, the human rights and citizenship approach facilitates a delineation of the responsibilities of the state and stakeholders to the child affected by AIDS premised on the interdependency and reciprocities of the child and society. However, getting states and the global community to embrace their obligations is a complex matter. In the next section, we will initiate this discussion by examining how responsibilities have evolved over the course of the epidemic. We will then review how the norma-tive assumptions of our overarching framework are being realized in the roles currently assumed by key stakeholders.

EVOLVING ROLES DURING VARIOUS PHASES OF THE GLOBAL AIDS RESPONSE

The course of the epidemic, since the first confirmed case in Los Angeles in 1981, has been characterized by distinct phases in the response. Initially viewed as a disease primarily affecting sexually active groups in the West, the true impact, particularly in poor countries and on families and children, slowly emerged over the course of the 1980s and early 1990s. By the 1990s, the HIV response had shifted from the public health and biomedical approach that predominated in the 1980s to one that recognized its developmental and human rights dimensions. With the establishment of the Joint United Nations Program on HIV and AIDS (UNAIDS) in 1997, the subsequent United Nations General Assembly Special Session (UNGASS) on AIDS, and the setting up of the Global Fund, an era of global, scaled-up action was ushered in at the turn of the century. The concerted global effort produced several successes but also demonstrated that the HIV epidemic remains a global challenge for the foreseeable future—a long-term challenge that will require a sustained response.

As discussed in Chapter 2, family-based care is the preferred choice, generating the best outcomes for children affected by HIV. Early in the epidemic, families were solely responsible for care, often supported by community contributions. Community groups, faith-based organizations, and other local organizations were and continue to be at the front line of support to families. Advocacy for children was usually undertaken by local civil society groups campaigning on behalf of children who were denied access to schools or health services because of their HIV status. With some exceptions, governments were slow to respond; political leadership was a critical determinant of government responsibility. Reflecting the global picture, aside from a few dedicated child advocacy groups, children's issues were on the periphery of the HIV response.

The global phase of the response emphasized joint action and shared responsibility, aspiring to link local and global efforts. It could be argued that this reflected the stronger grounding of the response within a rights-based approach. International organizations and donor governments played an increasing role in the delivery of care and advocacy, customarily funding state programs and partnering with local organizations. Global and national advocacy campaigns worked together to call on governments to fulfill their obligations to provide essential pediatric care and antiretroviral drugs to pregnant women.

As the next phase of the HIV response is charted, the responsibilities of governments, civil society, and international stakeholders remain urgent. However, the last three decades have highlighted that defining lines of responsibility is essential.

Building a long-term, sustainable response is a formidable challenge, but it is clear that, regardless of how the burden is shared, the responsibility of government, civil society, and the international community is to create an enabling environment in which families can thrive and care for their children. The next section will review the roles and responsibilities of these stakeholders in more depth, assessing the extent to which some of the theoretical underpinnings of the framework already discussed have been brought about.

ROLES AND RESPONSIBILITIES OF STAKEHOLDERS

Many stakeholders have played or should be playing significant roles in the response to children affected by HIV, including children, families, community members, civil society, governments, and the international community.

We earlier argued that children are citizens and bearers of rights. The realization of their rights as citizens is intrinsic to their development and upbringing. As such, they must be given the space to become active participants in decisions that affect their lives, supported by adults and enabled by the state. However, children have largely been passive recipients in the response to the HIV epidemic. Their role has been determined by the socioeconomic and cultural contexts in which they live, summed up traditionally as "children should be seen and not heard." This is especially the case for the most marginalized children, those disabled or living with HIV, whom stigma and discrimination has excluded even further. Ironically, perhaps the most seriously affected—double orphans, who have lost both of their parents—have been required to play the most active role, as many have taken over full responsibility for their siblings as heads of households.[11]

In recent years, gradually more efforts have been made to encourage children to be more active participants in the response. These efforts have been led by civil society actors and mobilized community members who have encouraged children to speak out about their needs and wishes. There has been an increasing transformation of the role of children, largely achieved through the empowerment of children and community members through training on children's rights and responsibilities. The tangible signs of this more active role can be found in the proliferation of children's groups, child parliaments, and opportunities for children to participate in local, national, and international decision-making forums. Described in Box 11.1, child parliaments in one province in Mozambique offer a strong illustration of how opening political spaces for children has not only demonstrated that children and young people are capable of taking on the mantle of responsibility, but also that their participation has raised the level of stakeholder engagement and standards of care for orphans and vulnerable children (OVCs).

BOX 11.1

MOZAMBIQUE: POLITICAL SPACES FOR CHILDREN AFFECTED BY AIDS

The active participation of children affected by AIDS has generally been low. However, there have been a number of good experiences, such as the Child Parliament initiative in Zambézia, Mozambique, set up in partnership with the Provincial AIDS Council, World Vision, and other stakeholders. In the Child Parliament, a project funded by the Provincial AIDS Council in Zambézia, young Members of Parliament (MPs) have conducted HIV/AIDS-related activities on their own initiative. The following are some of the Child Parliament's interventions and accomplishments:

- Focus Group Discussions are conducted with local leaders, parents, and youth to discuss how the needs and rights of children affected by AIDS in their areas are being addressed, or where gaps in care and support exist.
- District child parliaments identify households with children affected by AIDS who live in extreme poverty. Lists of names are then submitted to local nongovernmental organizations (NGOs) and governments to ensure that such households are assisted.
- The young MPs visit schools and participate in community meetings to disseminate existing HIV/AIDS-related policies and laws that are in

place to raise awareness among community leaders, other children, and adults.

The identified challenge of such approaches is that they are often project-based and not fully institutionalized and financed by "domestic" district or provincial government budgets. But experiences from this approach in Mozambique related to enhancing stakeholder responsibilities to children affected by AIDS have been very encouraging. Child Parliaments have been involved in planning for orphan and vulnerable child (OVC) care and support, and in particular, for the six basic services defined by the OVC National Plan of Action. Their engagement in areas like tracking government obligations to providing minimum standards of service for OVCs helps to ensure that governments are more accountable. The provision of services is also facilitated by providing a space for all partners to contribute good practices. In addition, stakeholders benefit from being part of a multisectoral coordination mechanism for OVC interventions that includes governments, civil society institutions, and community and faith-based organizations with the aim of ensuring complementarity, reducing duplication and competition, and promoting mutual learning.

Although challenges remain, and there is still a long way to go, the positive steps taken in Zambézia are prompting replication of the approach in other provinces.

Articulated within the model of the ecology and rights of the child, government, community, and family are *collectively* duty bearers. However, in most cases, the reality is very different. Families have long carried the principal burden of caring for and protecting children. In many cultures, these responsibilities are bound up in kinship ties based on long-established cultural values and extend well beyond the responsibilities of the nuclear family. The HIV epidemic has hit hard at the resource and asset base that has enabled families to care for children, and both nuclear and extended families have been overstretched to provide the level of care and protection they have historically provided, particularly to vulnerable children. The situation now is that, in some communities in high prevalence contexts, 60%[12] of the principal caregivers of OVCs are grandparents, many of whom live in extreme poverty. The role of caregivers of children and adults made vulnerable by HIV/AIDS has been largely ignored by policy-makers, in spite of a commitment to universal access to care and support, alongside prevention and treatment. Specific state measures could safeguard family-based care, such as social protection programs supported by or in partnership with donors, civil society, and international stakeholders.[13]

Where governments have abrogated their share of the responsibility, community members and civil society organizations have by necessity increasingly come together to discuss how best to respond to the inability of extended families to cope with the increasing demands placed on them by children made vulnerable by the HIV epidemic. The efforts of traditional community structures and organizations, especially faith-based organizations, have been greatly enhanced in recent years by additional efforts of civil society organizations already working to support communities. Collectively, these initiatives have generated—from within the local community—the bulk of the resources required to care for and protect vulnerable children, in some cases as much as 90% of said resources.[14] Civil societies (nongovernmental organizations [NGOs], foundations, and international NGOs [INGOs]) have helped local community members to come together and to build their organizational capacity, as well as to identify resources, thereby enabling them to sustain their efforts to regularly visit households with vulnerable children. Governments, which are formal duty bearers and crucial to creating an enabling ecosystem for the child, must participate in these relationships and not operate in isolation from them. In some countries, such as Kenya, these community-level care and protection structures have been integrated with government structures (e.g., Area Advisory Councils).[15] Some of these community-level structures have recently started engaging in advocacy with local authorities to change local attitudes and behaviors that make children vulnerable—for example, early marriage, female genital mutilation, and property disinheritance—and have also been holding local services providers (government and private) to account for the quality of essential services being provided to children. The experiences of addressing the issue of children and AIDS in Switzerland (Box 11.2) illustrate a discussion about how civil society can complement and enhance the efforts of governments, often resulting in innovative and leading-edge approaches. In collaboration with the Swiss government, the importance of psychosocial support for children made vulnerable by the AIDS epidemic was recognized. Furthermore, the partnership introduced cash transfers to affected families well before such social protection measures were more broadly appreciated.

Box 11.2

CHILDREN & AIDS IN SWITZERLAND: CIVIL SOCIETY COMPLEMENTING
GOVERNMENT EFFORTS[16]

The Swiss Aids Federation, and its network of regional centers, were created in 1985. These concentrated on the support to and care of those affected by HIV/AIDS, as well as on prevention. It was only in a few large towns that they were in contact with children affected by the illness, and they set up special services for this group. At that time, many of the children died before their tenth birthday. The first protease medicine became widely available only in 1995.

The Swiss Federal Office of Public Health based its activity against AIDS on the law dealing with epidemics. It supported prevention with national campaigns, helped in the fight against the illness being transmitted from mother to child, and also promoted the pediatric mother–child cohort study. The psychosocial support of children and young adults has until now not been one of the aims of this federal office.

In 1987, mother-to-child infection was estimated by many scientists to be at nearly 80%. This information led Linus G. Jauslin and others to set up the AIDS & Child (AIDS & Kind) foundation in 1988. In the planning stage, the welfare of the child and the complex situation of children affected by HIV were taken into consideration. From the very beginning, the psychosocial support of children was regarded as extremely important, together with medical care, finding answers to legal problems, fighting against discrimination and for social integration, and other issues. It is interesting to note that social transfers, in the form of cash transfers to children and youth affected by or living with HIV and their families was one of the first services facilitated by AIDS & Kind. This was particularly important because most families affected by AIDS at that time had a history of poor social structure, often weakened by a history of parental drug use. This was more than 20 years before the Joint Learning Initiative on Children and HIV/AIDS (JLICA)'s research efforts made the case for such social protection measures at a global level, as a mitigation effort in resource-constrained settings. A milestone for AIDS & Kind was the Third European Meeting for Young People affected by HIV/AIDS, in 2002. This led the youth delegates from AIDS & Kind to form their own support group, and today the AIDS & Child Swiss Youth + Group is a leading peer group worldwide.

The experience from Switzerland highlights the importance of partnerships and collaboration. Gaps in government efforts during the AIDS response have been complemented by responsive civil society groups, who then lobbied the government to address such gaps either within the government's own responses or via co-financing civil society efforts to sustain such responses.

Underscored by the human rights approach and international law, governments are the primary duty-bearers for their citizens. Most governments have signed international conventions, such as the CRC, as well as a plethora of international policies that oblige them to care for and protect children. Their role as duty bearers for children is outlined through constitutions, laws, and policies. In practice, the ability of most governments to provide adequate education, health, and social welfare services has been woefully inadequate, as evidenced by poor performance in reaching many of the UN's Millennium Development Goals (MDGs). Over the last decade, following the 2001 HIV/AIDS UNGASS, there has been increasing international attention to the needs of children affected by HIV; within high-prevalence countries in particular, this has become apparent through the creation by most countries of national plans of action for OVC, as well as the revision and consolidation of laws related to children generally and vulnerable children in particular. It is still too early to say whether these policy initiatives will result in the allocation of increased resources for the provision of essential services for children, particularly the enforcement of laws to care for and protect children. Many governmental social welfare services, which are charged with responsibility for protecting vulnerable children, are in fact among the most underfunded and marginalized government departments. There are encouraging signs that, with significant support from international donors, social protection services, particularly those providing social transfers (e.g., child grants) are receiving more resources.

A conceptualization of citizenship that transcends national boundaries has a bearing on the solidarity of the international community toward children affected by AIDS. The international community and donor governments were slow to recognize the importance of issues related to children affected by HIV/AIDS. For example, it was only in 2004 that the U.K. Government AIDS Strategy for developing countries first included children.

Few international agreements rise to the level of legal enforceability. The responsibility of the international community to children, especially those made vulnerable by the AIDS pandemic, relies largely on political will and on the mobilization of global civil society responses. The publication of the "Framework for the Protection,

Care and Support of Children Living in a World with HIV & AIDS"[17] provided a major opportunity to mobilize international support and resources for the issue. Subsequently, many donors, including G8 governments, gave increasing attention to the issue. The 2005 G8 Summit at Gleneagles, the 2006 UNGASS Political Declaration, and the 2007 G8 Summit at Heiligendamm gave much greater prominence to issues related to children and HIV. The U.S. government (through its President's Emergency Plan for AIDS Relief [PEPFAR] program), the Global Fund, the World Bank Multi-Country HIV/AIDS Program, and other bilateral donors have also allocated significant resources to children affected by HIV/AIDS. Similarly, UN agencies, notably UNICEF and UNAIDS, have played very significant roles in raising the profile of the issue of children affected by HIV, and UNICEF's "Unite for Children Unite Against AIDS" campaign has kept the issue high on the international development agenda. The challenge now is for the international community to continue to provide the significant amount of resources required to meet the needs of children made vulnerable by HIV/AIDS at a time of financial stringency and when donors want to refresh the appearance of their development priorities.

CONCLUSION

The crisis of orphans and other children made vulnerable by HIV/AIDS is enormous in scope, complex in impact, and lengthy in duration. There is no easy solution to this global crisis, but there is an urgent need to increase our collective efforts and use research findings to generate an adequate, sustained response over the long term. Presently, most responses are still NGO- and community-driven, and it almost appears that governments in many low-income countries believe that the problem will be adequately addressed by NGOs and community-based organizations. Although many national OVC policies have been put in place, they are often under-resourced and there is a need to move beyond rhetoric and toward action. The actual response to date in most countries is still limited in scale, fragmented, and shamefully short of what is required to sufficiently mitigate the impact of AIDS on children.

Responses must be brought to a scale that adequately ensures the protection, care, and support of all children made vulnerable by HIV/AIDS in highly affected countries. To succeed requires all stakeholders, from the local level to the global level, to take on their due responsibility and fulfill collectively our obligations toward children. In the words of Graça Machel, "we must do anything and everything to protect children, to give them priority and a better future. This is a call to action and a call to embrace a new morality that puts children where they belong—at the heart of all agendas."[18]

NOTES
   1. Bronfenbrenner, U. (1979). *The ecology of human development: Experiments by nature and design.* Cambridge, MA: Harvard University Press.
   2. United Nations. (1989). *The United Nations Convention on the Rights of the Child.* New York: United Nations General Assembly.
   3. Dolan, P. (2008). Prospective possibilities for building resilience in children, their families and communities. *Child Care in Practice, 14,* 83–91.

4. Germann, S. (2005). *An exploratory study of quality of life and coping strategies of orphans living in child-headed households in the high HIV/AIDS prevalent city of Bulawayo, Zimbabwe.* Pretoria: UNISA.
5. World Vision. (2009). *Integrated ministry framework.* Nairobi: World Vision.
6. Byrne, I. (1988). *The human rights of street and working children–A practical manual for advocates.* London: IT Publications.
7. Ooms, G. (2008). *The right to health and the sustainability of health care: Why a new global health aid paradigm is needed.* Ghent: International Center for Reproductive Health.
8. Dominelli, L. (1999). Empowering children: The end-point for community approaches to child welfare. In L. Dominelli (Ed.), *Community approaches to child welfare–International perspectives.* Aldershot, UK: Ashgate, 1999.
9. Germann, S. (2005). *An exploratory study of quality of life.*
10. Dominelli. (1999). Empowering children.
11. Germann. (2005). *An exploratory study of quality of life.*
12. HelpAge International. (2005). *MDGs must target poorest say older people: Supplement to Ageing and Development.* London: HelpAge International.
13. Richter, L.M., & Sherr, L. (2009). Editorial: Strengthening families: A key recommendation of the Joint Learning Initiative on Children and AIDS (JLICA). *AIDS Care, 21*, 1–2.
14. Joint Learning Initiative on Children and AIDS (JLICA). (2009). *Home truths: Facing the facts on children, AIDS, and poverty.* Final report of the Joint Learning Initiative on Children and AIDS. Boston: JLICA.
15. Republic of Kenya. (2007). *Training resource manual for area advisory councils.* Nairobi: World Vision Kenya and Irish Aid.
16. Joint Learning Initiative on Children and AIDS (JLICA). (2009). *Home truths*; Jauslin, L.G. (2010). *AIDS & Child "Positiv im Leben stehen."* Zurich: Rex Verlag.
17. UNICEF. (2004). *The Framework for the protection, care and support of orphans and vulnerable children living in a world with HIV and AIDS.* New York: UNICEF.
18. Machel, G. (2001). *The impact of war on children.* London: Hurst and Company.

View 4: The Responsibility Not to Turn Away

CHRIS DESMOND ■

Children experience many negative consequences as a result of HIV/AIDS. They can be infected and face illness and death. Their caregivers may be infected, leading to illness and death within the home, both of which have consequences for children. The consequences that flow from illness and death include impacts on children's education and health, their emotional well-being, their sense of security, and many others. These consequences are, however, not all inevitable, and steps can be taken to prevent and mitigate many of them.[1] Unfortunately, prevention and mitigation efforts are often under-resourced or absent. As a result, it is not simply HIV that is to blame for the negative consequences children experience; indeed, a share of blame must be reserved for those who should, and can, prevent or mitigate these conse-quences but fail to do so.

To suggest that there is blame to be apportioned implies that people are failing to meet their responsibilities. It is difficult to blame someone for not doing what they had no duty to do. It is also difficult to assign a duty to someone who does not have the capacity to fulfill it. Asking who is to blame for the current failure then is akin to identifying those who have a responsibility and the ability to prevent and mitigate the impacts of HIV/AIDS on children. Who carries responsibility may differ depend-ing on the situation. For example, someone may only become responsible when someone else has failed.

When looking for someone to blame, you need not look far. You are to blame. You have a responsibility to affected children, and you failed to meet it. I am also to blame, so don't feel lonely. Indeed, a case can be made that we all share a duty to respond to those most in need regardless of our genetic, social, or physical distance from them. The basis of this case, and how the degree of responsibility varies depend-ing on the actor, will be discussed shortly. This discussion, although interesting, is, from a practical point of view, not very useful. For this reason, a second, and argu-ably more useful, approach to the blame/responsibility discussion will also be exam-ined. This approach focuses on who is likely to take responsibility and how this might be influenced.

IDENTIFYING RESPONSIBILITIES OR APPORTIONING BLAME

This discussion can be framed in terms of responsibility or blame. I shall frame it in terms of responsibility. Although it is good to keep blame in mind, the responsibility formation is perhaps more useful as it allows for an important distinction to be made. Blame can only be assigned when duty, ability, and failure coincide. When a duty is not met because the actor was not able to meet it, then it is hardly appropriate to assign blame to that actor. For example, families have a responsibility to their children; if they fail to provide adequate care for their children because they are not able to, then they are not to blame for the negative consequences that their children experience. If, however, they fail to meet their responsibility because they don't want to, then they are to blame. Being able to make the distinction between failing to meet a duty because of an inability to meet it and failing to meet a duty because of a voluntary decision to ignore it is very helpful.

That parents have a special responsibility to their children is generally accepted and often legislated. That this responsibility extends to other family members is less clear. Many social norms are certainly based on the belief that families have a special responsibility to their children. Responsibility for children in the family context should, however, not be considered only in terms of biological relatedness. Parents of adopted children have a special duty toward their children. Caregivers, related or otherwise, are assuming a special duty when they accept a child into their care. The extent of these special responsibilities can be debated; such a debate, however, is not necessary for the present discussion. That families have responsibilities as a result of their relationship with children is sufficient.

The majority of children affected by HIV/AIDS live with related adults, most often with a parent.[2] This proximity means that families are typically in the best position to prevent and mitigate negative consequences for children. The family, therefore, has a role to play in the response to children not only because of their relationship with them, but because of their ability to do so. However, the family's obligation to be the center of an effective response is very different from the family's obligation to be the sole responder. Even the most resourced families need some support if they are to protect children from the preventable impacts of HIV/AIDS. Health and education services, for example, need to be available. Resource-poor families, however, need far more than available basic services. The question is: Who is responsible for providing this support to families?

Communities have often been among the most significant providers of support to families. It is not clear, however, that they have a responsibility to provide the level of support they are currently providing. Certainly, it can be argued that they have a responsibility to help because of a shared humanity, but this could be argued for all of us. Arguments that they have greater responsibility because of a shared history and lineage can be made, but it should be remembered that these same arguments could be made to support nationalism or even racism. Community members may be better placed to respond to the needs of other community members. This arguably does leave them with a greater responsibility.[3] This responsibility must, however, be limited by their ability to provide support. If the cost to the helper is greater than could reasonably be expected given the resources they have, others have a responsibility to help those community members who have taken on more than their share.

There has been much discussion of how much someone should be expected to help another person in need. Singer's strong version of the principle of preventing bad occurrences is one of the most demanding arguments in terms of how much it argues should be given.[4] The principle states that people should prevent bad things from happening to the point that they would be sacrificing something of comparable moral significance if they did more. For Singer's audience, he argues, this would mean a great deal of helping. For a member of a poor community helping another member of that community, it will not require much before they are sacrificing something of similar moral significance. It is not my purpose here to argue for or against Singer's principles. The point is that even when judged against the most demanding criteria, many people in poor communities are doing more than their duty.

Although the key point here is that community members are often expected to do more than they should, two caveats need to be noted. First, not all HIV-affected families are in poor communities. I focus here on poor communities as this is the setting in which it is most likely that the family will not be able to meet its responsibilities and will need significant support from others. The responsibility of community members in wealthy communities to help affected families in their midst is somewhat different. The need for help is likely to not be as great, but the ability of community members to provide support is likely to be greater (in terms of resources). The second caveat is that, although the discussion here is of the responsibility to help, the responsibility not to harm also needs to be kept in mind. For example, community members certainly have a responsibility not to contribute to stigma and discrimination.

That community members are doing more than should be expected, and often not being supported for doing so, is of great concern. That there seems to be an expectation that they do more is also of concern. Having so many responses to HIV-affected families in poor communities that are based on volunteer labor is troubling, and I would argue, exploitative. I am sure that many people in poor and rich communities value the opportunity to assist a person in need. I am, however, equally sure that there are people who will take on volunteer work in the hope that they will get some personal benefit from doing so. They may hope to benefit from a basic stipend, that they will work their way into a paid position in the organization providing the service, or that their experience will help them get work elsewhere. I believe that many poor people only accept such minimal reward for their work because of the desperate situations in which they find themselves. That the acceptance of the reward is contingent on the extremity of their situation is what makes it exploitation.

Discussions of responsibility often skip from community to government. Such a jump is problematic because the definition of community is typically so narrow. The community is most often a reference to people living in the same location as affected families. It does not encompass broader society in a given country. As poverty and HIV interact, the worst impacts, and therefore the greatest need for support, typically occur in poor communities. Because of the severity of the situation, discussions of community responses typically focus on poor communities. Wealthy citizens of affected countries, however, also have a responsibility to help because of a shared humanity and the ability to effectively respond that comes with proximity. Some would argue that they also have a responsibility because of shared citizenship or nationality, but there is much disagreement on this topic.[5] In addition to wealthy citizens, social responsibility also falls to the private sector that operates within each country.

It is interesting that the responsibilities of wealthy citizens to poor families who are struggling to respond to HIV/AIDS are so often forgotten. The skipping of this group makes me wonder if the poor are sometimes viewed in a way such that they take on the expectations typically associated with family. The poor appear to be seen by some as a related group with responsibility for each other flowing from that relatedness. Then again, maybe this perception that the poor should sacrifice for each other is a good thing. Maybe the problem is seeing this responsibility as special rather than general. It is not that too much is expected of the poor, but that too little is expected of the wealthy.

Governments certainly have a responsibility to respond to children affected by HIV/AIDS. The signing of the Convention of the Rights of the Children (CRC) in and of itself commits governments to respond. By signing the CRC, government responsibility extends beyond the provision of basic public services. They have a duty to prevent the violation of children's rights, and if this requires more than services—which it does—then they are obligated to provide what is needed. Social protection and other supports to the family would seem an important area of responsibility that is often missed. Governments, however, have limited resources, and although they have a responsibility to do everything they can, they have to balance this with their responsibility to future generations. For example, it would not be appropriate for governments, in an effort to meet their duty to children, to take on levels of debt that would compromise future governments' ability to do the same.

Aside from the CRC, past failures to lead countries out of poverty place a responsibility on governments stemming from principles of corrective justice. Governments have a duty to correct the wrongs that have occurred because of their actions or omissions. In many countries, if governments had done their job better in the past, and had not been so corrupt and self-serving, families would now be better resourced to respond to the challenges associated with the HIV epidemic. Government failure, negligence, and malice have led to wrongs that they have a duty to put right.

Thus far, I have not mentioned nongovernmental organizations (NGOs). This is because I see no special moral duty for them to respond. They are delivery agents. They may well at times be more efficient than private citizens or governments at providing particular types of support. As such, they certainly have a role to play in the response. However, that an agent is more efficient than the principal does not mean that they assume the principal's duty in the moral sense. The NGOs have a contractual duty to deliver what they have committed to do, but this is a different type of responsibility altogether. This distinction can be very important. Responding NGOs should expect support because the moral responsibility has not shifted, only the task of implementation. Those that have a moral duty to respond, such as wealthy citizens and governments, should support NGOs as they work to deliver what is the duty-bearer's responsibility to ensure.

There has been considerable debate in the literature on the extent of responsibility of foreign states and citizens to alleviate the suffering of distant others. There are those who argue that distance does not matter and the duty to respond is great,[6] and there are others who argue against this view.[7] Arguments that people should help distant others have been made along a variety of lines, such as shared humanity and corrective justice.[8] Arguments based on shared humanity suggest that international borders, physical distance, and genetic differences do not negate the duties people have to each other, which stem simply from all being human. Arguments based on corrective justice suggest that many of those who now have means have them because of past (or current) crimes and have a duty to correct this wrong. There are, however, those who believe that arguments in favor of assistance break down when you consider the effectiveness (or lack thereof) of foreign assistance.[9] They suggest that if people distant from the problem are not able to help because aid does not work, then they have no duty to give up their resources. Still others have argued that international responsibilities are limited as people first have an obligation to help their fellow citizens.[10]

For the most part, arguments have concerned the positive duty to help—that is, these arguments are based on what duty the citizens of one country have to provide help to reduce the suffering of those in other countries. There are, however, commentators who argue that the wealthy world is in violation of the negative duty not to do harm.[11] Although positive duties are duties to do something, negative duties are duties not to do something—in this case, something that harms people from other countries. The argument is that the current situation of continuing poverty is a result of unjust events in the past and the maintenance of unjust institutions in the present. As wealthy countries committed these acts and maintain these institutions, they have violated their negative duty not to harm. As a result, they have a duty to stop maintaining these unjust institutions because they are still harming poor countries. Moreover, given the role of wealthy countries in creating the current unjust system, they also have a duty to correct the damage they have done.[12]

Although there is much debate to be had on the level of responsibility distant people have to protect children affected by HIV/AIDS, it is difficult to argue that they have none. Similarly, the case can be made that they are falling far short of any reasonable assessment of that responsibility—although how short is up for discussion.[13]

A number of international institutions have special responsibilities. For multilateral organizations, such as the World Bank and UNICEF, these are mandated responsibilities. Major pharmaceutical companies have responsibilities stemming from their ability to help and the way in which they came about that ability. The extent of these responsibilities is a specialized area of debate and beyond the scope of the current discussion.

The above discussion highlights the responsibility of parents, communities, wealthy citizens of affected countries, governments, and everyone else in the world, particularly those with means. Apportioning responsibility or blame, however, is of limited practical significance. The limitations can already be seen at the level of the family. That families have a special responsibility is academic. The reality of the situation is that some family members, often young women, take on a far greater role in providing care to children affected by HIV/AIDS than do other members.[14] Perhaps a more practical approach would be to ask why some family members are not more involved, and how they could be brought into the response. Similar questions, regarding who will respond, and how more people can be brought into the response, could be raised at every level, from families to foreign citizens.

WHO TAKES RESPONSIBILITY?

We know that the more people who are able to help, the less likely that anyone will.[15] Research on this issue started many years ago with the development of the Bystander

Theorem.[16] Essentially, the argument was made that, although an individual may perceive the need for help, he may opt not to provide it if he feels that he is not able to, that the victim does not deserve his help, or that others are present who can provide the assistance.[17] I would add a layer to this theorem. I would suggest that individuals do not always make disinterested assessments of the situation before deciding if they should or should not provide help. Arguably, individuals do not want to feel that they should help, so they will try to convince themselves that victims are not deserving of their help, that others can help more easily than they, or that they are unable to respond. Individuals may well be limited in the extent to which they are able to achieve this denial of responsibility, but I am fairly sure that they try.

Families are responding to children affected by HIV/AIDS.[18] Social norms, however, often mean that male and female family members are expected to take on different roles in this response. Women are more often expected to provide physical care, whereas men are more likely to be expected to provide financially. Although men and women often act contrary to these expectations, the existence of these expectations has an impact on how people respond. For example, because it is often assumed that men should not play a major role in providing physical care to children, they may not do so. They may not do so because they think that it would be embarrassing to do what is labelled as "women's work" or because they can excuse their inaction by telling themselves that it's not their job.

It was argued above that community members often respond more than their duty requires. It is difficult not to feel the need to help when the need is so obvious. Personal experience of similar suffering may also lead to an awareness of how the difficulties arise, which makes it hard to blame the victim. Wealthier people in the same country, on the other hand, are not typically face-to-face with the suffering, making it less obvious and easier to deny, or to blame victims. Although blaming HIV-affected children for their situation is difficult, blaming their parents can be quite easy. This may be why there is so much interest in ensuring that support goes only to the child.

What is central for governments is not convincing themselves, but convincing others that they have discharged their responsibilities. This, to some extent, explains the emphasis on antiretrovirals (ARVs) and prevention of mother-to-child transmission (PMTCT) rather than HIV prevention. Outcomes that can be clearly measured make for better public relations than does arguing about difficult-to-measure successes. Similarly, there may be some reluctance to admit certain responsibilities. Admitting a role in social protection can, for example, have significant implications as governments will then have to be seen to try to meet this responsibility. That said, many governments in Africa are increasingly willing to accept social protection and other relevant interventions as their responsibility.

Distance helps in shaping your view of reality, such that you avoid the pressure to help. It becomes much easier to deny responsibility.[19] Even so, it is difficult to portray children affected by HIV/AIDS as undeserving or somehow at fault. Moreover, many organizations maintain that they could help, if only they had the money. The difficulty in denying need or apportioning fault is arguably why children are so often used to front fundraising efforts. Furthermore, it may explain why, to avoid the argument from potential donors that responding to the child is the family's responsibility, it is useful to focus on orphans or child-headed households. This presentation of the problem helps potential responders. If they can maintain the belief that they only have to respond to children without family, then their exposure to what they consider legitimate demands is limited. The numbers of child-headed households or orphans are far smaller than the number of children or families living in poverty. It is comforting to feel that your responsibility to help extends only to a few. Besides, it is much harder to make a case for family support as it is so easy to argue that they are at fault. Distinctions between the "deserving" and "undeserving" poor have long been recognized as important in determining the level of support.[20]

RECOMMENDED ACTIONS

Trying to identify whose responsibility it is to respond to children affected by HIV/AIDS does not lead to many recommendations. Considering who takes responsibility, and how more people could be encouraged to do so, on the other hand, does.

Identifying responsibilities suggests that volunteers should be paid. Not only is this the right thing to do, it will likely create more stability in the response and inject much-needed funds into poor communities. We do not want the response to shrink, so paying volunteers requires new money, not redirection of old. Beyond the need to pay volunteers, the conclusion that everyone is responsible to some degree does not help us identify what actions need to be taken.

Examining who provides support, however, does help identify the actions that need to be taken to expand and improve the response. A lot can be learned from the fact that some community members provide help to their neighbors even when they themselves are living in difficult situations. It demonstrates the capacity of people to help one another when excuses don't get in the way. It suggests that what is needed at all levels is to break down the excuses used to deny the duty to provide support. Counteracting excuses will hopefully help release the potential of people to give of themselves in response to the suffering of others. The potential of internal motivations to prompt help is far greater than any external force. This means that we have to try to understand what excuses people make to themselves and concentrate on how these can be challenged. Moreover, we need to ensure that we are careful not to inadvertently reinforce excuses or provide material for their construction. Unduly negative perceptions of fathers, poor people, HIV-positive people, and governments, for example, all need to be combated, so that they cannot be used as excuses to not provide help. It is true that those who really don't want to help might find more excuses, but for some, changing the perception may lead to a change of behavior and to more help being provided. To be clear, this is not a problem only for distant responders. Excuses are made, and need to be addressed, by family members, neighbors, wealthy citizens, governments, and many others.

Negative perceptions are often supported by those who wish to garner resources for the response. Although focusing on the problem of child-headed households and other particularly moving subpopulations may be good for fundraising, it helps to limit the exposure of those asked for support. The images of usually dirty and uncared-for looking children may help fund organizations in the good work they do. At the same time, however, it supports the view that the family has failed, and that outsiders have to step in to save the children. In the long term, this may make it more difficult to demand support for the family—the only institution capable of responding on the scale needed.

Far more excuses can be broken down if more people are involved. The greatest resource in efforts to improve the uptake of responsibility is the people whose right it is to be supported. If those living in poverty are of the mind that the help they receive is charity, they will feel the need to be grateful for what they get. If they are empowered with the knowledge that support is their right—they can demand what is owed.

CONCLUSION

Everyone is to blame for the fact that so many children are so badly affected by HIV/AIDS. Indeed, everyone is to blame for all unnecessary suffering resulting from extreme poverty and preventable illness. Identifying who carries greater responsibility, and therefore greater blame, is an important exercise. It is, however, rather academic unless we also identify ways to ensure that actors at all levels take on more responsibility. This includes the wealthy of affected countries, governments, and the wealthy of the world. It is not allocating the parts which is difficult—it is getting people to play theirs.

Notes

1. Desmond, C. (2009). Consequences of HIV for children: Avoidable or inevitable? *AIDS Care, 21*, S1, 98–104.
2. Hosegood, V. The demographic impact of HIV and AIDS across the family and household life-cycle: Implications for efforts to strengthen families in sub-Saharan Africa. *AIDS Care, 21*, S1, 13–21.
3. Godwin, R. (1988). What is so special about our fellow countrymen? *Ethics, 98*, 4, 663–686.
4. Singer, P. (1972). Famine, affluence, and morality. *Philosophy and Public Affairs, 1*, 1, 229–243.
5. Waldron, J. (2003). Who is my neighbour?: Humanity and proximity. *The Monist, 86*, 3, 333–354; Arneson, R. (2005). Do patriotic ties limit global justice duties? *The Journal of Ethics, 9*, 1/2, 127–150.
6. Singer. (1972). Famine, affluence, and morality.
7. Narveson, J. (2003). We don't owe them a thing! A tough-minded but soft-hearted view of aid to the faraway needy. *The Monist, 86*, 3, 419–433.
8. Operskin, B. (1996). The moral foundations of foreign aid. *World Development, 24*, 1, 21–44.
9. Easterly, W. (2007). *The white man's burden*. New York: Penguin.
10. Reader, S. (2003). Distance, relationship and moral obligation. *The Monist, 86*, 3, 367–381.
11. Pogge, T. (2005). Real world justice. *The Journal of Ethics, 9*, 1/2, 29–53.
12. Ibid.
13. Operskin. (1996). The moral foundations of foreign aid.
14. Desmond, C., & Desmond, C. (2005). HIV/AIDS and the crisis of care for children. In L. Richter & R. Morrell (Eds.), *Baba: Men and fatherhood in South Africa*. Cape Town: HSRC Press.
15. With the exception that one person being able to help will lead to a higher probability of help than if no one was able to help.

16. Latane, B., & Darley, J. (1968). Group inhibition of bystander intervention in emergencies. *Journal of Personality and Social Psychology, 10*, 3, 215–221.

17. Latane, B., & Darley, J. (1970). *The unresponsive bystander: Why doesn't he help?* New York: Appleton Century Crofts.

18. Hosegood, V. (2009). The demographic impact of HIV and AIDS across the family and household life-cycle.

19. Cohen, S. (2005). *States of denial: Knowing about atrocities and suffering.* Cambridge: Polity Press.

20. Katz, M. (1989). *The undeserving poor.* New York: Pantheon.

Social Cash Transfer Scheme (Malawi), 30, 85, 240–42. *See also* Cash transfer programs
Social protection. *See* Targeting: social protection
Social Protection Committee, 241–42
Social security, 29
Social services, 234–35. *See also under* Targeting
Social support, 84–85, 125. *See also* Psychosocial support
  increasing, 131
Social transfer programs. *See* Targeting: social transfers
Solution-focused stories, 127
Soul Buddyz clubs (South Africa), 128
South Africa
  community-based home visiting in, 31–32
  means tests and categorical targeting in, 244–48
  National Infant feeding policy, 201
  proportions of children in the clinical range in, 120, 121f
  psychosocial interventions for school-aged children in, 128, 132–33
  training of lay counselors in, 210–11
Speak for the Child project (Kenya), 83, 86
STI. *See* Sexually transmitted infection
Stakeholders, roles and responsibilities of, 270, 279–84
Stigma, AIDS-related, 125, 231–32
  reducing, 130
STRIVE. *See* Support to Replicable, Innovative Village/Community Level Efforts
Street-children, 124, 133
Support to Replicable, Innovative Village/Community Level Efforts (Zimbabwe), 61–62
Sustainable interventions, 37–41, 64, 113
SWAP. *See* Sector-wide approach
Swaziland, 103t, 108–9
Swiss Aids Federation, 282

Swiss Federal Office of Public Health, 282
Switzerland, 282–83

Tanzania, 103t, 105, 109–10
  psychosocial and income support to aged caregivers and vulnerable families in, 35–36
Targeting, 248–49. *See also* Cash transfer programs
  assumptions underlying, 225
  cash transfers to poor and vulnerable or AIDS-affected families, 226–27. *See also* Cash transfer programs.
  conceptual dilemmas, evidence, and arguments about, 227–32
  definition of, 225
  food transfers, livelihoods programs, and social services for AIDS-affected families, 232–35
  geographic, 236, 237t
  poverty vs. AIDS-affected, 227–231
  social protection
    challenges in, 248
    definition of, 225–26
    methods, evidence, and policy debates, 226, 235-39
  social transfers, methods for, 235–36, 237–38t, 239–40
Targeting approaches in AIDS-affected contexts
  community-based targeting in eastern and southern Africa, 240–44
  means tests and categorical targeting in South Africa, 244–48
Task shifting, 202–3
T cells (lymphocytes), 186–87
Teachers, impact of HIV/AIDS on, 95–96
Thailand, free schooling for vulnerable children in, 102t, 104
Therapeutic storytelling, 127
Transmission, 24. *See also* Antiretroviral prophylaxis for prevention of postnatal transmission; Prevention of mother-to-child